A Text Book Of

MEDICINAL CHEMISTRY - III

As Per PCI Regulations

THIRD YEAR B. PHARM.
Semester VI

Dr. Sanjay G. Walode
M. Pharm., Ph.D. (Pharmaceutical Chemistry)
Principal & Professor
S.V.N.H.T's Collage of B. Pharmacy
Shrishivajinagar, Rahuri, Ahmednagar 413706, India

Dr. Chandan R. S.
M. Pharm., Ph.D. (Pharmaceutical Chemistry)
Assistant Professor
JSS College of Pharmacy
Mysuru 570015, India

Dr. Mrs. Alpana J. Asnani
M. Pharm., Ph.D. (Pharmaceutical Chemistry)
Professor & HOD
Priyadarshini J. L. College of Pharmacy
Nagpur 440016, India

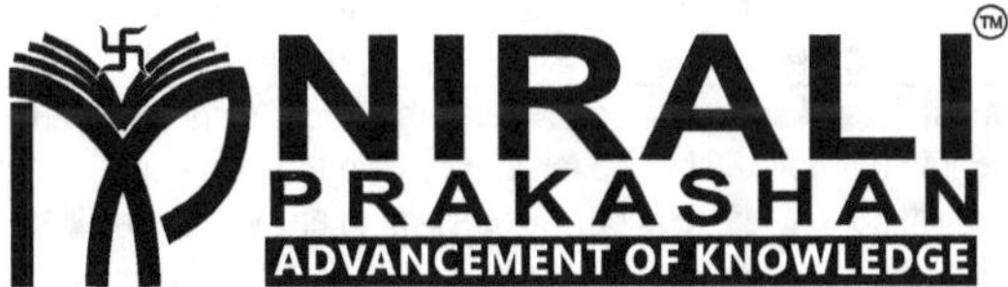

N4056

MEDICINAL CHEMISTRY-III
ISBN 978-93-89944-06-8

First Edition : **February 2020**
© : **Authors**

Published By :
NIRALI PRAKASHAN
Abhyudaya Pragati, 1312, Shivaji Nagar
Off J.M. Road, PUNE – 411005
Tel - (020) 25512336/37/39, Fax - (020) 25511379
Email : niralipune@pragationline.com

➤ DISTRIBUTION CENTRES

PUNE

Nirali Prakashan : 119, Budhwar Peth, Jogeshwari Mandir Lane, Pune 411002, Maharashtra
(For orders within Pune) Tel : (020) 2445 2044; Mobile : 9657703145
Email : niralilocal@pragationline.com

Nirali Prakashan : S. No. 28/27, Dhayari, Near Asian College Pune 411041
(For orders outside Pune) Tel : (020) 24690204; Mobile : 9657703143
Email : bookorder@pragationline.com

MUMBAI

Nirali Prakashan : 385, S.V.P. Road, Rasdhara Co-op. Hsg. Society Ltd.,
Girgaum, Mumbai 400004, Maharashtra; Mobile : 9320129587
Tel : (022) 2385 6339 / 2386 9976
Email : niralimumbai@pragationline.com

➤ DISTRIBUTION BRANCHES

JALGAON

Nirali Prakashan : 34, V. V. Golani Market, Navi Peth, Jalgaon 425001, Maharashtra,
Tel : (0257) 222 0395, Mob : 94234 91860; Email : niralijalgaon@pragationline.com

KOLHAPUR

Nirali Prakashan : New Mahadvar Road, Kedar Plaza, 1st Floor Opp. IDBI Bank, Kolhapur 416 012
Maharashtra. Mob : 9850046155; Email : niralikolhapur@pragationline.com

NAGPUR

Nirali Prakashan : Above Maratha Mandir, Shop No. 3, First Floor,
Rani Jhanshi Square, Sitabuldi, Nagpur 440012, Maharashtra
Tel : (0712) 254 7129; Email : niralinagpur@pragationline.com

DELHI

Nirali Prakashan : 4593/15, Basement, Agarwal Lane, Ansari Road, Daryaganj
Near Times of India Building, New Delhi 110002 Mob : 08505972553
Email : niralidelhi@pragationline.com

BENGALURU

Nirali Prakashan : Maitri Ground Floor, Jaya Apartments, No. 99, 6th Cross, 6th Main,
Malleswaram, Bengaluru 560003, Karnataka; Mob : 9449043034
Email: niralibangalore@pragationline.com

Other Branches : Hyderabad, Chennai

niralipune@pragationline.com | www.pragationline.com
Also find us on www.facebook.com/niralibooks

Acknowledgement

It is a matter of great pride and immense pleasure to extend our sincere regards and deepest sense of gratitude towards management of all three colleges of Pharmacy for their continuous encouragement, constructive criticism and invaluable support for the publication of this book.

It is a pleasure moment for all of us to gratefully acknowledge the constant co-operation of Principals, colleagues and friends of all the three pharmacy colleges for their inspiration, help and guidance, which provided us confidence during writing of this book.

We cordially acknowledge our family members who have not only endured but also encouraged, assisted and inspired throughout our writing endeavor.

The authors extend their due thanks to publishers Mr. Dineshbhai K. Furia and Mr. Jigneshbhai C. Furia of Nirali Prakashan, Pune, for their excellent support in the production of this book in a record time period.

We express our heartfelt thanks to Mrs. Roshan Khan, Mrs. Varsha Bodake, Mr. Akbar Shaikh, Mrs. Deepa Sawant and other supporting staff members of Nirali Prakashan, for their helpful suggestions and skilful supervision which helped us to mould the text in a beautiful book.

Last but not least, we would like to dedicate this book to our beloved parents, whose love and blessings provided us tremendous emotional support and the zeal to work hard towards our goal.

Dr. Sanjay G. Walode
Dr. Chandan R. S.
Dr. Alpana J. Asnani

■■■

Preface

As per the need of students and instructors, we have been engaged in writing and compiling the data based on Pharmacy Council of India regulated syllabus. It gives us immense pleasure to introduce "Text Book of Medicinal Chemistry-III" in continuation with "Text Book of Medicinal Chemistry-I" and "Text Book of Medicinal Chemistry-II". This book has been designed and arranged to provide the basic knowledge of chemistry, classification, mechanism of action and uses of the drugs mentioned in the course of study. The content is focused on synthesis and structure activity relationship of drugs which enable determination of chemical group responsible for evoking a target biological effect in the organism.

The contents of the book are structured as per Pharmacy Council of India regulated syllabus and will be more useful to undergraduate students pursuing carrier in Pharmaceutical Sciences in India.

Book is written in a simple and comprehensive manner along with the structures, schematic diagrams and tables that clearly demonstrate core concept of Medicinal Chemistry. The authentic text of the book will definitely furnish exhaustive information to the students with impressively and user-friendly style.

We will be grateful to all the students, teachers and readers for their constructive suggestions to improve the quality of content of this book. The suggestions from all the readers will be highly appreciated and will be incorporated in the next edition.

Dr. Sanjay G. Walode
Dr. Chandan R. S.
Dr. Alpana J. Asnani

■■■

Syllabus

UNIT- I   **[10 Hours]**

Antibiotics

Historical background, Nomenclature, Stereochemistry, Structure activity relationship, Chemical degradation, classification and important products of the following classes.

β-Lactam antibiotics: Penicillin, Cepholosporins, β-Lactamase inhibitors, Monobactams.

Aminoglycosides: Streptomycin, Neomycin, Kanamycin.

Tetracyclines: Tetracycline, Oxytetracycline, Chlortetracycline, Minocycline, Doxycycline.

UNIT- II   **[10 Hours]**

Antibiotics

Historical background, Nomenclature, Stereochemistry, Structure activity relationship, Chemical degradation, classification and important products of the following classes.

Macrolide: Erythromycin, Clarithromycin, Azithromycin.

Miscellaneous: Chloramphenicol*, Clindamycin.

Prodrugs: Basic concepts and application of prodrugs design.

Antimalarials: Etiology of malaria.

Quinolines: SAR, Quinine sulphate, Chloroquine*, Amodiaquine, Primaquine phosphate, Pamaquine*, Quinacrine hydrochloride, Mefloquine.

Biguanides and dihydro triazines: Cycloguanil pamoate, Proguanil.

Miscellaneous: Pyrimethamine, Artesunete, Artemether, Atovoquone.

UNIT- III   **[10 Hours]**

Anti-tubercular Agents

Synthetic anti-tubercular agents: Isoniozid*, Ethionamide, Ethambutol, Pyrazinamide, Para amino salicylic acid.*

Anti-tubercular Antibiotics: Rifampicin, Rifabutin, Cycloserine Streptomycine, Capreomycin sulphate.

Urinary Tract Anti-infective Agents

Quinolones: SAR of quinolones, Nalidixic Acid, Norfloxacin, Enoxacin, Ciprofloxacin*, Ofloxacin, Lomefloxacin, Sparfloxacin, Gatifloxacin, Moxifloxacin

Miscellaneous: Furazolidine, Nitrofurantoin*, Methanamine.

Antiviral Agents:

Amantadine hydrochloride, Rimantadine hydrochloride, Idoxuridine trifluoride, Acyclovir*, Gancyclovir, Zidovudine, Didanosine, Zalcitabine, Lamivudine, Loviride, Delavirding, Ribavirin, Saquinavir, Indinavir, Ritonavir.

UNIT- IV   **[08 Hours]**

Antifungal Agents:

Antifungal antibiotics: Amphotericin-B, Nystatin, Natamycin, Griseofulvin.

Synthetic Antifungal Agents: Clotrimazole, Econazole, Butoconazole, Oxiconazole Tioconozole, Miconazole*, Ketoconazole, Terconazole, Itraconazole, Fluconazole, Naftifine hydrochloride, Tolnaftate*.

Anti-protozoal Agents: Metronidazole*, Tinidazole, Ornidazole, Diloxanide, Iodoquinol, Pentamidine Isethionate, Atovaquone, Eflornithine.

Anthelmintics: Diethylcarbamazine citrate*, Thiabendazole, Mebendazole*, Albendazole, Niclosamide, Oxamniquine, Praziquantal, Ivermectin.

Sulphonamides and Sulfones

Historical development, chemistry, classification and SAR of Sulfonamides: Sulphamethizole, Sulfisoxazole, Sulphamethizine, Sulfacetamide*, Sulphapyridine, Sulfamethoxaole*, Sulphadiazine, Mefenide acetate, Sulfasalazine.

Folate Reductase Inhibitors: Trimethoprim*, Cotrimoxazole.

Sulfones: Dapsone*.

UNIT – V   **[07 Hours]**

Introduction to Drug Design

Various approaches used in drug design.

Physicochemical parameters used in quantitative structure activity relationship (QSAR) such as partition coefficient, Hammet's electronic parameter, Tafts steric parameter and Hansch analysis.

Pharmacophore modeling and docking techniques.

Combinatorial Chemistry: Concept and applications of combinatorial chemistry: solid phase and solution phase synthesis.

■■■

Contents

■■■

Unit I

Chapter ... 1

ANTIBIOTICS (1)

♦ LEARNING OBJECTIVES ♦

After completing this sub-unit the students should be able:

- *To learn historical background of antibiotics*

- *To study detail classification of antibiotics based on MOA and chemical nature.*

- *To study in brief nomenclature, MOA, SAR, stereochemistry, degradation profile and classification of Penicillin.*

- *To study in brief nomenclature, MOA, SAR, stereochemistry, degradation profile and classification of Cephalosporins.*

- *To learn the drugs belonging to monobactam antibiotics.*

- *To study history, chemistry, MOA, SAR and uses of various aminoglycoside antibiotics.*

- *To study in detail tetracyclines with respect to their structure, stereochemistry, classification, SAR, MOA and uses.*

1.1 INTRODUCTION

The term antibiotic was coined from the word 'antibiosis' which literally means 'against life'. Antibiotics are naturally produced substances of various microorganisms such as bacteria or fungi, which are able to inhibit the growth of other microorganisms and destroy their cells. With the production of semi-synthetic derivatives in modern era, the term "antibiotics" has been replaced by the term "antimicrobials" which refers to natural, semi-synthetic and synthetic substances capable of inhibiting the proliferation of microbes and thus leading them to apoptosis.

Some antibiotics are able to completely kill other bacteria; some are only able to inhibit their growth. Those that kill bacteria are termed as bactericidal, while those that inhibit bacterial growth are termed as bacteriostatic. Although antibiotics generally refer to antibacterial, antibiotic compounds are differentiated as antibacterials, antifungals and antivirals to reflect the group of microorganisms they antagonize.

Before the appearance of antibiotics, the human beings were almost completely exposed to various infectious diseases such as pneumonia, meningitis, or tuberculosis and were treated very difficult or not at all. Humanity lived under the fear of major epidemics. Specialties such as surgery, pediatrics and hematology had high mortality rates as a consequence of infections. Since then and for many years, medicine has changed the form. Without the stress of infection, physicians were able to broaden and advance their research. Specialties such as surgery and hematology flourished. Moreover, for several decades, mankind has been relieved of the fear of major pandemics (e.g., plague, syphilis) and diseases such as tuberculosis have been effectively treated. Antibiotic was slowly established for the awareness of the average human as medicine-salvation. Over the time, dozens of new antimicrobial agents have been discovered, with various mechanisms of action and uses. It has been well documented that the current discovery in the form of medicine provides complete protection against almost all pathogens. Now a days, antimicrobials are widely used drugs not only in medical practice, but also in agriculture, livestock farming, fish farming, as growth enhancers or as growth-protective agents.

1.2 HISTORICAL BACKGROUND

Over 2,500 years ago, a first known antibiotic was used by the ancient Chinese. Chinese had discovered the therapeutic properties of moldy soybeans and used this substance to cure furuncles (pimples), carbuncles and similar infections.

The history of antimicrobial drugs began in the late 1890s when two German researchers, Rudolph Emmerich and Oscar Low, discovered the first antibiotic, pyocyanase, derived from the cultivation of the microbe *Pseudomonas aeruginosa*, with dubious effectiveness and safety in the patient population used against cholera and typhus.

In 1877, French biologists Louis Pasteur and Jules Francois Joubert, discovered that *Anthrax bacilli* were killed when grown in culture in the presence of certain bacteria, along with similar observations by other microbiologists, led Vuillemin to define antibiosis (literally "against life") as the biological concept of survival of the fittest, in which one destroys another to preserve itself. The word antibiotic was derived from this root and the definition was proposed and widely cited by Waksman in 1942.

In 1909 Paul Ehrlich introduced the arsenic-based drug Salvarsan, which acted against *Treponema pallidum*, the bacterium, which is responsible for the disease of syphilis. This discovery laid the foundations for the further development of antimicrobial agents.

In 1932, the first commercially available antibacterial was Prontosil, a sulfonamide was discovered, by Bayer's research team and, Gerhard Domagk, proved its efficacy against major bacterial infections. However, the milestone in the development of antimicrobial drugs was the discovery of penicillin by Sir Alexander Flemming in 1928, which is used until today in clinical therapies. The antibiotic properties of Penicilium species was originally described in France by Ernest Duchesne in 1897. However, his work did not affect the scientific community until the discovery of penicillin by Sir Alexander Fleming.

Sir Alexander Fleming was a Scottish biologist and pharmacologist and he was involved in research of Bacteriology, Immunology and Chemotherapy. He has accidentally discovered the antibacterial properties of penicillin in 1928 and is largely credited with initiating the modern antibiotic era, for which he received the Nobel Prize in Physiology and Medicine in 1945, along with Florey and Chain.

The introduction of penicillin marked the beginning of the so-called "golden era" of antibiotics. The first antibiotic available to doctors in 1946 was penicillin. Its discovery was regarded as modern miracle, as penicillin could treat all types of infections caused by staphylococci and streptococci as these two pathogens cause the greatest number of known infections.

By the end of the 1940s and early 50s, the use of streptomycin and tetracycline was discovered and the era of antibiotic chemotherapy became well tolerated in clinical medicine. These antibiotics were effective against a range of pathogenic bacteria including bacillus tuberculosis

Between 1940 and 1962, most of the antibiotic classes we use as medicines today were discovered and introduced to the market. Each class typically contains several antibiotics that have been discovered over time or are modified versions of previous types.

Today, there are very few novel antibiotics under development. At the same time antibiotic resistant bacteria that survive antibiotic treatment are becoming more and more prevalent, making available antibiotics ineffective. Thus, we are inevitably facing a major health problem.

1.3 DRUG NOMENCLATURE

The names given to the antimicrobials and antibiotics are different as per their inventor's taste; however, some of them can be remembered precisely such as the penicillins are derived from fungi and have names ending in the suffix - cillin (i.e. ampicillin), whereas cephalosporins are fungal products, and their names mostly begin with the prefix - cef (i.e. cefodoxime). The synthetic fluoroquinolones mostly end in the suffix – floxacin (i.e. ciprofloxacin). Most of the antibiotics are produced by fermentation of soil microorganisms from several *Streptomyces* species. These antibiotics have names ending in the suffix – mycin (i.e. streptomycin), whereas some prominent antibiotics are produced by fermentation of various soil microbes known as *Micromonospora* species, have names ending in the suffix-micin, (i.e. gentamicin).

As many related substances possessing quite similar names, it is very difficult to remember the substances with consideration of such kinds of nomenclature.

The terms "broad spectrum" and "narrow spectrum" had specific clinical meaning depends on microbes resistant to single agents and to multiple agents. Some antimicrobial families have the potential of inhibiting a wide range of bacteria belonging to both Gram-positive and Gram-negative cultures and so are called broad spectrum (e.g. tetracyclines); while others inhibit only a few bacteria and are called narrow spectrum (e.g. vancomycin, exclusively used for few Gram-positive and anaerobic microorganisms).

1.4 CLASSIFICATION OF ANTIBIOTICS AS PER MECHANISM OF ACTION

(A) Cell wall synthesis inhibitors:

  (a) Penicillins (Bactericidal**:** block cross linking via competitive inhibition of transpeptidase enzyme)**:**

    1. **Penicillin:** Penicillin-G, Penicillin-V.

    2. **Aminopenicillins:** Ampicillin, Amoxicillin.

    3. **Penicillinase-resistant-penicillins:** Methicillin, Nafcillin, Oxacillin, Cloxacillin, Dicloxacillin.

    4. **Antipseudomonal penicillins:** Carbenicillin, Ticarcillin, Piperacillin.

  (b) Cephalosporines: (Bactericidal: inhibits bacterial cell wall synthesis via competitive inhibition of transpeptidase enzyme)**:**

    1. **1st generation:** Cefazolin, Cephalexin.

    2. **2nd generation:** Cefoxitin, Cefaclor, Cefuroxime.

    3. **3rd generation:** Ceftriaxone, Cefotaxime, Ceftazidime.

    4. **4th generation:** Cefepime.

  (c) Other cell wall inhibitors:

    1. **Vancomycin** (Bactericidal: disrupts peptioglycan cross-linkage)**:** Vancomycin.

    2. **Beta-lactamase Inhibitors** (Bactericidal**:** blocking cross linking)**:** Clavulanic Acid, Sulbactam, Tazobactam.

    3. **Carbapenems:** Imipenem, Meropenem, Doripenem, Ertapenem.

    4. **Aztreonam:** Aztreonam.

    5. **Polymyxins:** Polymyxin-B, Polymyxin-E.

    6. **Bacitracin:** Bacitracin.

(B) Protein Synthesis Inhibitors:

  (a) Anti-30S ribosomal subunits:

    1. **Aminoglycosides** (Bactericidal**:** irreversible binding to 30S)**:** Gentamicin, Neomycin, Amikacin, Tobramycin, Streptomycin.

    2. **Tetracyclines** (Bacteriostatic**:** blocks tRNA)**:** Tetracycline, Doxycycline, Minocycline, Demeclocycline.

  (b) Anti-5OS ribosomal subunits:

    1. **Macrolides** (Bacteriostatic**:** reversibly binds 50S)**:** Erythromycin, Azithromycin, Clarithromycin.

    2. **Chloramphenicol** (Bacteriostatic)**:** Chloramphenicol.

    3. **Lincosamide** (Bacteriostatic**:** inhibits peptidyl transferase by interfering with amino acyl-tRNA complex)**:** Clindamycin.

    4. **Streptogramins:** Quinupristin, Dalfopristin.

(C) DNA Synthesis Inhibitors:
- (a) **Fluoroquinolones** (Batericidal: inhibit DNA gyrase enzyme, inhibiting DNA synthesis)
    1. **1st generation:** Nalidixic acid.
    2. **2nd generation:** Ciprofloxacin, Norfloxacin, Enoxacin, Ofloxacin, Levofloxacin.
    3. **3rd generation:** Gatifloxacin.
    4. **4th generation:** Moxifloxacin, Gemifloxacin.

(D) Other DNA Inhibitors (Bacteridical: metabolic byproducts disrupt DNA)**:** Metronidazole.

(E) RNA Synthesis Inhibitors (Bactericidal: inhibits RNA transcription by inhibiting RNA polymerase)**:** Rifampin.

(F) Mycolic Acid Synthesis Inhibitors: Isoniazid.

(G) Folic Acid Synthesis Inhibitors (Bacteriostatic: inhibition with PABA)**:** Sulfisoxazole, Sulfadiazine, Trimethoprim /Sulfamethoxazole.

1.5 CLASSIFICATION OF ANTIBIOTICS BASED ON CHEMICAL NATURE/ STRUCTURE

1. **β-Lactam Antibiotics:**
   (A) Penicillins:
   - (a) **Natural:** Penicillin-G, Penicillin-V.
   - (b) **Penicillinase resistant:** Methicillin, Nafcillin, Oxacillin, Cloxacillin.
   - (c) **Aminopenicillins:** Ampicillin, Amoxicillin.
   - (d) **Carboxypenicillins:** Carbenicillin, Ticarcillin.
   - (e) **Ureidopenicillins:** Pepericillin, Meclocillin.

   (B) Cephalosporins:
   - (a) **1st generation:** Cefadroxil, Cephalexin, Cephaloridine, cephalothin, Cefazolin, Cephradine.
   - (b) **2nd generation:** Cefaclor, Cefprozil, Cefuroxime, Cefotoxitin, Cefotetan, Cefmetazole.
   - (c) **3rd generation:** Cefixime, cefodoxime, cefotaxime, Ceftriaxone, Ceftazidime.
   - (d) **4th generation:** Cefepime, Cefozopran, Cefclidine, Cefpirome, Cefoselis.

   (C) Monobactams: Aztreonam, Nocardicin-A, Tabtoxin.

   (D) Carbapenems: Biapenem, Eratapenem, Imipenem, Meropenem.

2. **Quinolones:**
   - (a) **1st generation:** Nalidixic acid, Cinoxicin.

3. **Fluoroquinolones:**
   - (a) **2nd generation:** Norfloxacin, Ofloxacin, Lomefloxacin, Fleroxacin.
   - (b) **3rd generation:** Ciprofloxacin.
   - (c) **4th generation:** Levofloxacin, Balofloxacin, Temafloxacin, Sparfloxacin.

4. **Phenazine Derivative:** Clofazimine.

5. **Nitrofurans:** Nitrofurantoin, Nifuroxazide, Nitroimidazoles (Metronidazole, Ornidazole, Tinidazole, Secnidazole).
6. **Sulphonamides:** Prontosil (1st antibacterial drug).
    (a) **Short acting:** Sulfacetamide, Sulfadiazine, Sulfadimidine, sulfafurazole.
    (b) **Intermediate acting:** Sulfadoxime, Sulfamethoxazole, Sulfamoxole.
    (c) **Long lasting:** Sulfanitran, Sulfadimethoxine, sulfamethoxypyridazine.
    (d) **Ultra long-acting:** Sufamethoxydiazine.
    (e) **Paediatric Antibacterial:** Sulfadoxine, Sulfametopyrazine, Pediazole.
    (f) **Cotrimoxazole:** (Sulphonamide + Trimethoprime).
7. **Tetracyclines:**
    (a) **Natural:** Tetracycline, Chlortetracycline, Oxytetracycline, Demeclocycline.
    (b) **Semisynthetic:** Meclocycline, Methacycline, Minocycline, Rolitetracycline.
8. **Aminoglycosides:**
    (a) **Mycins (From *Streptomyces*):** Streptomycin, Neomycin, Kanamycin, Tobramycin.
    (b) **Micins (From *Micromonospora*):** Gentamicin, Verdamicin, Astromicin, Netilmicin.
9. **Oxazolidinone:** Eperezolid, Linezolid, Ranbezolid, Sutezolid, Tedizolid.
10. **Macroloides:** Azithromycin, Clarithromycin, Erythromycin, Roxithromycin.
11. **Ketolides:** Telithromycin, Cethromycin, Solithromycin.
12. **Aminophenicols:** Chloramphenicol, Thiamphenicol.
13. **Pleuromutiline:** Retapamulin, Tiamulin.
14. **Lincosamides:** Clindamycin, Lincomycin.
15. **Streptogramins:** Prinstinamycin, Quinupristin.
16. **Steroid Antibiotics:** Fusidic acid.
17. **Glycopeptides:**
    (a) **Natural:** Vancomycin, Ramoplanin, Bleomycin.
    (b) **Semisynthetic:** Telavancin, Delbavacin, Oritavacin.
18. **Lipopeptides:** Daptomycin, Bacillomycin, Mycosubtilin.
19. **Polyene Antibiotics:** Amphoterecin-B, Nystatin, Natamycin, Candicin.
20. **Peptide antibiotics:** Polymyxins, Octapeptins, Circulins.
21. **Phosphoric acid:** Tobramycin, Fosfomycin.

1.6 β-LACTAM ANTIBIOTICS

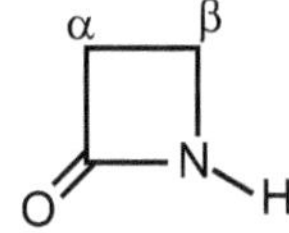

Fig. 1.1: Chemical structure of a β-lactam ring (Azetidinone)

β-lactam is a cyclic amide with four atoms (3-carbon and 1-nitrogen) in its ring named as azetidinone. β-lactam ring is much more reactive and, therefore, more sensitive to nucleophilic attack when compared with normal planar amides.

Penicillin-G or benzyl penicillin (natural) and a close biosynthetic relative, phenoxymethyl penicillin (penicillin-V) remain the agents of choice for the treatment of infections caused by most species of Gram-positive bacteria. Cephalosporin is the discovery of a second major group of β-lactam antibiotics. Chemical modifications of naturally occurring penicillins and cephalosporins have provided semisynthetic derivatives that are effective against various bacterial species known to be resistant to penicillin, in particular, penicillinase-producing staphylococci and Gram-negative bacilli. Thus, apart from a few strains that have either inherent or acquired resistance, almost all bacterial species are sensitive to one or more of the available antibiotics.

Mechanism of action of β-Lactam antibiotics:

β-Lactam antibiotics act by interfering with proteins essential for synthesis of bacterial cell wall, and in the process either kills or inhibits their growth. Bacterial enzymes, penicillin-binding protein (PBP) are responsible for cross linking peptide units during synthesis of peptidoglycan that provide strength and rigidity to the cell wall. Members of β-lactam antibiotics are able to bind themselves to these PBP enzymes, and in the process, they interfere with the synthesis of peptidoglycan resulting to lysis and cell death.

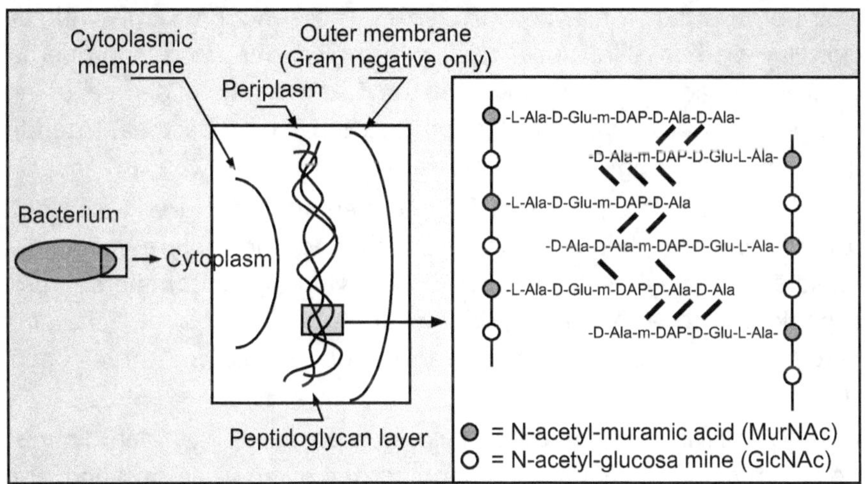

Fig. 1.2

The most prominent representatives of the β-lactam class include Penicillins, Cephalosporins, Monobactams and Carbapenems.

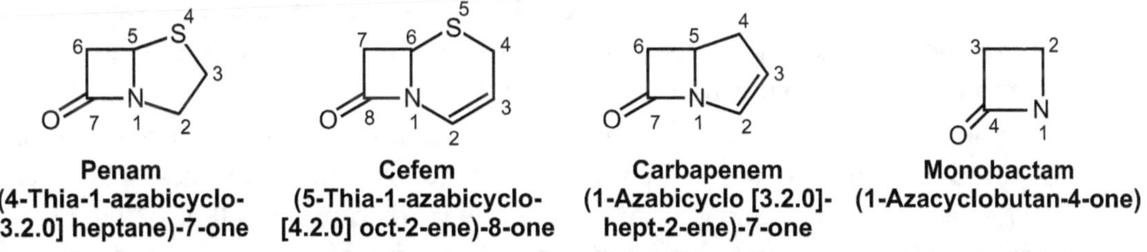

Fig. 1.3: Ring and numbering system of clinically available β-lactum antibiotics

1.7 PENICILLINS

The first antibiotic, penicillin, which was first discovered and reported in 1929 by Sir Alexander Fleming, was later found to be among several other antibiotic compounds called the penicillins. Penicillins are involved in a class of diverse group of compounds, most of which end in the suffix-cillin. They are β-lactam compounds containing a nucleus of 6-animopenicillanic acid (lactam plus thiazolidine) ring and other ring side chains. The side chain determines, in large part, the antibacterial spectrum and pharmacologic properties.

An expanded role for the penicillins came from the discovery that natural penicillins can be modified chemically by removing the acyl group to leave 6-aminopenicillanic acid and then adding acyl groups that confer new properties. These modern semi-synthetic penicillins such as Ampicillin, Carbenicillin, and Oxacillin have various specific properties such as, resistance to stomach acids so that they can be taken orally, a degree of resistance to penicillinase (a penicillin-destroying enzyme produced by some bacteria) extended range of activity against some Gram-negative bacteria.

Over 30 penicillins have been isolated from fermentation mixtures. Some of these occur naturally; others have been biosynthesized by altering the culture medium to provide certain precursors that may be incorporated as acyl groups. Commercial production of biosynthetic penicillins today depends chiefly on various strains of *Penicillium notatum* and *P. chrysogenum*. In recent years, many more penicillins have been prepared semi-synthetically.

Although the penicillins are still used clinically, their value has been diminished by the widespread development of resistance among target microorganisms and also by some people's allergic reaction to penicillin.

1.7.1 Mechanism of Action

The penicillins cause the lysis of growing bacteria. They bind to the enzymes involved in the biosynthesis of the bacterial cell wall. Since eukaryotes do not have cell walls, this is a particularly convenient and safe target for antimicrobial chemotherapy. Thus, the β-lactam antibiotics, as a group, are the most widely prescribed antibiotics.

The penicillins and the other β-lactam antibiotics have a structure that closely resembles that of acylated D-alanyl-D-alanine. Penicillins bind to a number of receptor proteins, transpeptidases and carboxypeptidases called penicillin binding proteins (PBPs), the enzymes that catalyze the synthesis of peptidoglycan, which is a critical component of the bacterial cell wall. This leads to the interruption of cell wall synthesis, consequently leading to bacterial cell growth inhibition and cell lysis.

Different microorganisms vary in the affinity of their PBPs for penicillin. In addition, some organisms, particularly Gram-positive bacteria, are able to mutate their PBPs to provide targets with significantly less affinity (resistance) for penicillin binding. Some of the PBPs are essential, and are present in low amounts. Other PBPs are not essential, and thus, are less desirable targets for antibiotics.

Differences in the "activity" i.e. the amount of a particular penicillin needed to kill an organism are also related to the ability of the penicillin to go through the outer wall of a bacterium. This usually depends on charge properties of the molecule and the affinity of that penicillin for PBPs involved in cell wall biosynthesis.

1.7.2 Nomenclature

The nomenclature of the penicillins as with most antibiotics is complex and cumbersome. Two numbering systems for the fused heterocyclic system exist.

The Chemical Abstracts initiate the numbering with the sulfur atom and assigns the ring nitrogen at the 4 position. Thus penicillins are named as 4-thia-1-azabicyclo [3.2.0] heptanes, according to this system. The numbering system adopted by the USP is the reverse of the Chemical Abstracts procedure, assigning number 1 to the nitrogen atom and number 4 to the sulfur atom.

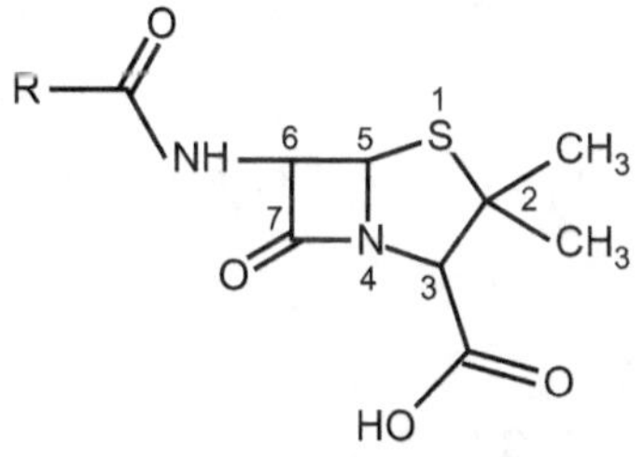

Chemical abstracts 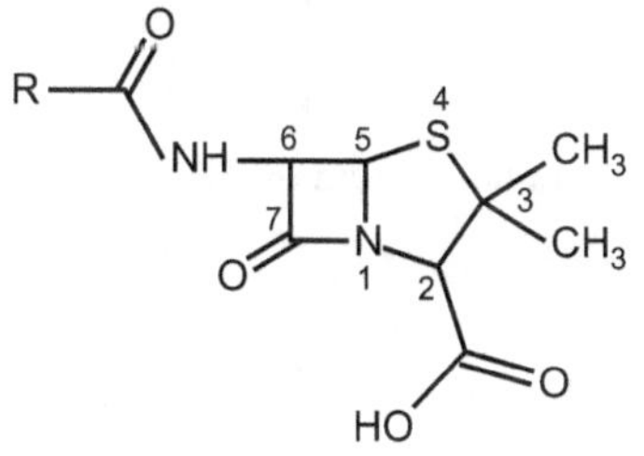   **USP**

Three simplified forms of penicillin nomenclature have been adopted for general use:

1. One uses the name "penam" for the unsubstituted bicyclic system, including the amide carbonyl group. Thus, generally are designated according to the Chemical Abstracts system as 5-acylamino-2,2-dimethylpenam-3-carboxylic acids.

2. The second, uses the name "penicillanic acid" to describe the ring system with substituent that are generally present (i.e., 2,2-dimethyl and 3-carboxyl).

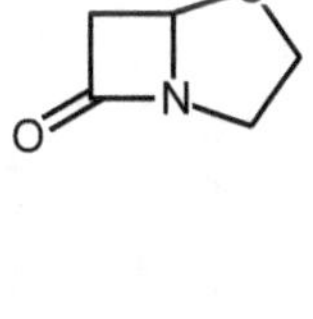

Penam 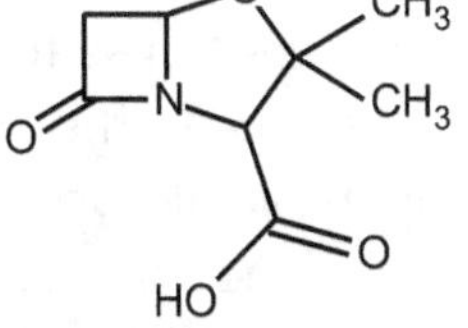   **Penicillanic acid** 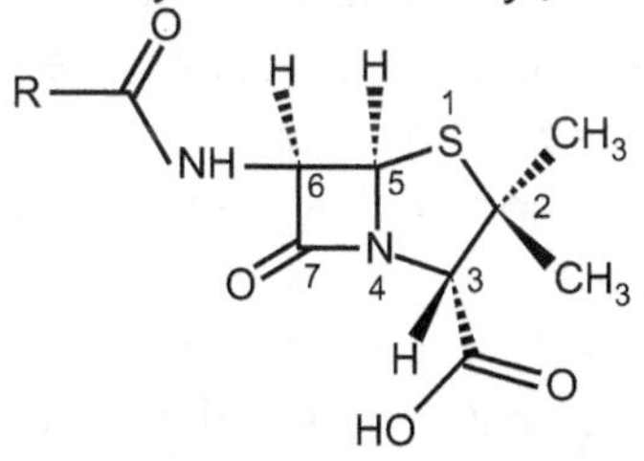   **Chemical abstracts**

3. A third form, to name the entire 6-carbonylaminopenicillanic acid portion of the molecule penicillin and then distinguishes compounds on the basis of the R-group of the acyl portion of the molecule. Thus, penicillin-G is named benzylpenicillin, penicillin-V is phenoxymethyl penicillin, methicillin is 2, 6-dimethoxyphenylpenicillin and so on.

For the most part, the later two systems serve well for naming and comparing closely similar penicillin structures, but they are too restrictive to be applied to compounds with unusual substituents or to ring-modified derivatives.

1.7.3 Synthesis of Penicillin Analogues

Penicillin analogues were originally synthesized by a fermentation process, in which different carboxylic acid derivatives were added to yield penicillins containing different 6-amido derivatives. The principle disadvantage of this approach was that not all carboxylic acids were biologically acceptable, and thus only a limited number of analogues could be prepared. The semi-synthetic approach relies on the isolation of 6-aminopenicillanic acid (6-APA) from fermentation media. A large number of 6-amido derivatives can then be prepared by chemical reaction with acyl chlorides.

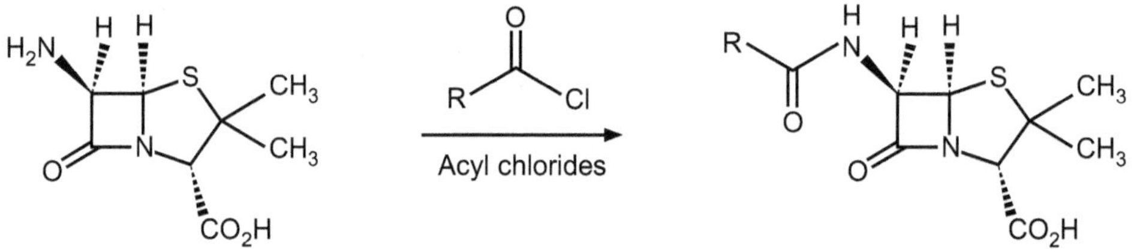

6-Aminopenicillanic acid (6-APA)   **Penicillin derivatives**

1.7.4 Stereochemistry

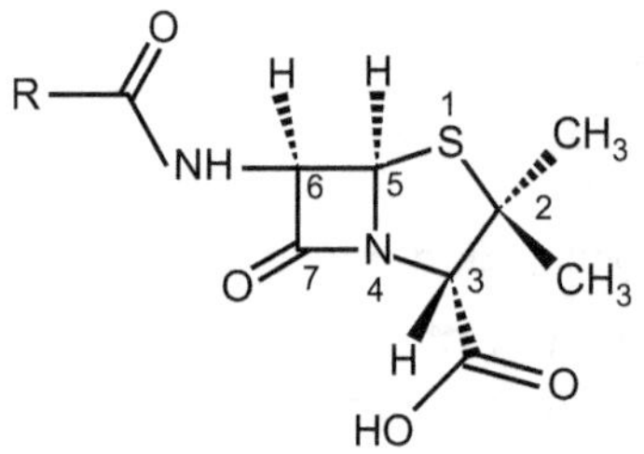

- Three chiral carbon atoms i. e. C-3, C-5 and C-6 are present in the penicillin molecule.
- All naturally occurring, synthetic and semi-synthetic penicillins possess the same absolute contiguration about these three centers for antimicrobial activity.
- The carbon atom bearing the acylamino group (C-6) has the L-configuration, whereas the carbon to which the carboxyl group is attached has the D-configuration.
- Thus, the acylamino and carboxyl groups are transe to each other, with the former in the α and the later in the β orientation relative to the penam ring system.
- The atoms composing the 6-aminopenicillanic acid portion of the structure are derived biosynthetically from two amino acids, L-cysteine (S-1, C5, C-6, C-7 and 6-amino) and L-valine (2,2-dimethyl, C-2, C-3, N-4 and 3-carboxyl).

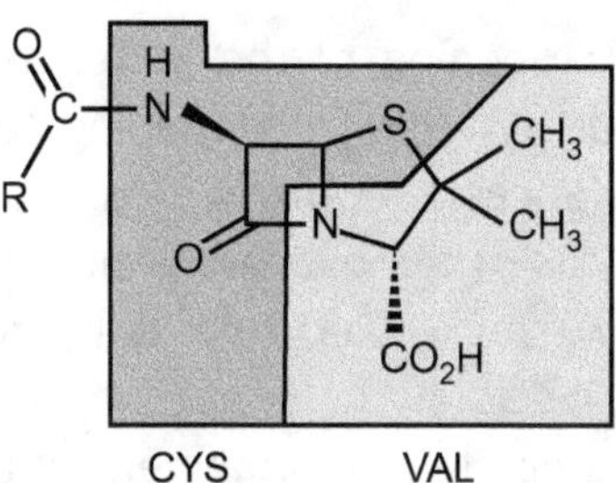

- The absolute stereochemistry of the penicillins is designated 3S : 5R : 6R.

1.7.5 Physicochemical Properties

The early commercial penicillin was a yellow to brown amorphous powder that was so unstable that refrigeration was required to maintain a reasonable level of activity for a short time. Improved purification procedures provided the white crystalline material in use today. Crystalline penicillin must be protected from moisture, but when kept dry, the salts will remain stable for years without refrigeration. Many types of penicillin have an unpleasant taste, which must be overcome in the formation of pediatric dosage forms. All of the natural penicillins are strongly dextrorotatory.

The solubility and other physicochemical properties of the penicillins are affected by the nature of the acyl side chain and by the cations used to make salts of the acid. Most penicillins are acids with pKa values in the range of 2.5 to 3.0, but some are amphoteric. The free acids are not suitable for oral or parenteral administration. The sodium and potassium salts of most penicillins, however, are soluble in water and readily absorbed orally or parenterally.

Salts of penicillins with organic bases, such as benzathine, procaine, and hydrabamine have limited water solubility and are, therefore, useful as depot forms to provide effective blood levels over a long period in the treatment of chronic infections. Some of the crystalline salts of the penicillins are hygroscopic and must be stored in sealed containers.

1.7.6 Chemical Degradation

The deterioration of penicillin occurred due to reactivity (hydrolysis) of the strained lactam ring and is influenced by the pH of the solution. The β-lactam carbonyl group of penicillin readily undergoes nucleophilic attack by water (-OH⁻) to form the inactive penicilloic acid, which is reasonably stable in neutral to alkaline solutions, but readily undergoes decarboxylation and further hydrolytic reactions in acidic solutions. Other nucleophiles, such as hydroxylamines, alkylamines, and alcohols, open the β-lactam ring to form the corresponding hydroxamic acids, amides, and esters.

It has been speculated that one of the causes of penicillin allergy may be the formation of antigenic penicilloyl proteins *in vivo* by the reaction of nucleophilic groups (e.g., α-amino) on specific body proteins with the β-lactam carbonyl group.

In strongly acidic solutions (pH < 3), penicillin undergoes a complex series of reactions leading to a variety of inactive degradation products. The first step appears to involve rearrangement to the penicillanic acid. This process is initiated by protonation of the β-lactam nitrogen, followed by nucleophilic attack of the acyl oxygen atom on the β-lactam carbonyl carbon. The subsequent opening of the β-lactam ring destabilizes the thiazoline ring, which then also suffers acid-catalyzed ring opening to form the penicillanic acid. The later is very unstable and experiences two major degradation pathways. The most easily understood path involves hydrolysis of the oxazolone ring to form the unstable penamaldic acid. Because it is an enamine, penamaldic acid easily hydrolyzes to penicillamine (a major degradation product) and penaldic acid.

The second path involves a complete rearrangement of penicillanic acid to a penillic acid through a series of intramolecular processes that remain to be elucidated completely. Penillic acid (an imidazoline-2-carboxylic acid) readily decarboxylates and suffers hydrolytic ring opening under acidic conditions to form a second major end product of acid-catalyzed penicillin degradant, penilloic acid.

Penicilloic acid, the major product formed under weakly acidic to alkaline hydrolytic conditions, cannot be detected as an intermediate under strongly acidic conditions. It exists in equilibrium with penamaldic acid, however, and undergoes decarboxylation in acid to form penilloic acid. The third product of the degradation is penicilloaldehyde formed by decarhoxylation of penaldic acid.

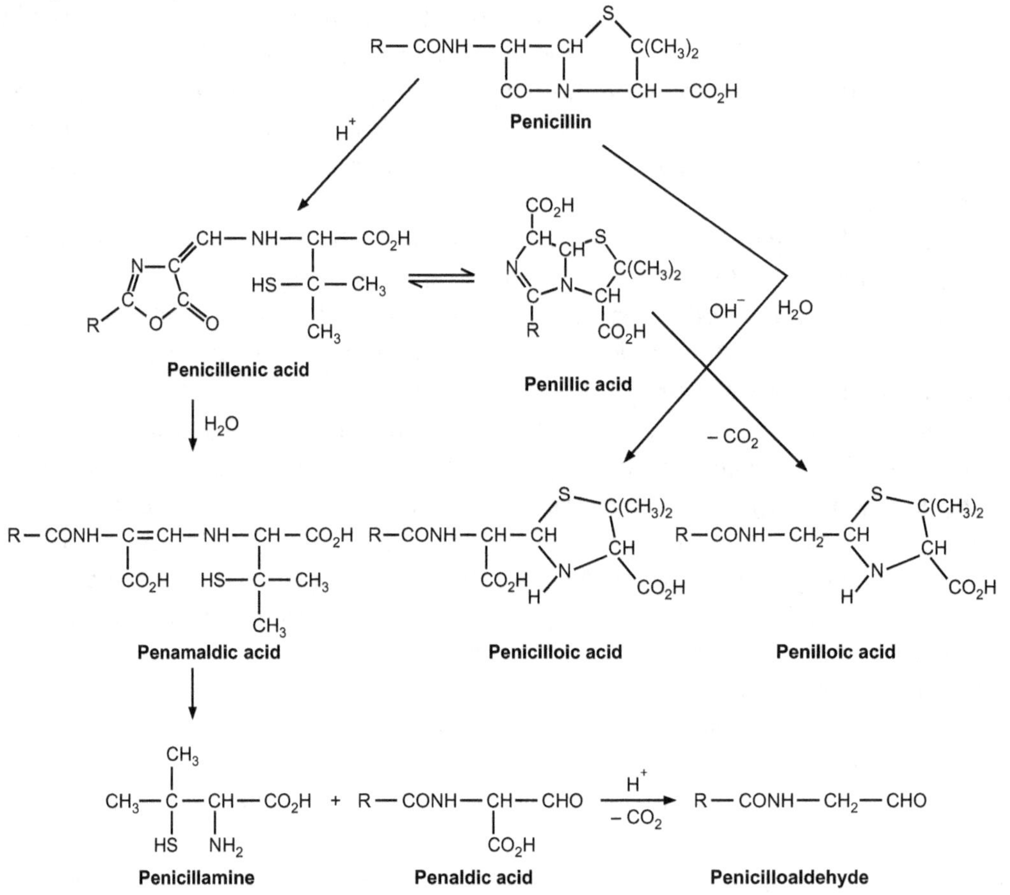

Fig. 1.4: Degradation pathway of Penicillin

Oxidizing agents also inactivate penicillins, but reducing agents have little effect on them. Temperature affects the rate of deterioration: although the dry salts are stable at room temperature and do not require refrigeration, prolonged heating inactivates the penicillins.

Acid-catalyzed degradation in the stomach contributes strongly to the poor oral absorption of penicillin. Thus, efforts to obtain penicillins with improved pharmacokinetic and microbiological properties have focused on acyl functionalities that would minimize sensitivity of the β-lactam ring to acid hydrolysis while maintaining antibacterial activity.

1.7.7 Structure Activity Relationship

Penicillin molecules contain a highly strained 4-membered β-lactam ring fused to a 5-membered thiazolidene ring. The β-lactam ring is unstable and is primarily responsible for the antibiotic potency of these molecules.

- The bicyclic ring system containing the β-lactam is crucial, as are the cis relationship between the two hydrogens at positions 5 and 6, a free 3-carboxylate and a 6-amide. Changing one or more of these results in a loss of activity.
- The side chain determines, in large part, the antibacterial spectrum and pharmacologic properties.
- The chemical substituent attached to the penicillin nucleus can greatly influence the stability of the penicillins as well as the spectrum of activity.

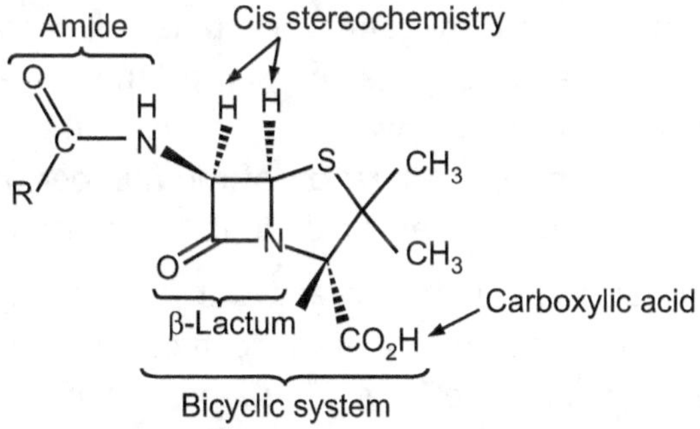

- The substitution of a side-chain 'R' group on the primary amine with an electron-withdrawing group decreases the electron density on the side-chain carbonyl and protects these penicillins, as they passage through the stomach better and many can be given orally for systemic purpose.
- The more lipophilic the side chain of penicillin, the more serum protein bound is the antibiotic.
- Stability of the penicillin towards β-lactamase is influenced by the bulk in the acyl group attached to the primary amine.

- β-lactamase stability of penicillin increases, when the aromatic ring is attached directly to the side-chain carbonyl and both ortho positions are substituted by methoxy groups.
- Changing of one of the methoxy groups to the para position, or replacing one of them by hydrogen, resulted in an analogue sensitive to β-lactamases.
- Putting in a methylene between the aromatic ring and 6-APA likewise produced a β-lactamase–sensitive agent.

1.7.8 Bacterial Resistance

Gram-negative bacteria are more prone to resistant to the action of penicillins. Other sensitive species can develop penicillin resistance through mutation. The most important biochemical mechanism of penicillin resistance is the bacterial elaboration of enzymes (penicillinase) that inactivate penicillins. There are two general types of penicillinase i.e. β-lactamases and acylases.

β-lactamase, catalyze the hydrolytic opening of the β-lactam ring of penicillin to produce inactive penicilloic acids. Acylase can hydrolyze the acylamino side chain of penicillins, have been obtained from species of Gram-negative bacteria. These enzymes find some commercial use in the preparation of aminopenicillanic acid (6-APA) for the preparation of semi-synthetic penicillins. 6-APA is less active and hydrolyzed more rapidly than penicillin.

Another important resistance mechanism in Gram-negative bacteria is by decreasing permeability to penicillins. The cell envelope (linked by lipoprotein bridges to the peptido-glycan cell wall) in most Gram-negative bacteria is more complex than in Gram-positive bacteria. It creates a physical barrier to the penetration of hydrophobic antibiotics. Small hydrophilic molecules, however, can traverse the outer membrane through pores formed by proteins called porins. Alteration of the number or nature of porins in the cell envelope could be an important mechanism of antibiotic resistance.

Bacterial resistance can also result from changes in the affinity of PBPs for penicillins. Certain strains of bacteria are resistant to the lytic properties of penicillins, but remain susceptible to their growth inhibiting effects. Thus, the action of the antibiotic has been converted from bactericidal to bacteriostatic. This mechanism of resistance is termed as tolerance and apparently results from impaired autolysin activity in the bacterium.

1.7.9 Allergic Reaction Associated with Penicillins

Different allergic reactions associated with various penicillins, such as variety of skin and mucous membrane rashes, fever and anaphylaxis. Occasionally, the reaction is immediate and profound. It may include cardiovascular collapse and shock and can even result in death. Sometimes, penicillin allergy can be anticipated by taking a medication history, and often, the patients who are likely to be allergic are those with a history of hypersensitivity to a wide variety of allergens.

1.7.10 Chemical Classification of Penicillins

Name of drugs	R_1
Fermentation Derived Penicillins	
Aminopenicillanic acid	H
Benzylpenicillin (Penicillin-G)	$-CH_2-$ (benzyl)
Phenoxymethylpenicillin (Penicillin-V)	$-O-CH_2-$ (phenoxymethyl)
Semi-synthetic penicillinase-resistant (Parenteral Penicillins)	
Methicillin	2,6-dimethoxyphenyl (OCH_3, OCH_3)
Nafcillin	2-ethoxynaphthyl (OC_2H_5)
Semi-synthetic penicillinase-resistant (Oral Penicillins)	
Oxacillin (X = Y = H)	3-phenyl-5-methylisoxazol-4-yl (CH_3)
Cloxacillin (X = Cl, Y = H)	
Dicloxacillin (X = Y = Cl)	

Semi-synthetic penicillinase-sensitive (Broad Spectrum Parenteral Penicillins)	
Carbenicillin	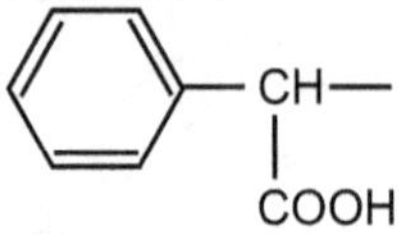
Ticarcillin	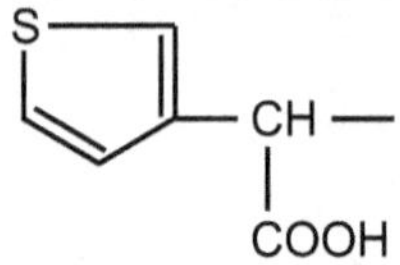
Semi-synthetic penicillinase-sensitive (Broad Spectrum Oral Penicillins)	
Ampicillin (X = H)	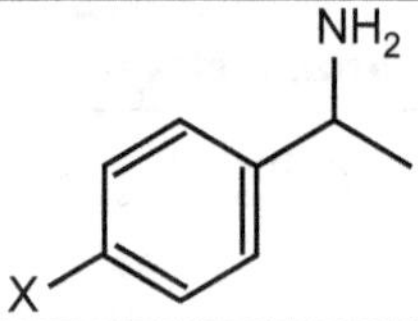
Amoxycillin (X = OH)	

1.7.11 Drug Profile

1. Penicillin-G (Benzylpenicillin):

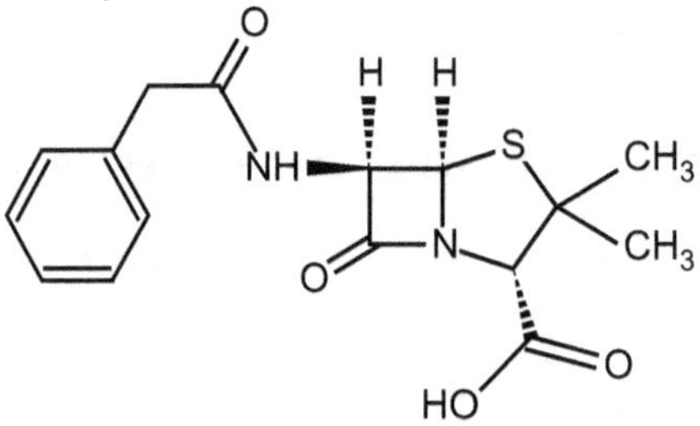

Penicillin-G (Benzylpenicillin)

- Penicillin-G or benzylpenicillin is a broad-spectrum, β-lactam naturally occurring penicillin antibiotic with antibacterial activity.
- It is chemically, (2S,5R,6R)-3,3-dimethyl-7-oxo-6-[(2-phenylacetyl)amino]-4-thia-1-azabicyclo [3.2.0]heptane-2-carboxylic acid.
- It acts as given in mechanism of action of penicillin.
- Penicillin-G is unstable under the acidic conditions of the stomach.
- As it is not β-lactamase stable, and organisms are developing altered targets (PBPs), it is less likely to remain the drug of first choice for many infections.
- The widely used amine salt of penicillin-G was made with procaine with and N, N'-benzathine.

Uses:

- Penicillin-G remains a remarkably useful agent for the treatment of diseases caused by susceptible microorganisms.
- It is the prototypic penicillin with activity against a variety of organisms such as the streptococci, treponemes and meningococci.

2. Penicillin-V (Phenoxymethylpenicillin):

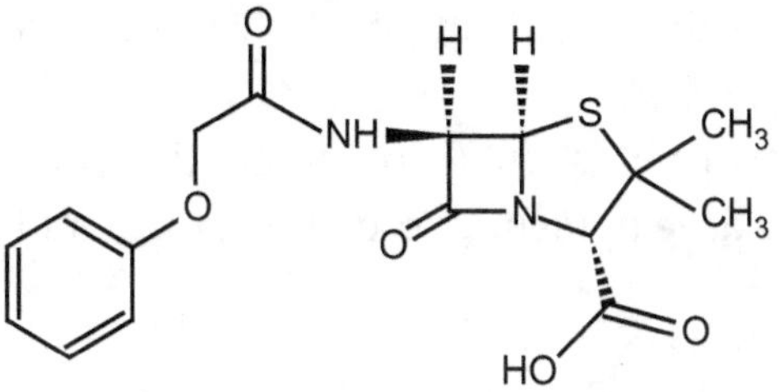

Penicillin-V (Phenoxymethylpenicillin)

- Penicillin-V or phenoxymethylpenicillin is a broad-spectrum β-lactam antibiotic produced by either fermentation or by semisynthesis.
- It is chemically, (2S, 5R, 6R)-3,3-dimethyl-7-oxo-6-[(2-phenoxyacetyl)amino]-4-thia-1-azabicyclo [3.2.0]heptane-2-carboxylic acid.
- The electronegative oxygen atom in the C-7 amide side chain inhibits participation in β-lactam bond hydrolysis.
- It acts as given in mechanism of action of penicillin.
- It is considerably more acid stable than benzylpenicillin.
- Penicillin-V was the first of the so-called oral penicillins, giving higher and more prolonged blood levels than penicillin-G itself.
- Its antimicrobial, clinical spectrum sensitivity to β-lactamases and allergenicity is same as penicillin-G.

3. Methicillin

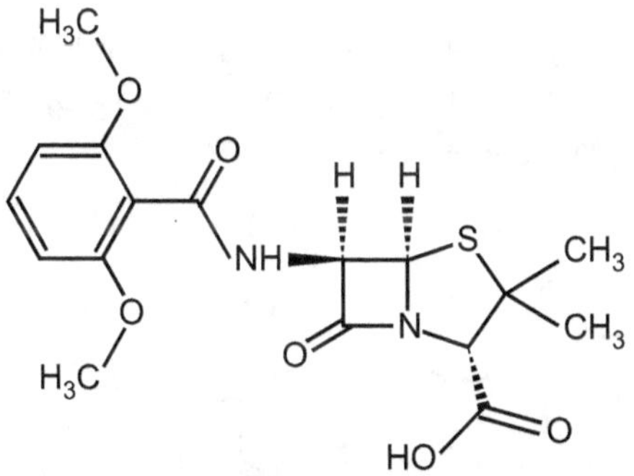

Methicillin

- Methicillin is a semisynthetic, narrow spectrum β-lactamase-resistant penicillin antibiotic with bactericidal activity.
- It is a 6-aminopenicillanic acid in which one of the amino hydrogens is replaced by a 2,6-dimethoxybenzoyl group.
- It is chemically, (2S, 5R, 6R)-6-[(2,6-dimethoxybenzoyl)amino]-3,3-dimethyl-7-oxo-4-thia-1-azabicyclo[3.2.0]heptane-2-carboxylic acid.
- It inhibits bacterial wall synthesis by a mechanism of action similar to penicillin.
- It is inactivated by gastric acid, so administered by injection.

Uses:

- Methicillin is used in the treatment of staphylococcal infections caused by strains resistant to other penicillins.
- It is recommended that it should not be used in general therapy, to avoid the possible widespread development of organisms resistant to it.

4. Nafcillin:

Nafcillin

- Nafcillin is a semi-synthetic naphthalene and β-lactam antibiotic with antibacterial activity.
- It is chemically, (2S, 5R, 6R)-6-[(2-ethoxynaphthalene-1-carbonyl)amino]-3,3-dimethyl-7-oxo-4-thia-1-azabicyclo[3.2.0]heptane-2-carboxylic acid.
- It inhibits bacterial wall synthesis by a mechanism of action similar to penicillin.

Uses:

- Nafcillin is a parenteral, second generation penicillinase-resistant penicillin antibiotic used largely to treat moderate to severe staphylococcal infections.

5. Oxacillin, Cloxacillin and Dicloxacillin:

Dicloxacillin

- Oxacillin (R_1 and R_2 = H), Cloxacillin (R_1 = Cl and R_2 = H) and Dicloxacillin (R_1 and R_2 = Cl) are semi-synthetic penicillinase-resistant and acid-stable penicillin with an antimicrobial activity.
- Replacement of bio-isosteric isoxazolyl ring and a methyl in place of benzene ring and a substituted benzene ring on the other in place of the methoxyls of methicillin produces the isoxazolyl penicillins.

- Steric effects of the 3-phenyl and 5-methyl groups of the isoxazolyl ring prevent the binding of this penicillin to the β-lactamase active site and, thereby, protect the lactam ring from degradation like methicillin.
- The chlorine atoms at ortho position of the phenyl ring to the isoxazole ring enhance the activity as well as stability.
- Oxacillin is chemically, (2S, 5R, 6R)-3,3-dimethyl-6-[(5-methyl-3-phenyl-1,2-oxazole-4-carbonyl) amino]-7-oxo-4-thia-1-azabicyclo[3.2.0]heptane-2-carboxylic acid.
- Cloxacillin is chemically, (2S, 5R, 6R)-6-[[3-(2-chlorophenyl)-5-methyl-1,2-oxazole-4-carbonyl]amino]-3,3-dimethyl-7-oxo-4-thia-1-azabicyclo[3.2.0]heptane-2-carboxylic acid.
- Dicloxacillin is chemically, (2S, 5R, 6R)-6-[[3-(2,6-dichlorophenyl)-5-methyl-1,2-oxazole-4-carbonyl]amino]-3,3-dimethyl-7-oxo-4-thia-1-azabicyclo[3.2.0]heptane-2-carboxylic acid.
- These penicillins are resistant to acid hydrolysis, therefore may be administered orally.
- These drugs inhibit bacterial wall synthesis by a mechanism of action similar to penicillin.

Uses:

- Oxacillin, Cloxacillin and Dicloxacillin are parenteral, second generation penicillin antibiotics that are used to treat moderate-to-severe, penicillinase-resistant staphylococcal infections.

6. **Carbenicillin:**

Carbenicillin

- Carbenicillin is a broad-spectrum, semi-synthetic penicillin antibiotic with bactericidal and β-lactamase resistant activity.
- It is chemically, (2S, 5R, 6R)-6-[(2-carboxy-2-phenylacetyl)amino]-3,3-dimethyl-7-oxo-4-thia-1-azabicyclo[3.2.0]heptane-2-carboxylic acid.
- It is a benzylpenicillin analogue in which one of the methylene hydrogens of the side chain has been substituted with a carboxylic acid moiety.
- The introduction of the side-chain carboxyl produces enhanced anti-Gram-negative activity.
- It acylates the penicillin-sensitive transpeptidase C-terminal domain by opening the lactam ring.

- The drug is susceptible to β-lactamases and is acid unstable, so it must be given by injection.

Uses:

- Carbenicillin is used for therapy of moderate to severe urinary, respiratory, gastrointestinal tract, skin, bone and joint infections.
- Oral prodrug ester indanyl carbenicillin is primarily used for oral treatment of urinary tract infections.

7. **Ticarcillin:**

Ticarcillin

- Ticarcillin is a broad-spectrum, semi-synthetic penicillin antibiotic with bactericidal activity.
- It is chemically, (2S, 5R, 6R)-6-[[(2R)-2-carboxy-2-thiophen-3-yl-acetyl]amino]-3,3-dimethyl-7-oxo-4-thia-1-azabicyclo[3.2.0]heptane-2-carboxylic acid.
- It inactivates the penicillin-sensitive transpeptidase C-terminal domain by opening the lactam ring.
- In combination with potassium clavulanate, it has enhanced anti-pseudomonas activity because of its enhanced stability to lactamases.

Uses:

- Ticarcillin is a sulfur-based bio-isostere of carbenicillin and more potent against pseudomonas compared with indanyl carbenicillin.
- It used to treat moderate-to-severe infections due to susceptible organisms.

8. **Ampicillin:**

Ampicillin

- Ampicillin is a broad-spectrum, semi-synthetic, β-lactam penicillin antibiotic with bactericidal activity.

- It is chemically, (2*S*, 5*R*, 6*R*)-6-[[(2*R*)-2-amino-2-phenylacetyl]amino]-3,3-dimethyl-7-oxo-4-thia-1-azabicyclo[3.2.0]heptane-2-carboxylic acid.
- It is a benzylpenicillin analogue in which one of the hydrogen atoms of the side-chain methylene has been replaced with a primary amino group to produce an *R*-phenylglycine moiety.
- It is stable against hydrolysis by a variety of β-lactamases, therefore, can be used in wide range of Gram-positive and Gram-negative infections.
- It inhibits bacterial wall synthesis by a mechanism of action similar to penicillin.

Uses:

- Ampicillin is used widely to treat mild-to-severe infections due to susceptible organisms.

9. Amoxicillin:

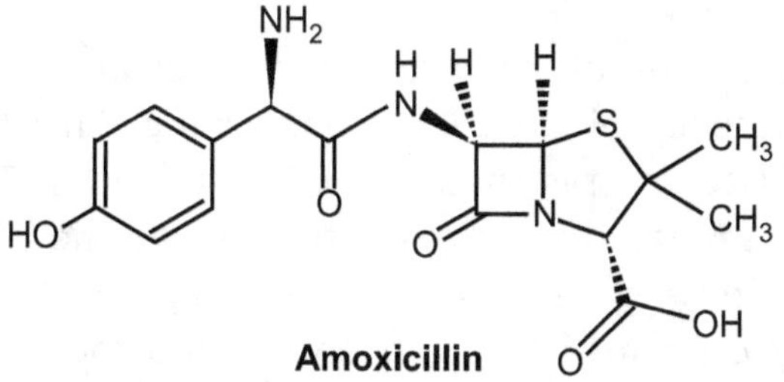

NH$_2$ H H H N S CH$_3$ CH$_3$ HO O O N OH O

Amoxicillin

- Amoxicillin is the anhydrous form of a broad-spectrum, semisynthetic aminopenicillin antibiotic with bactericidal activity.
- It is chemically, (2S, 5R, 6R)-6-[[(2R)-2-amino-2-(4-hydroxyphenyl)acetyl]amino]-3,3-dimethyl-7-oxo-4-thia-1-azabicyclo[3.2.0]heptane-2-carboxylic acid.
- It is a close analogue of ampicillin, in which a para-phenolic hydroxyl group has been introduced into the side-chain phenyl moiety.
- It inhibits bacterial wall synthesis by a mechanism of action similar to penicillin.

Uses:

- Amoxicillin is one of the most commonly prescribed antibacterial antibiotics.
- The antimicrobial spectrum and clinical uses of amoxicillin are approximately the same as those of ampicillin.

1.8 CEPHALOSPORINS

Members of this group of antibiotics are similar to penicillin in their structure and mode of action. They account for one-third of all antibiotics prescribed and administered.

The cephalosporins are β-lactam antibiotics isolated cephalosporium species or prepared semi-synthetically. Most of the antibiotics introduced since 1965 have been semi-synthetic cephalosporins. The first known member of this group of antibiotics was first isolated by Guiseppe Brotzu in 1945 from the fungus *Cephalosporium acremonium* which inhibited the growth of wide varieties of Gram-positive and Gram-negative bacteria.

Cephalosporins contain 7-aminocephalosporanic acid (7-ACA) nucleus and side chain containing 3,6-dihydro-2 H-1,3- thiazane ring. Cephalosporins are used in the treatment of bacterial infections and diseases arising from penicillinase-producing, methicillin-susceptible Staphylococci and Streptococci, *Proteus mirabilis*, some *Escherichia coli*, *Klebsiella pneumonia*, *Haemophilus influenza*, *Enterobacter aerogenes* and some *Neisseria*.

They are subdivided into generations (1st-5th) in accordance to their target organism, but later versions are increasingly more effective against Gram-negative pathogens. Cephalosporins have a variety of side chains that enable them to get attached to different penicillin-binding proteins (PBPs), to circumvent blood brain barrier, resist breakdown by penicillinase producing bacterial strains and ionize to facilitate entry into Gram-negative bacteria cells.

1.8.1 Nomenclature

The chemical nomenclature of cephalosporins is slightly more complex than the penicillins because of presence of a double bond in the dihydrothiazine ring. Chemical abstract designated the fused ring system as 5-thia-1-azabicyclo[4.2.0]oct-2-ene. Further the name is simplified for the saturated bicyclic ring system with the lactam carbonyl oxygen as *Cepham*. According to this system all commercially available cephalosporins and cephamycins are named 3-cephams (or Δ^3- cephams) to designate the position of the double bond. All known 2-cephams are inactive, because the β-lactam lacks the necessary ring strain to react sufficiently.

Cepham   **Cephalosporanic Acid**   **Structure of Cephalosporins**

Some cephalosporins are named as derivatives of cephalosporanic acids; this practice applies only to the derivatives that have a 3-acetoxymethyl group.

1.8.2 Chemical Degradation of Cephalosporins

Cephalosporins experience a variety of hydrolytic degradation reactions whose specific nature depends on the individual structure. Among 7-acylaminocephalosporanic acid (7-ACA) derivatives, the 3-acetoxylmethyl group is the most reactive site. In addition to its reactivity to nucleophilic displacement reactions, the acetoxyl function of this group readily undergoes solvolysis in strongly acidic solutions to form the des-acetylcephalosporin derivatives. The later lactonizes to form the desacetylcephalosporin lactones, which are virtually inactive.

The 7-acylamino group of some cephalosporins can also be hydrolyzed under enzymatic (acylases) and, possibly, non-enzymatic conditions to give 7-ACA (or 7-ADCA) derivatives. Following hydrolysis or solvolysis of the 3-acetoxymethyl group, 7-ACA lactonizes under acidic conditions.

The reactive functionality common to all cephalosporins is the β-lactam. Hydrolysis of the β-lactam of cephalosporins is believed to give initially cephalosporanic acids or possibly anhydro-desacetylcephalosporanic acids (for the 7-acylaminocephalosporanic acids). It has not been possible to isolate either of these initial hydrolysis products in aqueous systems. Apparently, both types of cephalosporanic acids undergo fragmentation reactions that have not been characterized fully.

1.8.3 Structure-Activity Relationship

As with the penicillins, various molecular changes in the cephalosporin can improve *in-vitro* stability, antibacterial activity, and stability towards β-lactamases.

- The addition of an amino and a hydrogen to the α and α′ position, respectively, results in a basic compound that is protonated under the acidic conditions of the stomach.
- The ammonium ion improves the stability of the β-lactam of the cephalosporin, leading to orally active drugs.
- The 7β-amino group is essential for antimicrobial activity (X = H), whereas replacement of the hydrogen at C-7 (X = H) with an alkoxy (X = OR) results in improvement of the antibacterial activity of the cephalosporin.
- Within specific cephalosporin derivatives, the addition of a 7α-methoxy also improves the drugs stability towards β-lactamase.
- The derivatives, where Y = S, exhibit greater antibacterial activity than if Y = O, but the reverse is true when stability towards β-lactamase is considered.
- The 6α-hydrogen is essential for biological activity.
- Finally, antibacterial activity is improved when Z is a 5-membered heterocycle versus a 6-membered heterocycle.
- In a study examining the stability of cephalosporins towards β-lactamase, it was noted that the following changes improved β-lactamase resistance:
    1. The L-isomer of an α-amino α′-hydrogen derivative of a cephalosporin was 30- to 40- fold more stable than the D-isomer.
    2. The addition of a methoxyoxime to the α and α′ positions increased stability nearly 100-fold.

Z-oxime   **E-oxime**

3. The Z-oxime was as much as 20,000-fold more stable than the E-oxime. These changes have been incorporated into a number of marketed and experimental cephalosporins (Cefuroxime, Ceftizoxime, Ceftazidime, and Cefixime).

1.8.4 Mechanism of Action

The cephalosporins are believed to act in a manner analogous to that of the penicillins. Cephalosporins bind with receptor proteins, transpeptidases and carboxypeptidases called penicillin binding proteins (PBPs), the enzymes that catalyze the synthesis of peptidoglycan, which is a critical component of the bacterial cell wall. This leads to the interruption of cell wall synthesis, consequently leading to bacterial cell growth inhibition and cell lysis.

1.8.5 Bacterial Resistance

Analogous to the penicillins, susceptible cephalosporins can be hydrolyzed by β-lactamases before they reach the penicillin binding proteins. Many β-lactamases are known. Some are more efficient at hydrolysis of penicillins, some at hydrolysis of cephalosporins and some are indiscriminate. Certain β-lactamases are constitutive (chromosomally encoded) in certain strains of Gram-negative bacteria (*Citrobacter, Enterobacter, Pseudomonas,* and *Serratia* sp.) and normally are repressed. These are induced (or derepressed) by certain β-lactam antibiotics (e.g., imipenem, cefotetam, and cefoxitin).

As with the penicillins, specific examples will be seen below wherein resistance to β-lactamase hydrolysis is conveyed by strategic steric bulk near the side-chain amide linkage. Recently, an increasing number of metallo- β-lactamases have been discovered. The mechanism of these enzymes is dependent on divalent metal ions, commonly zinc. These are both chromosomally and plasmids derived and are as yet confined to the Gram-negative rods. Commonly, these enzymes attack some penicillins, cephalosporins, and carbapenems.

1.8.6 Allergic Reactions Associated with Cephalosporins

Allergenicity is less commonly experienced and is less severe with cephalosporins than with penicillins. Cephalosporins frequently are administered to patients who have had a mild or delayed penicillin reaction. Cross-allergenicity is comparatively common, however, and cephalosporins should be administered with caution for patients who have a history of allergies. Patients who have had a rapid and severe reaction to penicillins should not be treated with cephalosporins.

1.8.7 Classification of Cephalosporins

Cephalosporins are divided into first, second, third, and fourth-generation agents, based roughly on their time of discovery and their antimicrobial properties. In general, progression from first to fourth generation is associated with a broadening of the Gram-negative antibacterial spectrum, some reduction in activity against Gram-positive organisms, and enhanced resistance to β-lactamases.

1. **First Generation Cephalosporins:**
   (a) **Oral:** Cephalexin, Cefadroxil
   (b) **Parenteral:** Cephalothin, Cephapirin, Cefazolin
   (c) **Oral and parenteral:** Cephradine
2. **Second Generation Cephalosporins**
   (a) **Oral:** Cefaclor, Cefprozil, Cefpodoxime

 (b) Parenteral: Cefamandole, Cefonicid, Ceforanide, Cefoxitin, Cefotetan, Cefmetazole

 (c) Oral and parenteral: Cefuroxime

3. **Third Generation Cephalosporins**
   (a) Oral: Cefixime, Ceftibuten
   (b) Parenteral: Cefoperazone, Cefotaxime, Ceftizoxime, Ceftazidime
4. **Third Generation Cephalosporins**
   (a) Parenteral: Cefepime, Cefpirome

1.8.8 Drug Profile

(A) First Generation Cephalosporins:

1. Cephalexin:

Cephalexin

- Cephalexin is a β-lactam, first-generation Cephalosporin antibiotic with bactericidal activity.
- It is chemically, (6R,7R)-7-[[(2R)-2-amino-2-phenylacetyl]amino]-3-methyl-8-oxo-5-thia-1-azabicyclo[4.2.0]oct-2-ene-2-carboxylic acid.
- The α-amino group of cephalexin renders it acid stable and reduction of the 3- acetoxymethyl to a methyl group circumvents reaction at that site.
- It inhibits bacterial wall synthesis by a mechanism of action similar to Cephalosporin.
- Compared to second and third generation cephalosporins, cephalexin is more active against Gram-positive and less active against Gram-negative organisms.

Uses:

Cephalexin is a widely used drug, particularly against Gram-negative bacteria causing urinary tract infections, Gram-positive infections (*Staphylococcus aureus, Streptococcus pneumoniae and Streptococcus pyogenes*) of soft tissues, pharyngitis, and minor wounds.

2. Cefadroxil:

Cefadroxil

- Cefadroxil is a semi-synthetic first-generation Cephalosporin with antibacterial activity.
- It is chemically, (6R,7R)-7-[[(2R)-2-amino-2-(4-hydroxyphenyl)acetyl]amino]-3-methyl-8-oxo-5-thia-1-azabicyclo[4.2.0]oct-2-ene-2-carboxylic acid.
- It is a cephalosporin bearing methyl and (2R)-2-amino-2-(4-hydroxyphenyl) acetamido groups at positions 3 and 7, respectively, of the cephem skeleton.
- It inhibits bacterial wall synthesis by a mechanism of action similar to Cephalosporin.
- It has some immunostimulant properties mediated through T-cell activation and that this is of material assistance to patients in fighting infections.

Uses:

Cefadroxil has a role as an antibacterial drug.

3. Cephalothin:

Cephalothin

- Cephalothin is a semi-synthetic, β-lactam, first-generation Cephalosporin antibiotic with bactericidal activity.
- It is chemically, (6R,7R)-3-(acetyloxymethyl)-8-oxo-7-[(2-thiophen-2-yl-acetyl)amino]-5-thia-1-azabicyclo [4.2.0]oct-2-ene-2-carboxylic acid.
- It has acetoxymethyl and (2-thienylacetyl)nitrilo moieties at positions 3 and 7, respectively, of the core structure.
- It inhibits bacterial wall synthesis by a mechanism of action similar to Celphalosporin.

Uses:

- Cephalothin has a role as an antimicrobial agent and an antibacterial drug.

4. Cephapirin:

Cephapirin

- Cephapirin is a semi-synthetic, broad-spectrum, first-generation Cephalosporin with antibacterial activity.
- It is chemically, (6R,7R)-3-(acetyloxymethyl)-8-oxo-7-[(2-pyridin-4-yl-sulfanylacetyl) amino]-5-thia-1-azabicyclo[4.2.0]oct-2-ene-2-carboxylic acid.
- It has acetoxymethyl and 2(pyridin-4-yl-sulfanyl) acetamido substituents at positions 3 and 7, respectively, of the cephem skeleton.
- It is not orally active.
- It inhibits bacterial wall synthesis by a mechanism of action similar to Cephalosporin.

Uses:

- Cephapirin is used (as its sodium salt) as an antibiotic, being effective against Gram-negative and Gram-positive organisms.
- It has a role as an antibacterial drug.

5. Cefazolin:

Cefazolin

- Cefazolin is a β-lactam antibiotic and first-generation Cephalosporin with bactericidal activity.
- It is chemically, (6R,7R)-3-[(5-methyl-1,3,4-thiadiazol-2-yl)sulfanylmethyl]-8-oxo-7-[[2-(tetrazol-1-yl)acetyl] amino]-5-thia-1-azabicyclo[4.2.0]oct-2-ene-2-carboxylic acid.
- It inhibits bacterial wall synthesis by a mechanism of action similar to Cephalosporin.

Uses:

- Cefazolin is widely used as broad spectrum antibiotics for moderate-to-severe infections with susceptible organisms.

6. Cephradine:

Cephradine

- Cephradine is a β-lactam, first-generation Cephalosporin antibiotic with bactericidal activity.
- It is chemically, (6R,7R)-7-[[(2R)-2-amino-2-cyclohexa-1,4-dien-1-yl-acetyl]amino]-3-methyl-8-oxo-5-thia-1-azabicyclo[4.2.0]oct-2-ene-2-carboxylic acid.
- It has methyl substituent at position 3, and a (2R)-2-amino-2-cyclohexa-1,4-dien-1-yl-acetamido substituent at position 7 of the cephem skeleton.
- It inhibits bacterial wall synthesis by a mechanism of action similar to Cephalosporin.
- It is comparatively acid stable and, therefore, is rapidly and nearly completely absorbed from the GI tract. It can be used both orally and IM.

Uses:

- Cephradine has a role as an antibacterial drug.

(B) Second Generation Cephalosporins:

1. Cefaclor:

Cefaclor

- Cefaclor is an orally active semi-synthetic Cephalosporin.
- It is chemically, (6R,7R)-7-[[(2R)-2-amino-2-phenylacetyl]amino]-3-chloro-8-oxo-5-thia-1-azabicyclo[4.2.0]oct-2-ene-2-carboxylic acid.
- It is synthesized from the corresponding 3-methylenecepham sulfoxide ester by ozonolysis, followed by halogenation of the resulting β-ketoester.
- It differs structurally from cephalexin in that the 3-CH_3 group has been replaced by a -Cl atom.
- It is a cephalosporin bearing chloro and (R)-2-amino-2-phenylacetamido groups at positions 3 and 7, respectively, of the cephem skeleton.
- It inhibits bacterial wall synthesis by a mechanism of action similar to Cephalosporin.

Uses:

- Cefaclor has a role as an antibacterial drug and a drug allergen.
- The antibacterial spectrum of activity is similar to that of cephalexin.
- The drug is recommended for the treatment of non-life-threatening infections caused by *H. influenza*.

2. Cefprozil:

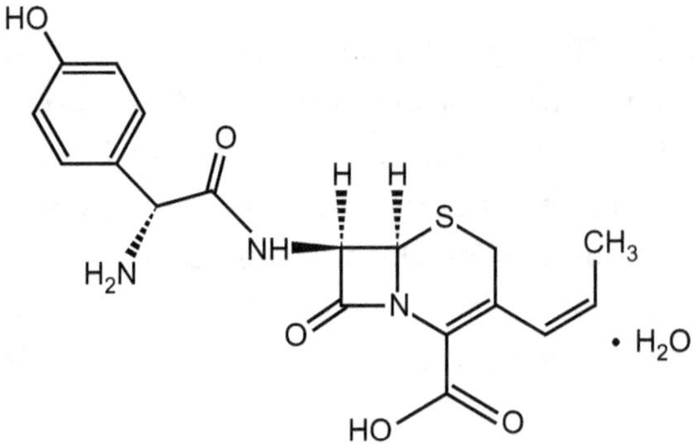

Cefprozil

- Cefprozil is a semi-synthetic, second-generation oral Cephalosporin.
- It most closely resembles with Cefaclor in its properties, but is a little more potent.
- It is chemically, (6R,7R)-7-[[(2R)-2-amino-2-(4-hydroxyphenyl)acetyl]amino]-8-oxo-3-[(E)-prop-1-enyl]-5-thia-1-azabicyclo[4.2.0]oct-2-ene-2-carboxylic acid.
- It has prop-1-enyl and (R)-2-amino-2-(4-hydroxyphenyl)acetamido groups at positions 3 and 7, respectively, of the cephem skeleton.
- It inhibits bacterial wall synthesis by a mechanism of action similar to Cephalosporin.
- It is more active than the first-generation Cephalosporins against members of the *Enterobacteriaceae* family.

Uses:

- Cefprozil has a role as an antibacterial drug and is used to treat bronchitis as well as ear, skin and other bacterial infections.

3. Cefamandole:

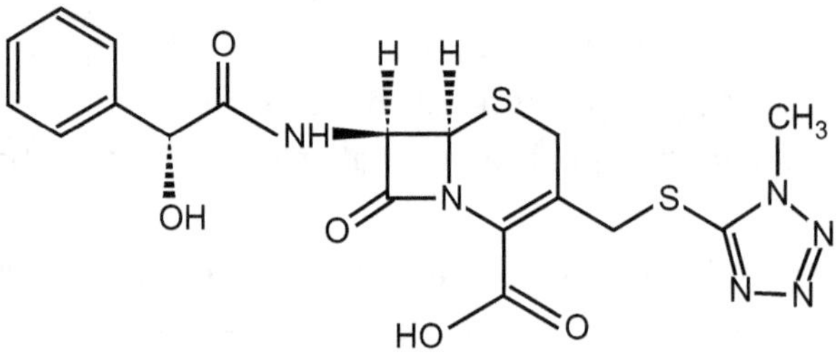

Cefamandole

- Cefamandole is a parenterally administered broad-spectrum Cephalosporin antibiotic.
- It is chemically, (6R,7R)-7-[[(2R)-2-hydroxy-2-phenylacetyl]amino]-3-[(1-methyl-tetrazol-5-yl) sulfanylmethyl]-8-oxo-5-thia-1-azabicyclo[4.2.0]oct-2-ene-2-carboxylic acid.
- It has (R)-mandelamido and N-methylthiotetrazole side-groups.

- The clinically used form of cefamandole is the formate ester cefamandole nafate, a prodrug which is administered parenterally.
- It binds to specific penicillin-binding proteins (PBPs) located inside the bacterial cell wall, causing the inhibition of the third and last stage of bacterial cell wall synthesis.

Uses:

- Cefamandole has a role as an antibacterial drug and active against some ampicillin-resistant strains of *Neisseria* and *Haemophilus* spp.
- It is active against *Haemophilus influenzae* and some Gram-negative bacilli as compared with the first-generation Cephalosporin.
- Clinically it is used for lower respiratory tract, skin, bone and joint infections as well as septicemia and urinary tract infections.

4. Cefonicid:

Cefonicid

- Cefonicid is a second-generation Cephalosporin administered intravenously or intramuscularly.
- It bears {[1-(sulfomethyl)-1H-tetrazol-5-yl]sulfanyl}methyl and (R)-2-hydroxy-2-phenylacetamido groups at positions 3 and 7, respectively, of the cephem skeleton.
- It is chemically, (6R,7R)-7-[[(2R)-2-hydroxy-2-phenylacetyl]amino]-8-oxo-3-[[1-(sulfomethyl)tetrazol-5-yl]sulfanylmethyl]-5-thia-1-azabicyclo[4.2.0]oct-2-ene-2-carboxylic acid.
- It inhibits bacterial wall synthesis by a mechanism of action similar to Cephalosporin.

Uses:

- Cefonicid is used for urinary tract infections, lower respiratory tract infections, and soft tissue and bone infections.

5. Ceforanide:

Ceforanide

- Ceforanide is a second-generation Cephalosporin antibiotic administered parenterally.
- It bears {[1-(carboxymethyl)-1H-tetrazol-5-yl]sulfanyl}methyl and 2-(aminomethyl) phenyl acetamido groups at positions 3 and 7, respectively, of the cephem skeleton.
- It is chemically, (6R,7R)-7-[[2-[2-(aminomethyl)phenyl]acetyl]amino]-3-[[1-(carboxy-methyl) tetrazol-5-yl]sulfanylmethyl]-8-oxo-5-thia-1-azabicyclo[4.2.0]oct-2-ene-2-carboxylic acid.
- It inhibits bacterial wall synthesis by a mechanism of action similar to Cephalosporin.

Uses:

- Ceforanide has excellent potency against most members of the *Enterobacteriaceae* family, especially *K. pneumoniae*, *E. coli*, *P. mirabilis*, and *Enterobacter cloacae*.
- It is less active than cefamandole against *H. influenza*.

6. Cefoxitin:

Cefoxitin

- Cefoxitin is a semi-synthetic, broad-spectrum Cephalosporin antibiotic for intravenous administration.
- It is derived from cephamycin-C, which is produced by *Streptomyces lactamdurans*.
- It is chemically, (6R,7S)-3-(carbamoyloxymethyl)-7-methoxy-8-oxo-7-[(2-thiophen-2-yl-acetyl) amino]-5-thia-1-azabicyclo[4.2.0]oct-2-ene-2-carboxylic acid.
- It inhibits bacterial wall synthesis by a mechanism of action similar to Cephalosporin.

Uses:

- Cefoxitin used in the treatment of certain anaerobic and mixed aerobic-anaerobic infections.
- It is also used to treat gonorrhea caused by β-lactamase producing strains.

7. Cefotetan:

Cefotetan

- Cefotetan is a second-generation semi-synthetic Cephamycin antibiotic that is administered intravenously or intramuscularly.
- It is chemically, (6R,7S)-7-[[4-(2-amino-1-carboxy-2-oxoethylidene)-1,3-dithietane-2-carbonyl] amino]-7-methoxy-3-[(1-methyltetrazol-5-yl)sulfanylmethyl]-8-oxo-5-thia-1-azabicyclo[4.2.0] oct -2-ene-2-carboxylic acid.
- It inhibits bacterial wall synthesis by a mechanism of action similar to Cephalosporin.

Uses:

- Cefotetan is highly resistant to a broad spectrum of β-lactamases.
- It is active against a wide range of both aerobic and anaerobic Gram-positive and Gram-negative microorganisms.
- It is more active against *S. aureus* and members of the *Enterobactcriaceae* family.
- It also exhibits excellent potency against *H. infineuzue* and *N. gonorrhoeae*.

8. Cefmetazole:

Cefmetazole

- Cefmetazole is a second-generation parenteral Cephalosporin antibiotic.
- It is chemically, (6R,7S)-7-[[2-(cyanomethylsulfanyl)acetyl]amino]-7-methoxy-3-[(1-methyl tetrazol-5-yl)sulfanylmethyl]-8-oxo-5-thia-1-azabicyclo[4.2.0]oct-2-ene-2-carboxylic acid.
- It inhibits bacterial wall synthesis by a mechanism of action similar to Cephalosporin.

Uses:

- Cefmetazole has broad spectrum of activity against both Gram-positive and Gram-negative microorganisms.
- It exhibits significantly higher potency against members of the *Enterobacteriaceae* family.
- It is highly active against *N. gonorrhaeae* including β-lactamase-producing strains.

9. Cefuroxime Axetil:

Cefuroxime Axetil

- Cefuroxime axetil is a second-generation semi-synthetic Cephalosporin which can be administered orally as well as parentrally.
- It is chemically, 1-acetyloxyethyl (6R,7R)-3-(carbamoyloxymethyl)-7-[[(2Z)-2-(furan-2-yl)-2-methoxyiminoacetyl]amino]-8-oxo-5-thia-1-azabicyclo[4.2.0]oct-2-ene-2-carboxylate.
- Its spectrum of antibacterial activity more closely resembles that of cefamandole.
- It inhibits bacterial wall synthesis by a mechanism of action similar to Cephalosporin.

Uses:

- Ceruroxime axetil is effective in meningitis caused by susceptible organisms.
- Axetil ester is used for the oral treatment of non-life-threatening infections caused by bacteria that are susceptible to cefuroxime.

(C) Third-Generation Cephalosporins:

1. Cefpodoxime proxetil:

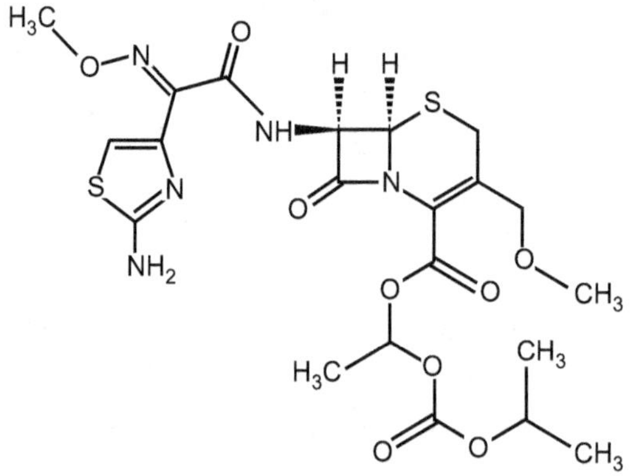

Cefpodoxime Proxetil

- Cefpodoxime Proxetil is a third-generation semi-synthetic Cephalosporin antibiotic with bactericidal activity.
- It is chemically, 1-propan-2-yl-oxycarbonyloxyethyl (6R,7R)-7-[[2-(2-amino-1,3-thiazol-4-yl)-2-methoxyiminoacetyl]amino]-3-(methoxymethyl)-8-oxo-5-thia-1-azabicyclo[4.2.0]oct-2-ene-2- carboxylate.
- It is orally active prodrug derivative and is hydrolyzed by esterases in the intestinal wall and in the plasma to provide cefpodoxime.
- It inhibits bacterial wall synthesis by a mechanism of action similar to Cephalosporin.

Uses:

- Cefpodoxime is a broad-spectrum cephalosporin used against a relatively wide range of and Gram-positive and Gram-negative bacteria.
- It is used in the treatment of upper and lower respiratory infections, such as pharyngilis, bronchitis, otitis media, and community-acquired pneumonia and gonorrhea.

2. Cefixime:

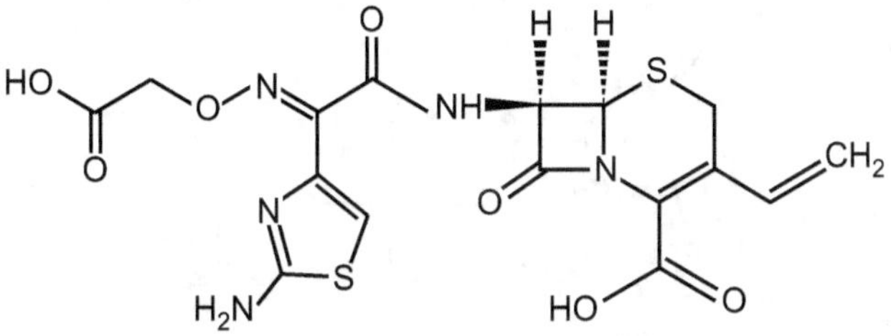

Cefixime

- Cefixime is a third-generation broad-spectrum Cephalosporin antibiotic.
- It is chemically, (6R,7R)-7-[[(2Z)-2-(2-amino-1,3-thiazol-4-yl)-2-(carboxy-methoxy-imino) acetyl] amino]-3-ethenyl-8-oxo-5-thia-1-azabicyclo[4.2.0]oct-2-ene-2-carboxylic acid.
- It is highly stable in the presence of β-lactamase enzymes.
- It acts by inhibition of mucopeptide synthesis in the bacterial cell wall.

Uses:

- Cefixime is used in the treatment of gonorrhoea, tonsilitis, pharyngitis, bronchitis, and urinary tract infections and gonorrhea caused by β-lactamase producing bacterial strain.
- It has a role as an antibacterial drug and a drug allergen.

3. Ceftibuten:

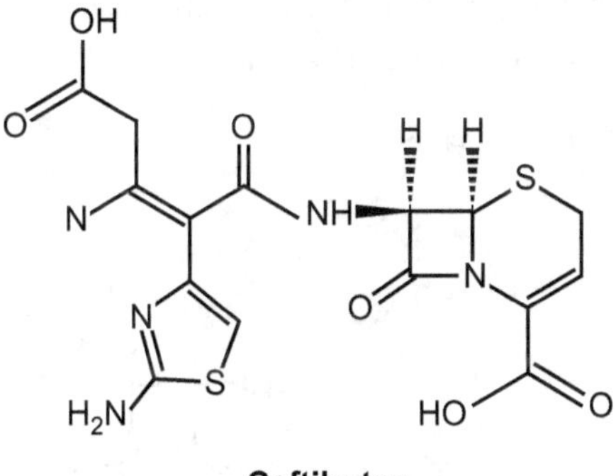

Ceftibuten

- Ceftibuten is orally-administered third-generation Cephalosporin antibiotic.
- It is chemically, (6R,7R)-7-[[(Z)-2-(2-amino-1,3-thiazol-4-yl)-4-carboxybut-2-enoyl]-amino]-8-oxo-5-thia-1-azabicyclo[4.2.0]oct-2-ene-2-carboxylic acid.
- It inhibits bacterial wall synthesis by a mechanism of action similar to Cephalosporin.
- It is orally active, chemically stable and highly stable in the presence of β-lactamase enzymes.

Uses:

- Ceftibuten is used as the dihydrate to treat urinary-tract, respiratory-tract infections and gynecological infections.
- It is typically used to treat acute bacterial exacerbations of chronic bronchitis (ABECB), acute bacterial otitis media, pharyngitis, and tonsilitis.

4. Cefotaxime:

Cefotaxime

- Cefotaxime is a third-generation broad spectrum Cephalosporin antibiotic given parentally.
- It is chemically, (6R,7R)-3-(acetyloxymethyl)-7-[[(2Z)-2-(2-amino-1,3-thiazol-4-yl)-2-methoxy iminoacetyl]amino]-8-oxo-5-thia-1-azabicyclo[4.2.0]oct-2-ene-2-carboxylic acid
- It has activity against Gram-positive and Gram-negative bacteria.
- It inhibits bacterial wall synthesis by a mechanism of action similar to Cephalosporin.

Uses:

- Cefotaxime possesses excellent broad-spectrum activity against Gram-positive and Gram-negative aerobic and anaerobic bacteria.
- It is effective in the treatment of meningitis.

5. Ceftizoxime:

Ceftizoxime

- Ceftizoxime is a semi-synthetic third-generation Cephalosporin antibiotic which can be administered intravenously or by suppository.
- It is chemically, (6R,7R)-7-[[(2Z)-2-(2-amino-1,3-thiazol-4-yl)-2-methoxyiminoacetyl]-amino]-8-oxo-5-thia-1-azabicyclo[4.2.0]oct-2-ene-2-carboxylic acid.
- It is highly resistant to a broad spectrum of β-lactamases.
- It inhibits bacterial wall synthesis by a mechanism of action similar to Cephalosporin.

Uses:

- Ceftizoxime is used in the treatment of Gram-negative or Gram-positive bacterial meningitis.

6. Ceftazidime:

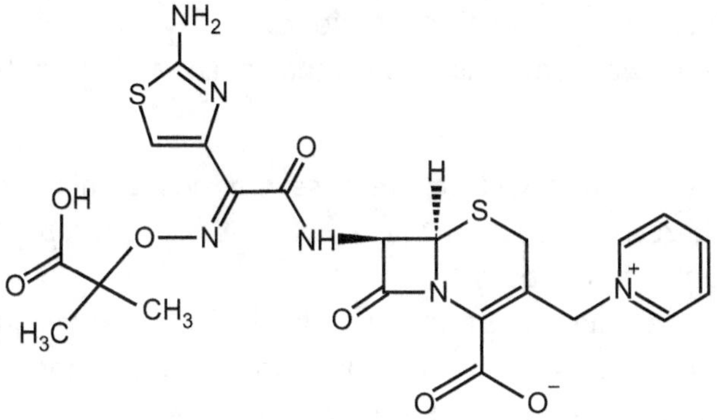

Ceftazidime

- Ceftazidime is a third-generation, semi-synthetic, broad-spectrum Cephalosporin antibiotic.
- It is chemically, (6R,7R)-7-[[(2Z)-2-(2-amino-1,3-thiazol-4-yl)-2-(2-carboxypropan-2-yloxyimino) acetyl]amino]-8-oxo-3-(pyridin-1-ium-1-ylmethyl)-5-thia-1-azabicyclo-[4.2.0]oct-2-ene-2-carboxylate.
- It inhibits bacterial wall synthesis by a mechanism of action similar to Cephalosporin.

Uses:

- Ceftazidime used especially for *Pseudomonas* and other Gram-negative infections in debilitated patients.
- It is noted for its anti-pseudomonal activity.
- It is active against some strains of *P. aeruginosa* as well as highly effective against β-lactamase producing strains of the *Enterobacteriaceae* family.

(D) Fourth-Generation Cephalosporins:

1. Cefepime:

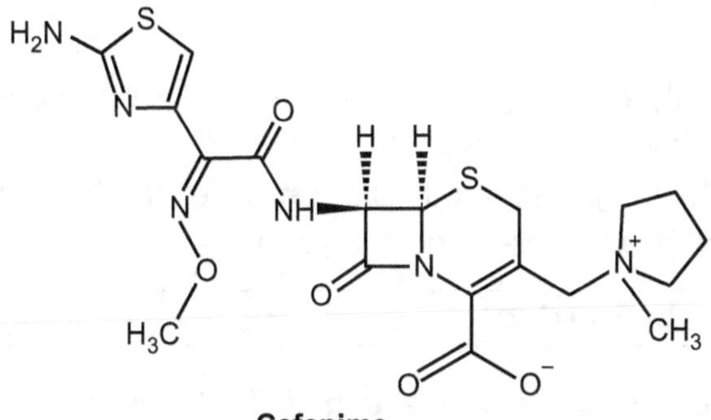

Cefepime

- Cefepime is a fourth-generation Cephalosporin antibiotic developed in 1994.
- It is chemically, (6R,7R)-7-[[(2Z)-2-(2-amino-1,3-thiazol-4-yl)-2-methoxyimino-acetyl]-amino]-3-[(1-methylpyrrolidin-1-ium-1-yl)methyl]-8-oxo-5-thia-1-azabicyclo[4.2.0]oct-2-ene-2-carboxylate.

- It is active against Gram-positive and Gram-negative bacteria, with greater activity against both than third-generation antibiotics.
- It inhibits bacterial wall synthesis by a mechanism of action similar to Cephalosporin.

Uses:

- Cefepime is usually reserved to treat severe nosocomial pneumonia, infections caused by multi-resistant micro-organisms (*Streptococci, Staphylococci, Pseudomonas species Enterobateriaceae strains*).
- It is used in the treatment of urinary tract infection, lower respiratory tract infections, skin infections, chronic osteomyelitis, and intra-abdominal and biliary infections.
- It is also used in the treatment of febrile neutropenia.

2. **Cefpirome:**

Cefpirome

- Cefpirome is a parentral fourth-generation Cephalosporin.
- It is chemically, (6R,7R)-7-[[(2Z)-2-(2-amino-1,3-thiazol-4-yl)-2-methoxyiminoacetyl]-amino]-3-(6,7-dihydro-5H-cyclopenta[b]pyridin-1-ium-1-ylmethyl)-8-oxo-5-thia-1-azabicyclo[4.2.0]oct-2-ene-2-carboxylate.
- It inhibits bacterial wall synthesis by a mechanism of action similar to Cephalosporin.

Uses:

- Cefpirome is highly active against Gram-negative bacteria, including *Pseudomonas aeruginosa*, and Gram-positive bacteria.
- It is also effective against, methicillin-sensitive *staphylococci*, penicillin resistant *pneumococci*, and β-lactamase-producing strain.

1.9 β-LACTAMASE INHIBITORS

β-lactamase-mediated resistance to β-lactam antibiotics is an increasing threat to clinical antimicrobial chemotherapy. Resistance to β-lactams is primarily because of bacterially produced β-lactamase enzymes that hydrolyze the β-lactam ring, thereby inactivating the drug. The newest effort to circumvent resistance is the development of novel broad-spectrum β-lactamase inhibitors that work against many problematic β-lactamases.

The discovery of the naturally occurring, mechanism based inhibitor clavulanic acid, which causes potent and progressive inactivation of β-lactamases, has created renewed interest in β-lactum combination therapy. This interest has led to the design and synthesis of additional mechanism based β-lactamase inhibitors, such as sulbactam and tazobactam and the isolation of naturally occurring β-lactums, such as the thienamycins, which both inhibit β-lactamases and interact with PBPs.

The combinations of β-lactam antibiotics and β-lactamase inhibitors (such as sulbactam, tazobactam and clavulanic acid) have been successfully used for β-lactamase-mediated resistance.

1.9.1 Drug Profile

1. Clavulanic Acid:

Clavulanic acid

- Clavulanic acid is a semi-synthetic β-lactamase inhibitor isolated from *Streptomyces clavuligerus*.
- It is chemically, (2R,3Z,5R)-3-(2-hydroxyethylidene)-7-oxo-4-oxa-1-azabicyclo[3.2.0]-heptane-2-carboxylic acid.
- It acts as a suicide inhibitor of bacterial β-lactamase enzymes.
- It contains a β-lactam ring and binds strongly to β-lactamase at or near its active site, thereby hindering enzymatic activity. This protects other β-lactam antibiotics from β-lactamase catalysis, thereby enhancing their antibacterial effects.

Uses:

- Clavulanic acid is used in conjunction with β-lactamase susceptible antibiotics, such as penicillins and cephalosporins, to treat infections caused by β-lactamase producing organisms.
- Combinations of amoxicillin and the potassium salt of clavulanic acid are available (Augmentin) in a variety of fixed-dose oral dosage forms intended for the treatment of skin, respiratory, ear, and urinary tract infection caused by β-lactamase producing bacterial strains.
- Combination of potassium clavulanate and the extended-spectrum penicillin, ticarcillin have been recommended for septicemia, lower respiratory tract infections, and urinary tract infections.

2. Sulbactum:

Sulbactam

- Sulbactam is a semi-synthetic β-lactamase inhibitor.
- It is chemically, (2S,5R)-3,3-dimethyl-4,4,7-trioxo-4λ^6-thia-1-azabicyclo[3.2.0] heptane-2-carboxylic acid.
- The β-lactam ring of sulbactam irreversibly binds to β-lactamase at or near its active site, thereby blocking enzyme activity and preventing metabolism of other β-lactam antibiotics by the enzyme.

Uses:

- Sulbactum, with a β-lactamase susceptible antibiotic, such as penicillins or a cephalosporin, is used to treat infections caused by β-lactamase producing organisms.
- The combination with ampicillin, it is recommended for the treatment of skin, tissue, Intra-abdominal, and gynecological infections caused by β-lactamase strains.

3. Tazobactam:

Tazobactam

- Tazobactam is a penicillanic acid sulfone derivative and β-lactamase inhibitor with antibacterial activity.
- It is chemically, (2S,3S,5R)-3-methyl-4,4,7-trioxo-3-(triazol-1-ylmethyl)-4λ^6-thia-1-azabicyclo [3.2.0]heptane-2-carboxylic acid
- It contains a β-lactam ring and irreversibly binds to β-lactamase at or near its active site. This protects other β-lactam antibiotics from β-lactamase catalysis.
- It is a more potent β-lactamase inhibitor than Sulbactam.

Uses:

- This drug is used in conjunction with β-lactamase susceptible penicillins to treat infections caused by β-lactamase producing organisms.
- In combination with broad-spectrum penicillins used in the treatment of appendicitis, postpartum endometritis, and pelvic inflammatory disease.
- In combination with ceftolozane sulfate, it is recommended for treatment of complicated intra-abdominal infections and complicated urinary tract infections.

1.10 CARBAPENEMS

Carbapenems occupy a very important place in our fight against bacterial infections. This is because they are able to resist the hydrolytic action of β-lactamase enzyme. Among the several hundreds of known β-lactams, carbapenems possess the broadest spectrum of activity and greatest potency against Gram-positive and Gram-negative bacteria. As a result, they are often called "antibiotics of last resort" and are administered when patients with infections become gravely ill or are suspected of harboring resistant bacteria.

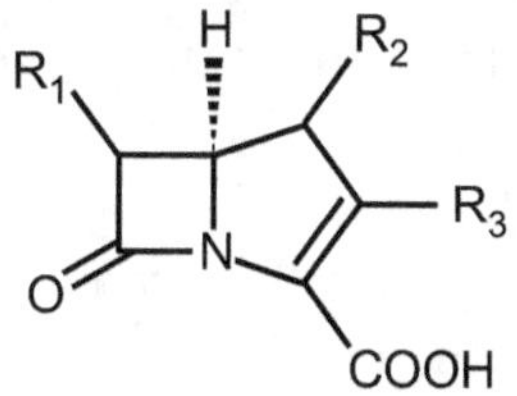

Structure of Carbapenem

Examples of Carbapenems are:

(i) Imipenem: A broad spectrum effective against aerobic and anaerobic pathogens, usually taken orally and active in low concentrations, with minimal allergy side effects.

(ii) Meropenem: A broad spectrum effective against non-fermentative Gram-negative bacilli particularly against acquired infections.

(iii) Ertapenem: A broad spectrum with limited activity against non-fermentative Gram-negative bacilli. Sadly, emergence of bacterial pathogens resistant to this life saving class of antibiotics has been reported.

More worrisome is the fact that bacterial resistance to carbapenems is on the increase globally and is fast becoming an international concern.

1.10.1 Drug Profile

1. Thienamycin:

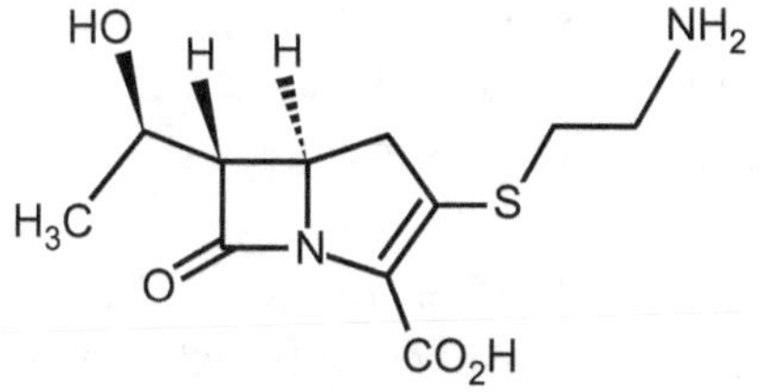

Thienamycin

- Thienamycin is isolated from *Streptomyces cattleya*. Thienamycin is reportedly considered to be the first "carbapenem" and serves as a standard for every other Carbapenem.
- It is chemically, (5R,6S)-3-(2-aminoethylsulfanyl)-6-[(1R)-1-hydroxyethyl]-7-oxo-1-azabicyclo [3.2.0]hept-2-ene-2-carboxylic acid.

- The bicyclic ring system consists of a Carbapenem containing a double bond between C_2 and C_3. Double bond in ring system creates considerable ring strain and increases the reactivity of the β-lactam to ring-opening reactions.
- Two unique side chains consisting of, 1-hydroxyethyl group (oriented to the bicyclic ring system) instead of the familiar acylamino side chain, and other, 2-aminoethylthioether function at C_2.
- The absolute stereochemistry of thienamycin has been determined to be 5R : 6S : 8S.

Uses:

1. Thienamycin has broad-spectrum antibacterial properties *in-vitro*.
2. It is highly active against most aerobic and anaerobic Gram-positive and Gram-negative bacteria, including *S. aureus*, *P. aeruginosa* and *B. fragilis*.
3. It is resistant to inactivation by most β-lactamases elaborated by Gram-negative and Gram-positive bacteria and, therefore, is effective against many strains resistant to penicillins and cephalosporins.

2. Imipenem:

Imipenem

- Imipenem is a broad-spectrum, semi-synthetic β-lactam carbapenem derived from thienamycin, produced by *Streptomyces cattleya*.
- It is chemically, (5R,6S)-3-[2-(aminomethylideneamino)ethylsulfanyl]-6-[(1R)-1-hydroxyethyl]-7-oxo-1-azabicyclo[3.2.0]hept-2-ene-2-carboxylic acid.
- It is an inhibitor of β-lactamases from certain Gram-negative bacteria resistant to other β-lactam antibiotics.
- It binds to and inactivates penicillin-binding proteins (PBPs) located on the inner membrane of the bacterial cell wall. This inactivation results in the weakening of the bacterial cell wall and eventually causes cell lysis.

Uses:

- Imipenem is active against a wide range of Gram-positive and Gram-negative organisms and is stable in the presence of β-lactamases.
- It is indicated for the treatment of a wide variety of bacterial infections of the skin and tissues, lower respiratory tract, bones and joints, and genitourinary tract, as well as of septicemia and endocarditis caused by β-lactamase producing strains of susceptible bacteria.
- It is given in combination with cilastatin, a DHP-I inhibitor which increases half-life and tissue penetration of imipenem.

1.11 MONOBACTAMS

Fermentation of unusual microorganisms led to the discovery of a class of monocyclic β-lactam antibiotics, named monobactams. The discovery of this class of antibiotics was first reported by Skyes and Co-workers. The antibiotic was obtained from the bacterium *Chromobacterium violaceum*. They are part of β-lactam compounds but unlike most other β-lactams, the β-lactam ring of monobactams stand alone and is not fused to another ring. The monobactams are not effective against Gram-positive bacteria or anaerobes. They are used as injectables and inhalers.

1.11.1 Drug Profile

1.   Aztreonam:

Aztreonam

- Aztreonam is the only commercially available parenteral monobactam antibiotic with a narrow spectrum of activity.
- It is isolated from *Chromobacterium violaceum*.
- It is chemically, 2-[[1-(2-amino-1,3-thiazol-4-yl)-2-[[(2S,3S)-2-methyl-4-oxo-1-sulfoazetidin-3-yl] amino]-2-oxoethylidene]amino]oxy-2-methylpropanoic acid.
- It preferentially binds to and inactivates penicillin-binding protein-3 (PBP-3), which is involved in bacterial cell wall synthesis, thereby inhibiting bacterial cell wall integrity and leading to cell lysis and death.

Uses:

- Aztreonam is active only against aerobic Gram-negative bacteria such as *Neisseria* and *Pseudomonas*; used for treating pneumonia, septicemia and urinary tract infections caused by these groups of bacteria.

1.12 AMINOGLYCOSIDES

1.12.1 History

Aminoglycoside antibiotics were the first drugs discovered by systematic screening of natural product sources for antibacterial activity. The laboratory of Waksman reported the discovery and isolation of the aminoglycoside antibiotic streptomycin from soil bacteria in 1944. Streptomycin was the first antibiotic effective against *Mycobacterium tuberculosis*. In the following two decades, many other aminoglycosides were isolated from soil bacteria including *Streptomyces* and *Actinomycetes* species. Despite their long history as antibacterial drugs, the present aminoglycosides remain important antibiotics for the treatment of serious Gram-negative pathogens. Resistance developed against the aminoglycosides as well as their relative toxicity has encouraged for the development of improved aminoglycoside derivatives.

1.12.2 Introduction

The aminoglycoside class of antibiotics contains a pharmacophoric 1,3-diaminoinositol moiety consisting of either streptamine, 2-deoxystreptamine, or spectinamine. Several of the alcoholic functions of the 1,3-diaminoinositol are substituted through glycosidic bonds with characteristic amino sugars to form pseudo-oligosaccharides.

Streptamine   **2-Deoxystreptamine**   **Spectinamine**

The chemistry, spectrum, potency, toxicity, and pharmacokinetics of these agents are a function of the specific identity of the diaminoinositol unit and the arrangement and identity of the attachments. These agents have intrinsically broad antimicrobial spectra, but their toxicity potential limits their clinical use to severe infections by Gram-negative bacteria. The aminoglycoside antibiotics are widely distributed (mainly in extracellular fluids) and have low levels of protein binding.

Because of their potent broad-spectrum antimicrobial activity, they are also used for the treatment of systemic infections. Their undesirable side effects, particularly ototoxicity and nephrotoxicity, have restricted their systemic use to serious infections or infections caused by bacterial strains resistant to other agents.

1.12.3 Chemistry of Aminoglycosides

Aminoglycosides are so named because their structures consist of amino sugars linked glycosidically. All have at least one aminohexose, and some have a pentose lacking an amino group (e.g.. Streptomycin, Neomycin and Paromomycin).

Additionally, each of the clinically useful aminoglycosides contains a highly substituted 1,3-diaminocyclohexane central ring: in Kanamycin, Neomycin, Gentamicin and Tobramycin, it is deoxystreptamine, and in Streptomycin, it is Streptidine.

1.12.4 Mechanism of Action

The aminoglycosides are bactericidal. They act directly on the bacterial ribosome to inhibit the initiation of protein synthesis and to interfere with the fidelity of translation of the genetic message. They bind to the 16S rRNA portion of the 30S ribosomal subunit to form a complex that cannot initiate proper amino acid polymerization and thus impairing function of the ribosome.

The binding of streptomycin and other aminoglycosides to ribosomes also causes misreading mutations of the genetic code, apparently resulting from failure of specific aminoacyl RNAs to recognize the proper codons on mRNA and hence incorporation of improper amino acids into the peptide chain.

1.12.5 Therapeutic Applications

Aminoglycosides have broad antibiotic spectra against aerobic Gram-positive and Gram-negative bacteria and are reserved for use in serious infections caused by Gram-negative organisms. Streptomycin is most commonly used for the treatment of tuberculosis, spectinomycin for treatment of gonorrhea and paromomycin is used primarily in the chemotherapy of amebic dysentery.

Under certain circumstances, aminoglycoside and β-lactam antibiotics exert a synergistic action *in vivo* against some bacterial strains when the two are administered jointly. Damage to the cell wall caused by the β-lactam antibiotic is believed to increase penetration of the aminoglycoside into the bacterial cell.

1.12.6 Structure Activity Relationship

Modification in ring 1: It is crucially important for characteristic broad-spectrum antibacterial activity, and it is the primary target for bacterial inactivating enzymes.

- Amino functions at 6′ and 2′ are particularly important as Kanamycin-B (6′- NH_2, 2′-NH_2) is more active than Kanamycin-A (6′- NH_2, 2′- OH), which in turn is more active than kanamycin-C (6′- OH, 2′-NH_2).

- Methylation at either the 6'- C or the 6'- NH_2 positions does not lower appreciably antibacterial activity and confers resistance to enzymatic acetylation of the 6'- NH_2 group.
- Removal of the 3'-OH or the 4'-OH group or both in the Kanamycins (e.g. 3',4'-Dideoxykanamycin-B or Dibekacin) does not reduce antibacterial potency.

Modifications of ring 2 (deoxystreptamine):

- 1- NH_2 group of Kanamycin-A can be acylates (e.g. Amikacin) with retention of activity.

Modifications of ring 3 in which functional groups appear to be somewhat less sensitive to structural changes than those of either ring 1 or ring 2.

- 2"-deoxygentamicins are significantly less active than their 2"-OH counterparts.
- 2"-NH_2 derivatives (seldomycins) are highly active.
- 3"- NH_2 of gentamicins may be primary or secondary with high antibacterial potency.
- 4"- OH group may be axial or equatorial with little change in potency.

1.12.7 Drug Profile

1. **Streptomycin:**

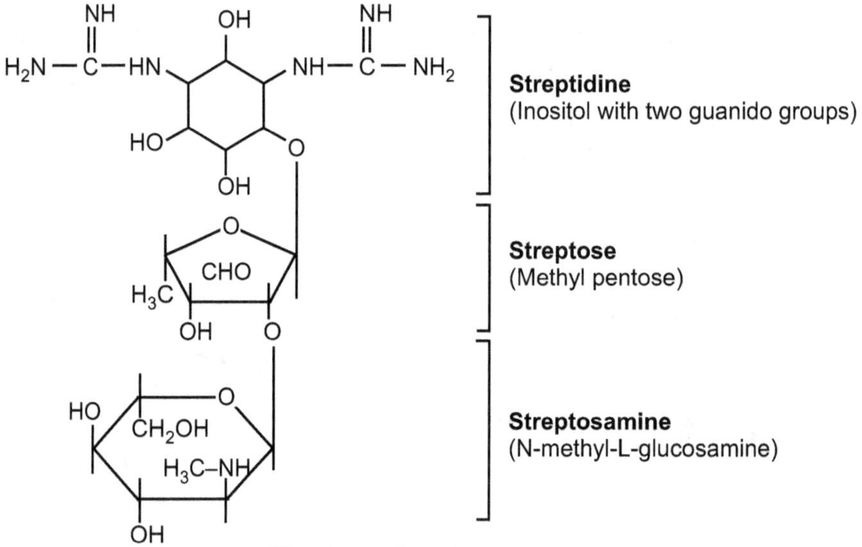

Streptidine
(Inositol with two guanido groups)

Streptose
(Methyl pentose)

Streptosamine
(N-methyl-L-glucosamine)

Streptomycin

- Streptomycin is an aminoglycoside antibacterial and antimycobacterial.
- It is biosynthesized by *Streptomyces griseus.*
- Streptomycin is an amino cyclitol glycoside that consists of streptidine having a disaccharyl moiety attached at the 4-position.
- It acts as a triacidic base through the effect of its two strongly basic guanidino groups and the more weakly basic methylamino group.

- Factors that limit the therapeutic use of streptomycin are,
    (i) Early development of resistant strains of bacteria.
    (ii) Neurotoxic reactions characterized by vertigo, disturbance of equilibrium and diminished auditory perception.
    (iii) Ototoxicity, the possible development of damage to the optic nerve by the continued use of streptomycin.
    (iv) Nephrotoxicity, need frequent checks of renal monitoring parameters.
- For systemic action, streptomycin usually is given by intramuscular injection.

Uses:

- Streptomycin is active against numerous Gram-negative and Gram-positive bacterias.
- It is a broad spectrum aminoglycoside antibiotic typically used for treatment of active tuberculosis (against the *tubercle bacillus, Mycobacterium tuberculosis*), always in combination with other antituberculosis agents.

2. Neomycin:

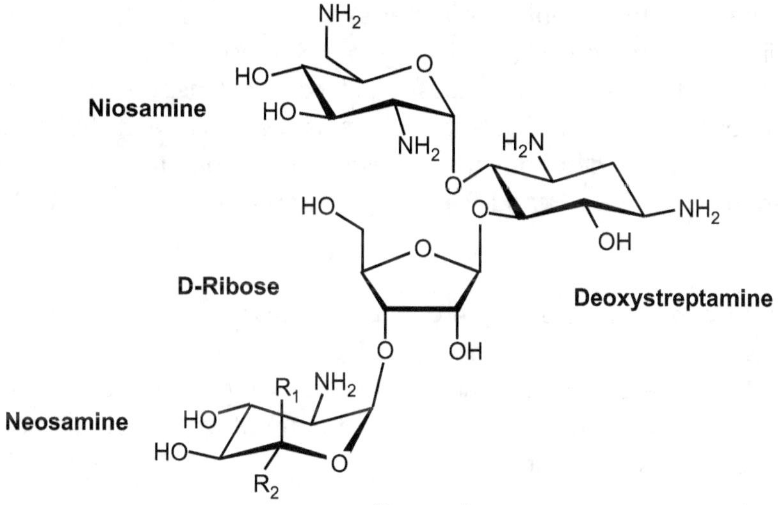

Niosamine

D-Ribose

Deoxystreptamine

Neosamine

Neomycin

- Neomycin is isolated from *Streptomyces fradiae.*
- Neomycin is a broad spectrum aminoglycoside antibiotic and shows a low incidence of toxic and hypersensitivity reactions.
- Neomycin-B (R_1 – CH_2NH_2 and R_2 - H) differs from Neomycin-C (R_1 = H and R_2 = CH_2NH_2) by the nature of the sugar attached terminally to D-ribose.

Uses:

- Neomycin considered one of the most useful antibiotics for the treatment of gastrointestinal infections, dermatological infections, and acute bacterial peritonitis.
- It is used in abdominal surgery to reduce infections from bacterial flora of the bowel.

3. Paromomycin:

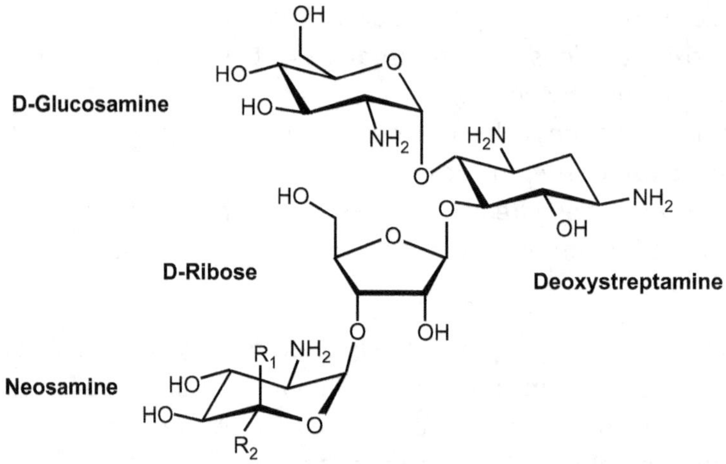

Paromomycin

- Paromomycin is oligosaccharide broad-spectrum antibiotic isolated in 1956 from fermentation with a *Streptomyces* species.
- It inhibits protein synthesis by binding to 16S ribosomal RNA.
- It binds to the A-site, which causes defective polypeptide chains to be produced. Continuous production of defective proteins eventually leads to bacterial death.
- Chromatographic determinations have shown paromomycin of two fractions, paromomycin-I (R_1 = H and R_2 = CH_2NH_2) and paromomycin-II (R_1 = CH_2NH_2 and R_2 = H).

Uses:

- Paromomycin more closely resembles Neomycin and Streptomycin in antibiotic activity.
- It is used for the treatment of acute and chronic intestinal protozoal infections.
- It has a role as an antibacterial drug, an antiprotozoal drug, an anthelminthic drug and an antiparasitic agent.

4. Kanamycin:

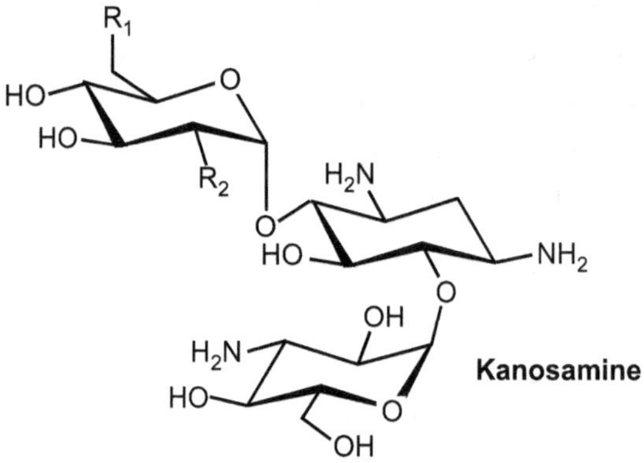

Kanamycin

- Kanamycin is an aminoglycoside bacteriocidal antibiotic isolated from the bacterium *Streptomyces kanamyceticus*.
- It comprises three components: Kanamycin-A (R_1 = NH_2 and R_2 = H) as the major component, and Kanamycin-B (R_1 = NH_2 and R_2 = NH_2) and Kanamycin-C (R_1 = OH and R_2 = NH_2) as the minor components.
- It irreversibly binds to specific 30S-subunit proteins and 16S rRNA.

Uses:

- Kanamycin is used in infections of the intestinal tract and to systemic infections arising from Gram-negative bacilli.
- It has also been recommended for preoperative antisepsis of the bowel.

5. Amikacin:

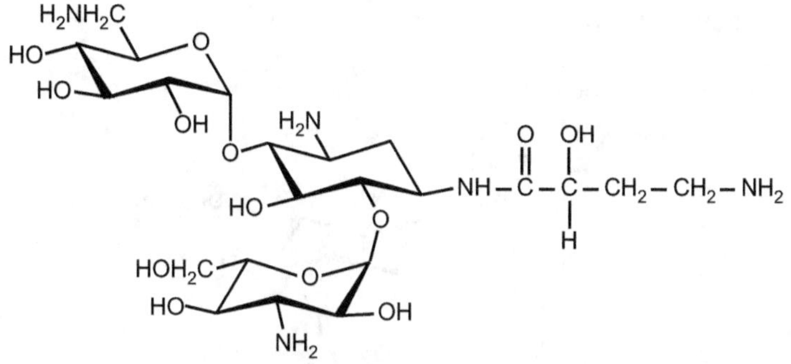

Amikacin

- Amikacin is a parenterally administered, broad spectrum aminoglycoside antibiotic.
- It resists attack by most bacteria-inactivating enzymes and therefore, is effective against strains of bacteria that are resistant to other aminoglycosides, including gentamicin and tobramycin.

Uses:

- Amikacin is typically used for severe Gram-negative infections.
- It has a role as an antimicrobial agent, an antibacterial drug and a nephrotoxin.

6. Gentamicin:

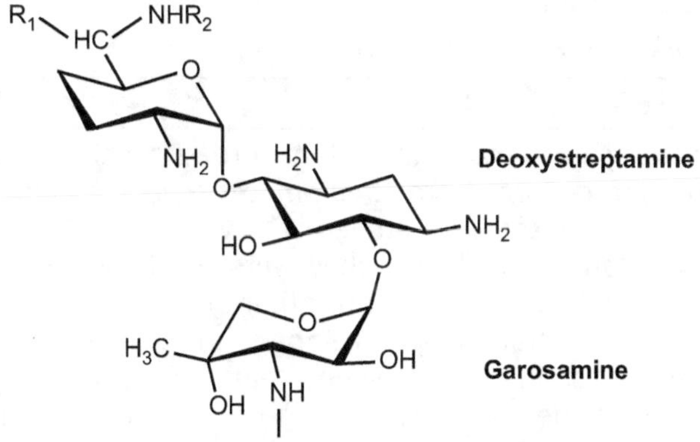

Gentamicin

- Gentamicin is a parenterally administered, broad spectrum aminoglycoside antibiotic.
- Gentamicin-C_1 (R_1 and R_2 = CH_3), Gentamicin-C_2 (R_1 = CH_3 and R_2 = H) and Gentamicin-C_{1a} (R_1 and R_2 = H), are obtained from *Micromonospora purpurea* and related species.
- They act to inhibit protein synthesis (genetic translation).
- They may cause ear and kidney damage.

Uses:

1. Gentamicin acts against many common pathogens, both Gram-positive and Gram-negative and having strong activity against *P. aeruginosa* and other Gram-negative enteric bacilli.
2. It is effective in the treatment of a variety of skin infections for which a topical cream or ointment may be used.

7. Tobramycin:

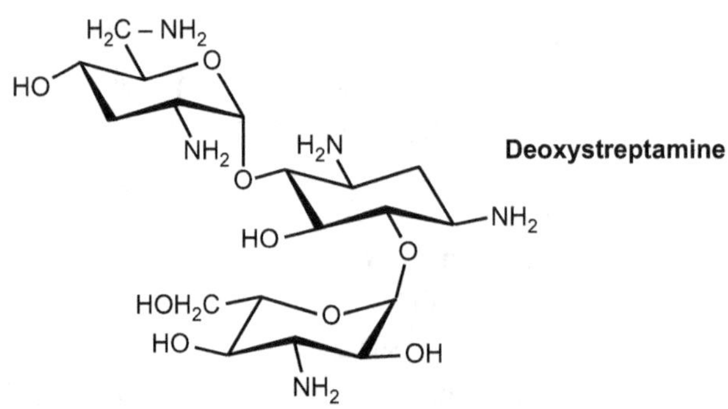

Tobramycin

- Tobramycin is a parenterally administered, broad spectrum aminoglycoside antibiotic.
- It is obtained from a strain of *Streptomyces tenebrains*.
- It more closely resembles with Kanamycin-B in structure (it is 3'-deoxykanamycin-B).
- It acts to inhibit protein synthesis (genetic translation).

Uses:

- Tobramycin is widely used in the treatment of moderate to severe bacterial infections due to sensitive organisms.
- It is active against most strains of *P. aeruginosa*.

1.13 TETRACYCLINES

Tetracyclins are among the most important broad-spectrum antibiotics. They are obtained by fermentation procedures from *Streptomyces spp.*, or by chemical transformations of the natural products. They possess a number of adverse effects, although most of them are annoying rather than dangerous. Earlier they were used widely because of their broad antimicrobial spectrum but due to the advent of other broad spectrum choices and the high incidence of resistance that tetracyclins developed, the use of tetracyclins has greatly decreased their medicinal prominence in recent years. Presently, they are recommended primarily for use against wide range of Gram-positive and Gram-negative bacteria, spirochetes, rickettsiae, chlamydiae, mycoplasma, anthrax, plague, and helicobacter organisms.

1.13.1 Structure of Tetracycline

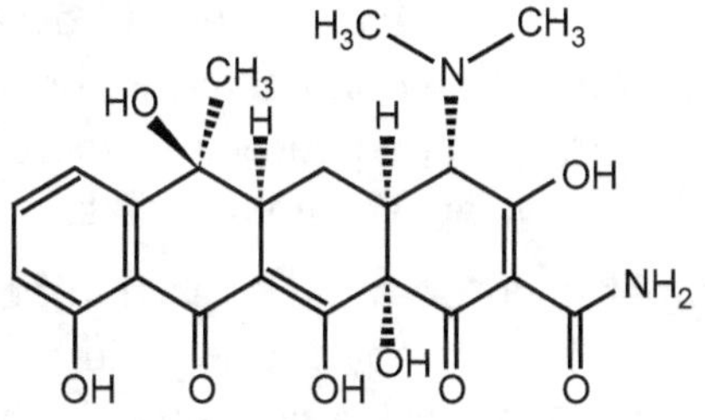

Tetracycline

This family of antibiotics is characterized by a highly functionalized, partially reduced octahydronaphthacene (four linearly fused, 6-membered rings) ring system, from which both the family name and the numbering system are derived.

The tetracyclines are amphoteric compounds, i.e., forming salts with either acids or bases. In neutral solutions these substances exist mainly as Zwitter ions. The hydrochloride salts are used most commonly for oral administration and usually are encapsulated owing to their bitter taste.

An interesting property of the tetracyclines is their ability to undergo epimerizaton at C-4 in solutions having intermediate pH range. These isomers are called epitetracyclines.

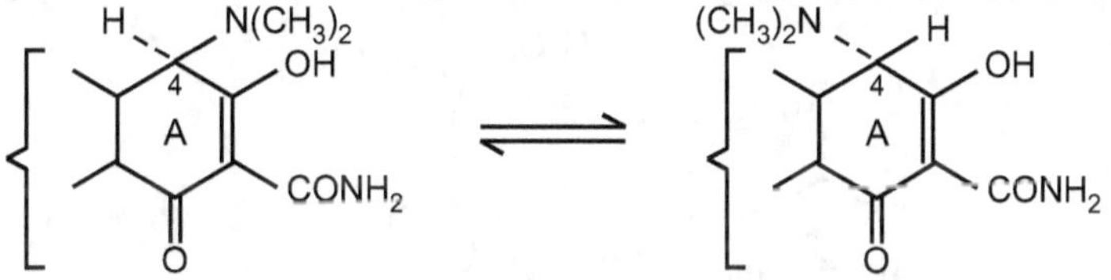

epi (less active)   **Natural** (more active)

It has been observed that the strong acids and bases attack the tetraclines having a hydroxy moiety at C-6, thereby causing a considerable loss in activity through modification.

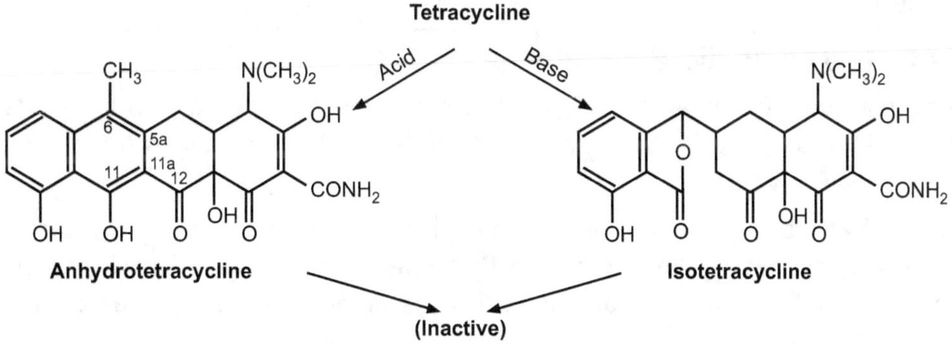

Tetracycline

Anhydrotetracycline   **Isotetracycline**

(Inactive)

Strong acids produce dehydration through a reduction involving the OH group at C-6 and the H atom at C-5a. The double bond thus generated between positions C-5a and C-6 induces a shift in the position of the double bond between the carbon atoms C-11 and C-11a thereby forming the relatively more energetically favoured resonant system of the naphthalene group found in the inactive anhydrotetracyclines.

The strong bases on the other hand promote a reaction between the hydroxyl group at C-6 and the carbonyl moiety at C-11, thereby causing the bond between C-11 and C-11a atoms to cleave and eventually form the lactone ring found in the inactive isotetracyclines.

The tetracyclines form stable chelate complexes with many metals, $e.g.$, Ca^{2+}, Mg^{2+}, Fe^{2+}, etc and are very insoluble in water, thus impaired absorption.

1.13.2 Stereochemistry

The stereochemistry of the tetracyclines is very complex. Carbon atoms 4, 4a, 5, 5a, 6, and 12a are potentially chiral, depending on substitution. Oxytetracycline and doxycycline, each with a 5α-hydroxyl substituent, have six asymmetric centers; the others, lacking chiralily at C-5, have only five.

1.13.3 Classification of Tetracyclines

Name of Compound	R_1	R_2	R_3	R_4	R_5
Tetracycline	H	OH	CH_3	H	H
Oxytetracycline	OH	OH	CH_3	H	H
Chlortetracycline	H	OH	CH_3	Cl	H
Minocycline	H	H	H	$N(CH_3)_2$	H
Doxycyclin	OH	H	CH_3	H	H

1.13.4 Structure-Activity Relationship

The large amount of research carried out to prepare semi-synthetic modifications of the tetracyclines and to obtain individual compounds by total synthesis revealed several interesting SARs.

1. All derivatives containing fewer than four rings are inactive or nearly inactive.
2. The simplest tetracycline derivative that retains the characteristic broad-spectrum activity associated with this antibiotic class is 6-dimethyl-6-deoxytetracycline.

3. The integrity of substituents at carbon atoms 1, 2, 3, 4, 10, 11, 11a, and 12, representing the hydrophilic "southern and eastern" faces of the molecule, cannot be violated drastically without deleterious effects on the antimicrobial properties of the resulting derivatives.

4. A-ring substituents can be modified only slightly without dramatic loss of antibacterial potency.

5. The enolized tricarbonylmethane system at C-I to C-3 must be intact for good activity.

6. Replacement of the amide at C-2 with other functions (e.g., aldehyde or nitrile) reduces or abolishes activity.

7. Monoalkylation of the amide nitrogen reduces activity proportionately to the size of the alkyl group.

8. Aminoalkylation of the amide nitrogen, accomplished by the Mannich reaction, yields derivatives that are substantially more water soluble than the parent tetracycline and are hydrolyzed to it *in vivo* (e.g. rolitetracycline).

9. The dimethylamino group at the 4 position must have the α-orientation; 4-epitetracyclines are very much less active than the natural isomers.

10. Removal of the 4-dimethylamino group reduces activity even further.

11. Activity is largely retained in the primary and N-methyl secondary amines, but rapidly diminishes in the higher alkylamines.

12. A cis A/B-ring fusion with a β-hydroxyl group at C-12a is apparently also essential.

13. Esters of the C-12a hydroxyl group are inactive, with the exception of the formyl ester, which readily hydrolyzes in aqueous solutions.

14. Alkylation at C-11a also leads to inactive compounds, demonstrating the importance of an enolizable β-diketone functionality at C-11 and C-12.

15. The importance of the shape of the tetracyclic ring system is illustrated further by substantial loss in antibacterial potency resulting from epimerization at C-5a.

16. Dehydrogenation to form a double bond between C-5a and C-11a markedly decreases activity, as does aromatization of ring C to form anhydrotetracyclines.

17. 5-hydroxyl group, as in oxytetracycline and doxycycline, may influence pharmacokinetic properties but does not change antimicrobial activity.

1.13.5 Adverse Effect

Tetracyclines have strong affinity for calcium which causes them to be incorporated into newly forming bones and teeth, as tetracycline-calcium orthophosphate complexes. Deposits of these antibiotics in teeth cause a yellow discoloration that darkens (a photochemical reaction) over time. Tetracyclines are distributed into the milk of lactating mothers and will cross the placental barrier into the fetus. The possible effects of these agents on the bones and teeth of the child should be considered before their use during pregnancy or in children less than 8 years of age.

1.13.6 Mechanism of Action

Tetracyclines are specific inhibitors of bacterial protein synthesis. They bind to the 30S-ribosomal subunit and, thereby, prevent the binding of aminoacyl tRNA to the mRNA-ribosome complex. Both the binding of aminoacyl tRNA and the binding of tetracyclines at the ribosomal binding site require magnesium ions. Tetracyclines also bind to mammalian ribosomes but with lower affinities, and they apparently do not achieve sufficient intracellular concentrations in interfere with protein synthesis.

The selective toxicity of the tetracyclines towards bacteria depends strongly on the self-destructive capacity of bacterial cells to concentrate these agents in the cell. Tetracyclines enter bacterial cells by two processes: passive diffusion and active transport. The active uptake of tetracyclines by bacterial cells is an energy dependent process that requires adenosine triphosphate (ATP) and magnesium ions.

1.13.7 Drug Profile

1.   Tetracycline:

Tetracycline

- Tetracycline is a broad-spectrum polyketide antibiotic produced by the *Streptomyces genus* of actinobacteria.
- It is chemically, (4*S*,4a*S*,5a*S*,6*S*,12a*R*)-4-(dimethylamino)-1,6,10,11,12a-pentahydroxy-6-methyl-3,12-dioxo-4,4a,5,5a-tetrahydrotetracene-2-carboxamide.
- The mechanism of action is similar to that of general MOA of Tetracycline.

Uses:

- Tetracycline has a role as an antimicrobial agent, an antibacterial drug, an antiprotozoal drug.
- A topical solution of tetracyclin is used for the management of acne vulguris.

2.   Oxytetracycline:

Oxytetracycline

- Oxytetracycline is isolated from *Streptomyces rimosus*.
- It is chemically, (4S,4aR,5S,5aR,6S,12aR)-4-(dimethylamino)-1,5,6,10,11,12a-hexa-hydroxy-6-methyl-3,12-dioxo-4,4a,5,5a-tetrahydrotetracene-2-carboxamide.
- The mechanism of action is similar to that of general MOA of Tetracycline.

Uses:

- Oxytetracycline is used for treatment of infections caused by a variety of Gram-positive and Gram-negative microorganisms including *Mycoplasma pneumoniae, Diplococcus pneumonia, Pasteurella pestis, Escherichia coli and Haemophilus influenzae (respiratory infections)*.

3. Chlortetracycline:

Chlortetracycline

- Chlortetracycline is isolated from *Streptomyces aureofaciens*.
- It is chemically, (4S,4aS,5aS,6S,12aR)-7-chloro-4-(dimethylamino)-1,6,10,11,12a-pentahydroxy-6-methyl-3,12-dioxo-4,4a,5,5a-tetrahydrotetracene-2-carboxamide.
- The mechanism of action is similar to that of general MOA of Tetracycline.

Uses:

1. Chlortetracycline has a role as an anti-protozoal drug and an antibacterial drug.
2. It is marketed in ointment forms for topical and ophthalmic use.

4. Minocycline:

Minocycline

- Minocycline is a tetracycline analogue having a dimethylamino group at position 7 and lacking the methyl and hydroxy groups at position 5.
- It is chemically, (4S,4aS,5aR,12aR)-4,7-bis(dimethylamino)-1,10,11,12a-tetrahydroxy-3,12-dioxo-4a,5,5a,6-tetrahydro-4H-tetracene-2-carboxamide.
- The mechanism of action is similar to that of general MOA of Tetracycline.

Uses:

1. Minocycline has activity towards Gram-positive bacteria, especially *staphylococci* and *streptococci*.
2. It is used for several bacterial infections as well as treatment of acne.
3. It has a role as an antibacterial drug and an *Escherichia coli* metabolite.
4. It is recommended for the treatment of chronic bronchitis and other upper respiratory tract infections and urinary tract infections.

5. Doxycycline:

Doxycycline

- Doxycycline is semi-synthetic tetracycline in which the 5β-hydrogen is replaced by a hydroxy group, while the 6α-hydroxy group is replaced by hydrogen.
- It is chemically, (4S,4aR,5S,5aR,6R,12aR)-4-(dimethylamino)-1,5,10,11,12a-penta-hydroxy-6-methyl-3,12-dioxo-4a,5,5a,6-tetrahydro-4H-tetracene-2-carboxamide.
- It is a second-generation tetracycline, exhibiting lesser toxicity than first-generation tetracyclines.
- The mechanism of action is similar to that of general MOA of Tetracycline.

Uses:

1. Doxycycline is broad-spectrum antibiotic and has a role as an antibacterial drug and an antimalarial.
2. It is used to treat non-gonococcal urethritis and cervicitis, exacerbations of bronchitis in patients with chronic obstructive pulmonary disease (COPD), and adult periodontitis.

QUESTIONS

Multiple Choice Questions:

1. Which of the following statements best describes structure-activity relationships (SAR)?
   - (a) The study of functional groups that are important to the chemical reactivity of the drug.
   - (b) The study of the physicochemical properties that are important to the absorption of a drug into the blood supply.
   - (c) The study of the structural features of a drug that are important to its biological activity.
   - (d) The study of the structural features of a drug that are important to its chemical stability.

2. A derivative of tetracycline which has a greater acidic and alkaline stability and slower rate of excretion, produces higher and more prolonged blood level. Identify.
    (a) Chlortetracycline   (b) Demeclocycline
    (c) Doxycycline   (d) Oxytetracycline

3. 1β-lactamase inhibitor clavulanic acid is ....
    (a) A-1,1-dioxo penicillanic acid
    (b) Δ2 carbapenam
    (c) Cepham
    (d) 1-oxapenam structure and has no 6-acyamino side chain of penicillin

4. Clavulanic acid has β-lactum ring fused to ....
    (a) Thienyl system   (b) Thiadiazole system
    (c) Thiazolidine system   (d) Oxazolidine system

5. Which of the following statements is true regarding the properties of benzylpenicillin?
    (a) It is a bacteriostatic agent.
    (b) It is active over a wide range of bacterial species.
    (c) It is resistant to β-lactamases.
    (d) Certain individuals may have an allergic response to it.

6. What crucial feature of a penicillin is involved in its mechanism of action?
    (a) Carboxylic acid   (b) β-lactam ring
    (c) Acyl side chain   (d) Thiazolidine ring

7. What reaction is catalysed by a β-lactamase enzyme?
    (a) The final cross-linking reaction to form the bacterial cell wall.
    (b) The hydrolysis of the acyl side chain from penicillin structures.
    (c) The hydrolysis of the four-membered ring present in penicillins.
    (d) The biosynthesis of the penicillin structure from the amino acids valine and cysteine.

8. What is the target for clavulanic acid?
    (a) The transpeptidase enzyme   (b) L-ala racemase
    (c) β-lactamase   (d) Penicillin acylase

9. Which of the following antibiotics is a tetracycline?
    (a) Chloramphenicol   (b) Doxycycline
    (c) Erythromycin   (d) Streptomycin

10. Amoxicillin is a .... type of antibiotic.
    (a) β-lactam   (b) Polypeptide
    (c) Macrolide   (d) Tetracyclines

11. Demeclocycline differs from chlortetracycline only by ....
    (a) Thienyl system   (b) Thiadiazole system
    (c) Thiazolidine system   (d) Oxazolidine system

12. Penicillin on hydrolysis with alkali gives ....
    (a) Penicilloic acid   (b) Penaldic acid
    (c) Penicillic acid   (d) Penicillamine

13. The penicillins have a carboxylic acid group placed at ....
    (a) C-3   (b) C-2
    (c) C-6   (d) C-7

14. The β-lactamase inhibitor with a 2-aminiethyl thio side chain is ....
    (a) Cephalexin   (b) Cefadroxil
    (c) Cefamandole   (d) Thienamycin

15. Which one of the following statements on the amino function in Penicillins is False?
    (a) The C-6 amine function is necessary for Antibacterial activity.
    (b) Sulphonation improves antibacterial activity.
    (c) Acylation of amino function improves antibacterial activity.
    (d) Carboxamido derivatisation are well tolerated.

16. The Cephalosporins are derivatives of ....
    (a) 7-amino cephalosporanic acid   (b) Amino glycoside
    (c) Tetracycline   (d) Penicilloic acid

17. The Macrolide antibiotics do not have ....
    (a) A large lactone ring   (b) Aglycosidically linked amino sugar
    (c) A spiro ketal group   (d) A ketone group

18. Dimethyl amino substituent is present in ....
    (a) Doxycycline   (b) Minocycline
    (c) Methacycline   (d) Demeclocycline

19. Neomycin A is a disaccharide, which is a common degradation product of ....
    (a) Neomycin D   (b) Neomycin B
    (c) Neomycin B & C   (d) Neomycin C

20. Which one of the following antibiotics produces concentration dependent bactericidal action and also possesses post-antibiotic effect?
    (a) Ceftazidime   (b) Azithromycin
    (c) Amikacin   (d) Piperacillin

21. Which one of the following is a β-lactamase inhibitor?
    (a) Penicillanic acid   (b) Embonic acid
    (c) Cephalosporanic acid   (d) Clavulanic acid

22. Of the four stereoisomers of chloramphenicol, which one is the biologically active isomer?
    (a) L-Erythro   (b) L-Threo
    (c) D-Erythro   (d) D-Threo

23. What role does the acetoxy group at the 3-position of cephalosporins have in enhancing antibacterial activity?
    (a) It acts as a steric shield and masks enzymatic attack at the β-lactam ring.
    (b) It acts as a good leaving group when the β-lactam ring is opened.
    (c) It takes part in a transesterification reaction with the carboxylic acid group at position 4.
    (d) It increases the reactivity of the β-lactam ring by neighbouring group participation.

24. The central bicyclic ring in penicillin is named as one of the following:
    (a) 1-Thia-4-azabicyclo[3.2.1] heptane
    (b) 4-Thia-1-azabicyclo[3.2.0] heptane
    (c) 4-Thia-1-azabicyclo[3.2] heptane
    (d) 1-Thia-4-azabicyclo[1.2.3] heptane

25. Penicillin ring system is derived from two of the following amino acids:
    (a) Alanine and methionine   (b) Cysteine and valine
    (c) Glycine and cysteine   (d) Methionine and leucine

26. Which one of the antifungal polyene macrolide antibiotic with seven conjugated double bonds, an internal eater, a free carboxyl group and a glycoside side chain with primary amino group.
    (a) Streptomycin   (b) Nystatin
    (c) Rifamycin   (d) Amphoterecin-B

27. Chemical name of amoxicillin is ....
    (a) 6-[D-(-) α-amino p-hydroxy phenyl acetamido] penicillanic acid
    (b) 4-[D-(-) α-amino p-hydroxy phenyl acetamido] penicillanic acid
    (c) β-OH analogue of benzyl penicillin
    (d) α-carboxy benzyl penicillin

28. Penicillinase resistant penicillin is ....
    (a) Amoxycillin   (b) Ampicillin
    (c) Penicillin-V   (d) Methicillin

29. Tetracyclines indergo epimerization at C4 between pH4 and 8 to give ....
    (a) Isotetracyclines   (b) Epitetracyclines
    (c) Nortetracyclines   (d) None of these

30. β-lactamase inhibitor clavulanic acid is ....
    (a) α-1,1-dioxo penicillanic acid
    (b) delta-2 carbapenam
    (c) Cepham
    (d) Oxapenam structure and has no 6-acylamino side chain of penicillin

31. The naturally occurring tetracyclines contain …………
     (a) α – C-4-dimethyl amino substituent
     (b) α – C-3-dimethyl amino substituent
     (c) α – C-3,C-4 keto enol group
     (d) α – C-3 dihydroxy substituents group
32. Which group of penicillins is responsible in determining the extent to which it is plasma protein binding?
     (a) β-lactam   (b) Thiazolidine
     (c) Acylamino   (d) Diethyl group

Answers :

1. (c)	2. (c)	3. (d)	4. (d)	5. (d)	6. (b)	7. (c)	8. (c)	9. (b)	10. (a)
11. (d)	12. (a)	13. (a)	14. (d)	15. (b)	16. (a)	17. (c)	18. (b)	19. (c)	20. (c)
21. (d)	22. (d)	23. (b)	24. (b)	25. (b)	26. (d)	27. (b)	28. (d)	29. (b)	30. (d)
31. (a)	32. (c)								

Answer the Following Questions:
1. Give the structure and chemical name of naturally occurring Penicillins.
2. Describe Polyene Antibiotics.
3. Give a brief account of the SAR of 'Tetracylines'.
4. What are 'Aminoglycoside Antibiotics'? Give structure and MOA of streptomycin.
5. Give classification of antibiotics based on chemical structure with suitable examples.
6. Discuss the salient features of the 'Tetracylines'.
7. Write a brief account of β-lactum antibiotics.
8. Discuss on chemical degradation of penicillins.
9. Define antibiotics. Give an account of SAR of penicillins.
10. Define antibiotics. Give an account of SAR of Cephalosporins.
11. Give an account of carbapenem.
12. Give an account of monobactams.
13. Give a comprehensive account of a 'cephalosporins' with suitable examples.
14. Define antibiotics with its historical background.
15. Discuss chemistry and mode of action of Aminoglycoside antibiotics.
16. Discuss mode of action and SAR of Aminoglycoside antibiotics.
17. Explain structure of tetracyclin. Give a note on MOA of tetracycline.
18. Describe stereochemistry and classification of tetracyclines.
19. Give in brief classification and mechanism of action of cephalosporins.
20. Give a short note on mechanism of action of β-lactam antibiotics.
21. Write a brief note on structure activity relationship of tetracyclines.
22. Discuss nomenclature of β-lactam antibiotics.
23. Classify antibiotics on the basis of mechanism of action with suitable examples.
24. Give an account of clavulanic acid, potent β-lactamase inhibitors.
25. Write chemical classification of penicillins with suitable examples.
26. Write a note on β-lactamase inhibitors.

■■■

Unit II

Chapter ... 2

ANTIBIOTICS (2)

2.1 MACROLIDES

The macrolide antibiotics are the group of chemically related compounds isolated from the actinomycetes species. The term "macrolide" is derived from the characteristic large lactone (cyclic ester) ring found in these antibiotics. In 1950, picromycin, was the first of this group to be identified as a macrolide compound which was first reported in 1952. Erythromycin and carbomycin were reported as new antibiotics, and they were followed in subsequent years by other macrolides.

Currently, more than 40 such compounds are known, and new ones are likely to appear in the future. Semisynthetic derivatives of erythromycin (e.g., clarithromycin and azithromycin), which have superior pharmacokinetic properties due to their enhanced acid stability and improved distribution properties.

2.1.1 Chemistry of Macrolide Antibiotics

The macrolide antibiotics have three common chemical characteristics:

(a) A large lactone ring (which prompted the name macrolide).

(b) A ketone group, and

(c) A glycosidically linked amino sugar.

Usually, the lactone ring has 12, 14, or 16 atoms in it, and it is often unsaturated, with an olefinic group conjugated with the ketone function. They are stable in aqueous solutions at or below room temperature but are inactivated by acids, bases and heat.

Chemical Properties

The early macrolides of the erythromycin class are chemically unstable because of rapid acid-catalyzed internal cyclic ketal formation, leading to inactivity. This reaction that occurs in the GI tract is clinically important. Most acid-susceptible macrolides are administered in coated tablets to minimize this effect. Semisynthetic analogues (i.e. clarithromycin, dirithromycin and azithromycin) have been prepared that are structurally incapable of undergoing this reaction and have become very popular.

Most of the macrolides have an unpleasant taste, which is partially overcome with water-insoluble dosage forms that also reduce acid instability and gut cramps. Enteric coatings are beneficial in reducing these adverse effects as well.

Mechanism of Action and Resistance:

The macrolides inhibit bacteria by interfering ribosomal protein biosynthesis. Macrolides bind selectively to a specific site on the 50S ribosomal subunit to prevent the translocation step of bacterial protein synthesis.

Spectrum of Activity:

The spectrum of antibacterial activity of the more potent macrolides, such as erythromycin, resembles to that of penicillin. They are frequently active against bacterial strains that are resistant to the penicillins. The macrolides are generally effective against most species of Gram-positive bacteria, both cocci and bacilli, and exhibit useful effectiveness against Gram-negative cocci, especially *Neisseria* spp.

Many of the macrolides are also effective against *Treponema pallidum*. In contrast to penicillin, macrolides are also effective against *Mycoplasma, Chlamydia, Campylobater,* and *Legionella* spp.

Therapeutic Application:

The macrolides are among the safest of the antibiotics in common use and often are used for the treatment of upper and lower respiratory tract and soft-tissue infections primarily caused by Gram-positive microorganisms like *Streptococcus pyogenes* and *Streptococcus pneumoniae*, Legionnaire's disease, prophylaxis of bacterial endocarditis by *Streptococcus viridians*. They are also used in upper and lower respiratory tract infections caused by *Haemophilus influenzae, mycoplasmal pneumonia*. In combination with rifabutin, macrolides are used in *Mycobacterium avium* complex infections in patients with AIDS. It also finds some use for certain sexually transmitted diseases, such as gonorrhea and pelvic inflammatory disease, caused by *Chlamydia trachomitis*.

2.1.2 Drug Profile

1. Erythromycin:

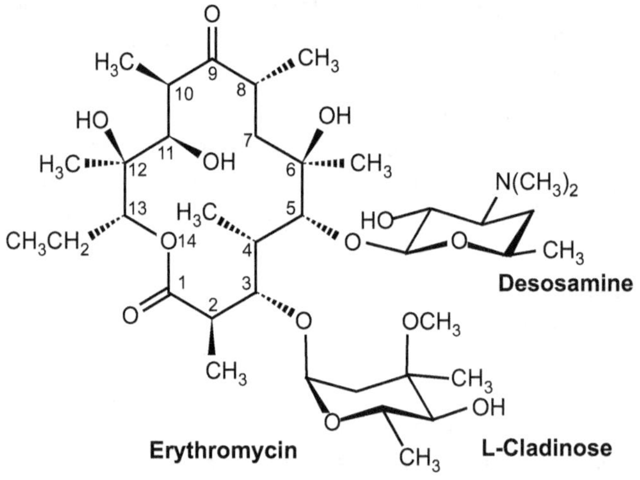

- Erythromycin is an orally and topically administered macrolide antibiotic.
- It is isolated from *Streptomyces erythraeus*.
- The amino sugar attached through a glycosidic link to C- 5 is desosamine which is a structure found in a number of other macrolide antibiotics.
- The tertiary amine of desosamine confers a basic character to erythromycin.
- The other carbohydrate structure linked as a glycoside to C-3 is called as L-cladinose and is unique to the erythromycin molecule.
- The mechanism of action is similar as given in the MOA of macrolide.

Uses:

- Erythromycin can be proved to be a useful alternative for the treatment of many infections in patients allergic to penicillins.
- It is used in the treatment of a variety of upper respiratory and soft-tissue infections caused by Gram-positive bacteria.
- It is also effective against many venereal diseases, including gonorrhea and syphilis.
- It is also effective against pneumonia (*Mycoplasm pneumoniea*) and veneral diseases caused by chlamydia.
- Also used for bacterial enteritis caused by *Campylobactor jejuni* and Legionnaires' disease.

2. **Clarithromycin:**

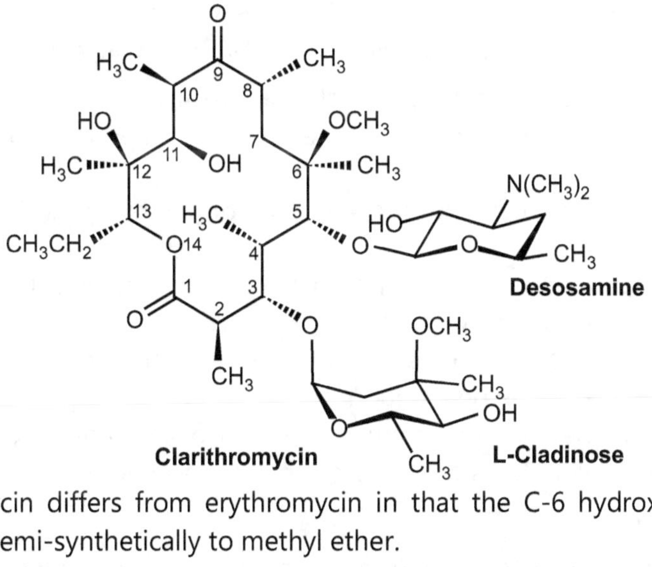

- Clarithromycin differs from erythromycin in that the C-6 hydroxy group has been converted semi-synthetically to methyl ether.
- Conversion of the molecule to its more lipophilic methyl ether prevents internal ketal formation, which not only gives better blood levels through chemical stabilization, but also results in less gastric upset.

- The enhanced lipophilicity of clarithromycin also allows lower and less frequent dosage for mild infections.
- The mechanism of action is similar as given in the MOA of macrolide.

Uses:

- Clarithromycin is a semi-synthetic macrolide antibiotic used for a wide variety of mild-to-moderate bacterial infections.
- It is used in the treatment of respiratory-tract, skin and soft-tissue infections.
- It is also used to eradicate *Helicobacter pylori* in the treatment of peptic ulcer disease.
- It has greater antimicrobial potency, especially against *Haemophilus influenzae*.

3. Azithromycin:

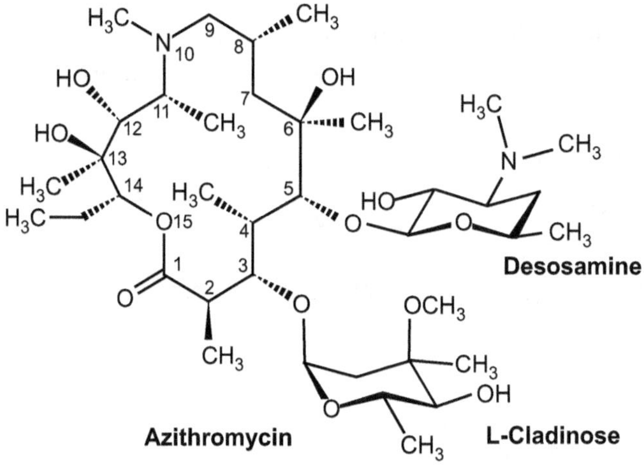

- Azithromycin is a semi-synthetic macrolide antibiotic.
- It contains 15 membered ring macrolides known as azalides. (15-membered lactone ring).
- It is formed by semi-synthetic conversion of erythromycin to a ring-expanded analogue in which,
  (i) N-methyl group has been inserted between carbons 9 and 10, and
  (ii) carbonyl moiety is absent.
- It is more stable to acid degradation than erythromycin, more lipid soluble and greater and longer tissue penetration.
- The drug should be taken on an empty stomach, once-a-day dosage.
- The mechanism of action is similar as given in the MOA of macrolide.

Uses:

- Azithromycin tends to be broader spectrum than either erythromycin or clarithromycin.
- It is primarily used for the treatment of respiratory, enteric and genitourinary infections, and other sexually transmitted infections.

2.2 LINCOMYCINS

The lincomycins are sulfur-containing antibiotics isolated from *Streptomyces lincolnensis*. Lincomycin is the most active and medically useful of the compounds obtained from fermentation. Extensive efforts to modify the lincomycin structure to improve its antibacterial and pharmacological properties resulted in the preparation of the 7-chloro-7-deoxy derivative clindamycin.

Mechanism of Action and Bacterial Resistance:

Lincomycins bind to the 50S ribosomal subunit to inhibit protein synthesis. Bacterial resistance and cross-resistance to lincomycins are similar to that observed with the macrolides.

Therapeutic Application:

Lincomycins have antibacterial spectrum and biochemical mechanisms of action similar to macrolides. Its action may be bacteriostatic or bactericidal depending on a variety of factors, including the concentration of the antibiotic.

They are primarily active against Gram-positive bacteria, particularly the cocci, but are also effective against non-spore-forming anaerobic bacteria, actinomycetes, mycoplasma, and some species of Plasmodium.

2.2.1 Drug Profile

1. Clindamycin:

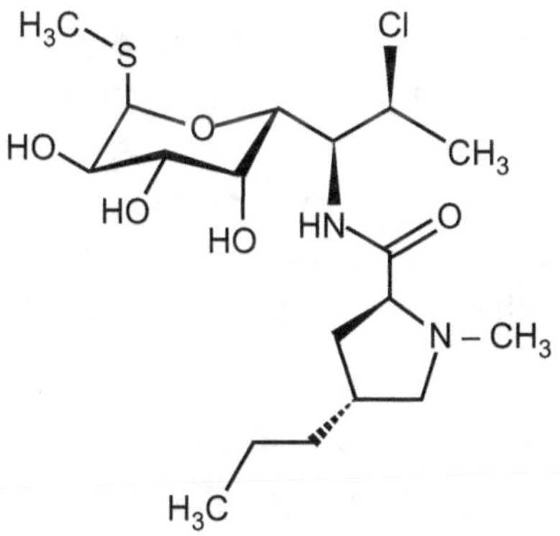

Clindamycin

- Clindamycin is a semi-synthetic lincosamide antibacterial.
- It is chemically, (2S,4R)-N-[(1S,2S)-2-chloro-1-[(2R,3R,4S,5R,6R)-3,4,5-trihydroxy-6-methyl sulfanyloxan-2-yl]propyl]-1-methyl-4-propylpyrrolidine-2-carboxamide.
- It inhibits bacterial protein synthesis by binding to bacterial 50S ribosomal subunits.

Uses:

- Clindamycin is a broad spectrum antibiotic used orally, topically and parenterally for bacterial infections.
- It is recommended for the treatment of a variety of upper respiratory, skin and tissue caused by susceptible bacteria.

2.3 MISCELLANEOUS DRUGS

2.3.1 Drug Profile

1. Chloramphenicol:

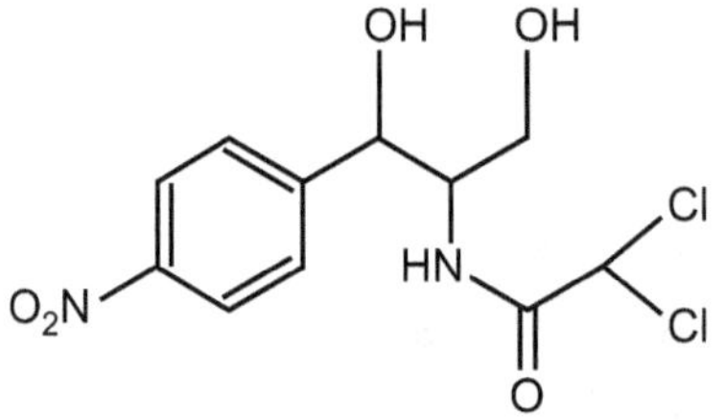

Chloramphenicol

- Chloramphenicol is an amphenicol-class antibacterial introduced into clinical practice in 1948.
- It is isolated from *Streptomyces venezuelae*, an organism found in a sample of soil collected in Venezuela. It is also synthesiezed for commercial production.
- It has dichloro-substituted acetamide containing a nitrobenzene ring, an amide bond and two alcohol functions.
- It possesses two chiral carbon atoms. Among four isomers, D-threo isomer is active, whereas, L-threo, D and L-erythro isomers are inactive.
- The most severe adverse effect associated with Chloramphenicol is bone marrow toxicity causing anemia and gray balsy syndrome.
- It causes serious and fatal aplastic anemia and is now used rarely and reserved for severe, life-threatening infections for which other antibiotics are not available.

Uses:

- Chloramphenicol has a role as an antimicrobial agent, an antibacterial drug, a protein synthesis inhibitor, an *Escherichia coli* metabolite and a *Mycoplasma genitalium* metabolite.
- It is recommended for the treatment of serious infections caused by strains of Gram-positive and Gram-negative bacteria that have developed resistance to penicillin-G and ampicillin.
- It is effective against *H. influenza, Salmonella typhi, S. pneumonia*.
- It is also recommended for meningitis and in the treatment of urinary tract infections.

SYNTHESIS

1. Chloramphenicol:

p-Nitroacetophenone — Br_2 / Bromination → (Bromo derivative) p-Nitrophenacyl bromide

(i) $(CH_2)_6N_4$ Hexamine
(ii) HCl / EtOH

→ α-Amino-p-nitroacetophenone hydrochloride

$(CH_3CO)_2O$ / Acetylation → p-Nitroacetamido-acetophenone

(i) HCHO
(ii) Na_2CO_3 (aq.)

→ Hydroxymethyl derivative

$[(CH_3)_2 — CHO]_3Al$ / Aluminium iso-propoxide → dl-form

HCl | $-CH_3COCl$ → DL-Form

(i) Resolution (with D-camphoric acid)
(ii) $Cl_2CH.COOCH_3$ Dichloromethylacetate (addition of the side chain)

→ **Chloramphenicol**

QUESTIONS

Multiple Choice Questions:

1. Erythromycin is an antibiotic. It belongs to the class of ....
   (a) β-lactum   (b) Aminoglycoside
   (c) Macrolide   (d) Peptide
2. The antibiotic with sulphur functionality is ....
   (a) Ampicillin   (b) Lincomycin
   (c) Doxycycline   (d) Chloramphenicol
3. Which of the following is the general mechanism of action for erythromycin?
   (a) Inhibition of a metabolic enzyme
   (b) Inhibition of cell wall synthesis
   (c) Disruption of protein synthesis
   (d) Inhibition of nucleic acid transcription and replication

4. Which of the following antibiotics is a macrolide?
    (a) Chloramphenicol   (b) Doxycycline
    (c) Erythromycin   (d) Streptomycin
5. Chloramphenicol is mainly synthesized from ....
    (a) o-nitro acetophenone   (b) m-nitro acetophenone
    (c) P-nitro acetophenone   (d) None of these
6. Chloramphenicol is isolated from ....
    (a) S. venezulae   (b) S. rimosus
    (c) S. natalensis   (d) S. aureofaciensis
7. Which of the following antibiotics is responsible for Gray Baby Syndrome?
    (a) Chloramphenicol   (b) Doxycycline
    (c) Erythromycin   (d) Streptomycin
8. Lincomycin binds to .... ribosomal subunit to inhibit protein synthesis.
    (a) 50S   (b) 30S
    (c) 40S   (d) 50 and 30S
9. Which of the following is the general mechanism of action for erythromycin?
    (a) Inhibition of a metabolic enzyme
    (b) Inhibition of cell wall synthesis
    (c) Disruption of protein synthesis
    (d) Inhibition of nucleic acid transcription and replication
10. Azithromycin is clinically administered once daily as compared to erythromycin which is administered after every 6 hours because azithromycin ....
    (a) penetrates into most tissues and is released very slowly.
    (b) has a methylated nitrogen in its latone ring which renders it much more potent than erythromycin.
    (c) is a very potent antibiotic but not tolerated well in gastrointestinal tract.
    (d) is usually presented in a sustained release dosage form.
11. Identify the antibiotic containing a big lactone ring (12, 14 or 16 membered), a ketone group and glycosidically attached one or more deoxysuder which act by inhibiting protein synthesis.
    (a) Ansamycins   (b) Tetracyclines
    (c) Macrolides   (d) Polypeptides

Answers :

1. (c)	2. (b)	3. (c)	4. (c)	5. (c)	6. (a)	7. (a)	8. (a)	9. (c)	10. (b)
11. (c)									

Answer the Following Questions:
1. Discuss the synthesis and chemical name of Chloramphenicol.
2. Discuss the SAR and stereochemistry of chloramphenicol.
3. Describe the synthesis of chloramphenicol from *p*-nitroacetophenone.
4. Write chemistry, mode of action and therapeutic applications of macrolides.
5. Write a note on lincomycins.
6. Write a note on macrolide antibiotics.

chapter ... 3

PRODRUGS

♦ LEARNING OBJECTIVES ♦

After completing this sub-unit the students should be able:

- *To know the basic concept of prodrug.*
- *To know the definition of prodrug, hard drug and soft drug.*
- *To study how to design prodrug and different functional groups used for design of prodrug.*
- *To study detail classification of prodrug.*
- *To learn objectives and applications of prodrug design.*

3.1 INTRODUCTION

The term prodrug or pro-agent was coined by Albert in 1958 which is referring to a pharmacologically inactive compound that is transformed by the mammalian system into an active substance by either chemical or metabolic means.

The term prodrug is applied to either an appropriate derivative of a drug that undergoes *in-vivo* hydrolysis to the parent drug, e.g., testosterone propionate, chloramphenicol palmitate and the like; or an analogue which is metabolically transformed to a biologically active drug,

Example: Phenylbutazone undergoes *in-vivo* hydroxylation to oxyphenbutazone.

The type of prodrug to be produced depends on the specific aspect of the drug's action that requires improvement and the type of functionality that is present in the active drug. Generally, prodrug approaches are undertaken to improve patient acceptability of the agent (i.e., reduce pain associated with administration), alter absorption, alter distribution, alter metabolism, or alter elimination.

The terms hard drugs and soft drugs were introduced recently. Hard drugs are the compounds that are designed to contain the structural characteristics necessary for pharmacological activity, but in a form that is not susceptible to metabolic or chemical transformation. In this way, the production of any toxic metabolite is avoided, and there is increased efficiency of action. Since the drug is not inactivated by metabolism, it may be less readily eliminated. On the other hand, soft drugs are active drugs that are designed to undergo a predictable and controllable deactivation or metabolism *in-vivo* after achieving their therapeutic effect. Thus soft drugs are considered to be the opposite of prodrugs.

3.2 BASIC CONCEPTS

A prodrug by definition is inactive and must be converted into an active species within the biological system. There are a variety of mechanisms by which this conversion may be accomplished. Generally, the conversion to an active form is most often carried out by metabolizing enzymes within the body. Conversion to an active form may be accomplished by chemical means (e.g., hydrolysis or decarboxylation), although this is less common. Chemical transformation does not depend on the presence or relative amounts of metabolizing enzymes.

The development of prodrugs established as a strategy to improve the physicochemical, biopharmaceutical or pharmacokinetic properties of pharmacologically potent compounds, and thereby increase the developability and usefulness of a potential drug. Prodrugs provide possibilities to overcome various barriers to drug formulation and delivery such as poor aqueous solubility, chemical instability, insufficient oral absorption, rapid pre-systemic metabolism, inadequate brain penetration, toxicity and local irritation.

3.3 DESIGN OF PRODRUG

Design of an appropriate prodrug structure should be considered at the early stages of preclinical development, bearing in mind that prodrugs might alter the tissue distribution, efficacy and the toxicity of the parent drug.

Factors needed to be considered while designing a prodrug structure:

- **Parent drug:** Which functional groups are amenable to chemical prodrug derivatization?
- **Promoiety:** This should ideally be safe and rapidly excreted from the body. The choice of promoiety should be considered with respect to the disease state, dose and the duration of therapy.

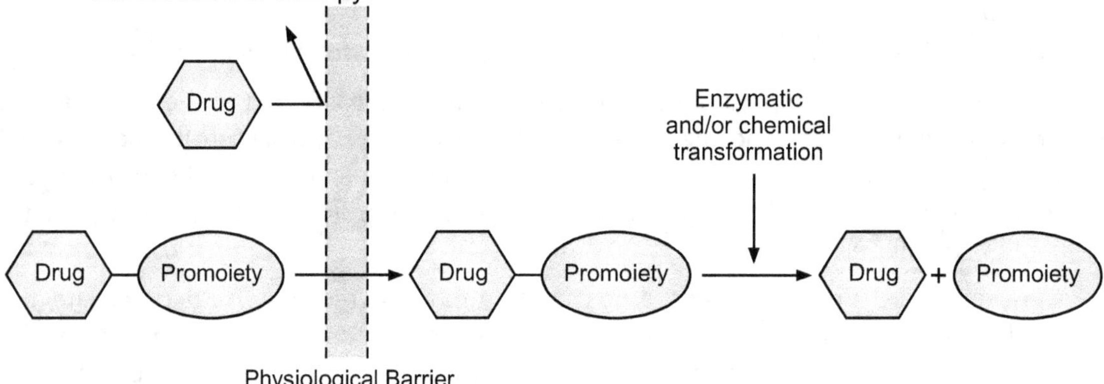

Fig. 3.1

- **Parent and prodrug:** The absorption, distribution, metabolism, excretion (ADME) and pharmacokinetic properties need to be comprehensively understood.
- **Degradation by-products:** These can affect chemical and physical stability and lead to the formation of new degradation products.

3.4 FUNCTIONAL GROUPS THAT ARE AMENABLE TO PRODRUG DESIGN

Most common functional groups such as, carboxylic, hydroxyl, amine, phosphate/phosphonate and carbonyl groups are amenable for designing the prodrugs. Prodrugs typically produced via the modification of these groups include esters, carbonates, carbamates, amides, phosphates and oximes. However, other uncommon functional groups have also been investigated as potentially useful structures in prodrug design. For example, thiols react in a similar manner to alcohols and can be derivatized to thioethers and thioesters. Amines may be derivatized into imines and N-Mannich bases.

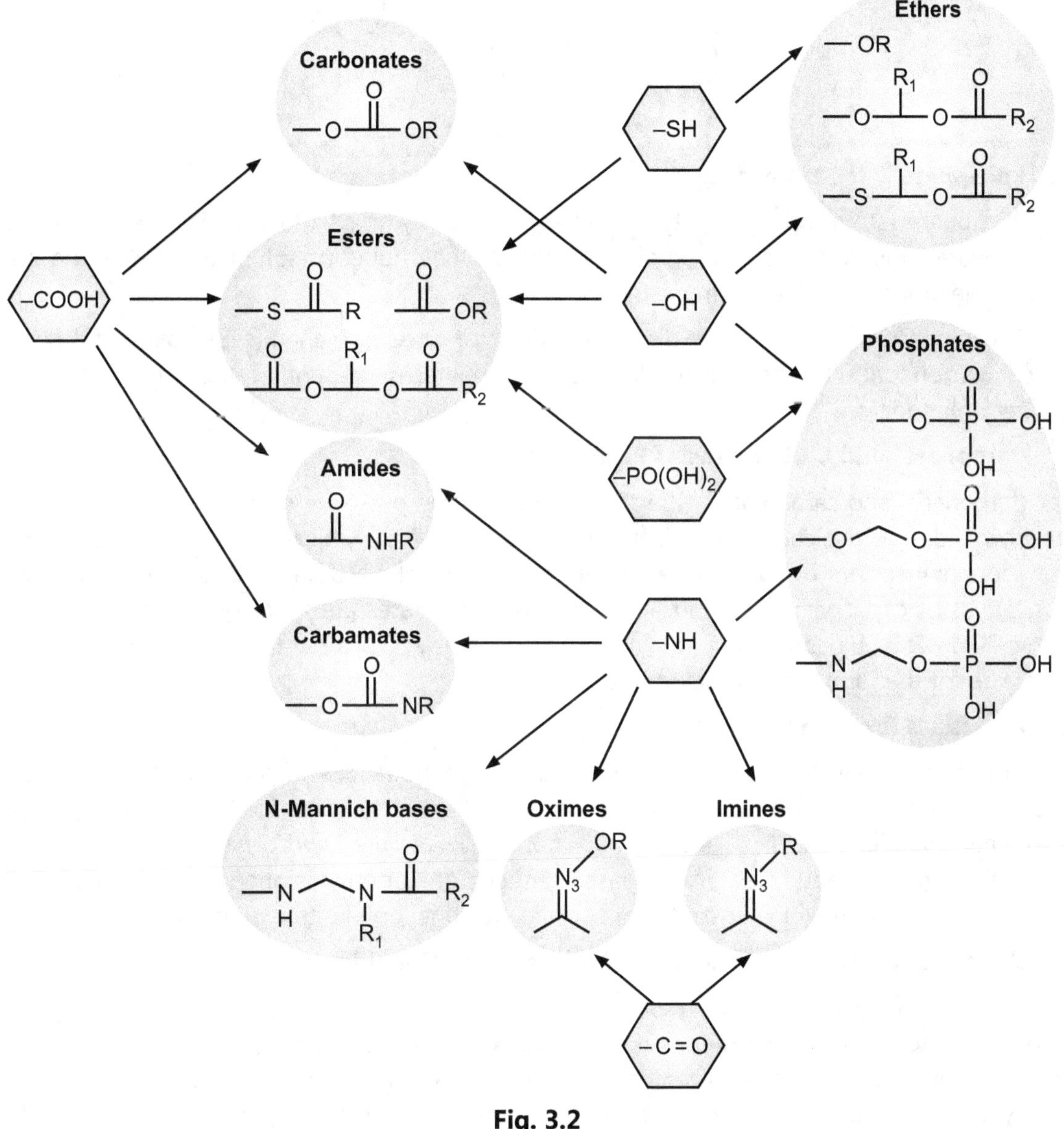

Fig. 3.2

1. Ester as Prodrugs:

Esters are the most common prodrugs used, and it is estimated that approximately 49% of all marketed prodrugs are activated by enzymatic hydrolysis. Ester prodrugs are most often used to enhance the lipophilicity. In the body, the ester bond is readily hydrolyzed by ubiquitous esterases found in the blood, liver and other organs and tissues.

Several alkyl and aryl ester prodrugs are in clinical use, of which angiotensin-converting enzyme (ACE) inhibitors are some of the most successful.

Monoethyl ester of Enalapril

2. Phosphate Ester as Prodrugs:

Phosphate ester prodrugs are typically designed for hydroxyl and amine functionalities of poorly water-soluble drugs with an aim to enhance their aqueous solubility to allow a more favourable oral or parenteral administration.

Phosphate prodrugs typically display excellent or adequate chemical stability and rapid bioconversion back to the parent drug by phosphatases present at the intestinal brush border or in the liver.

3. Carbonates and Carbamates as Prodrugs:

Carbonates and carbamates differ from esters by the presence of an oxygen or nitrogen on both sides of the carbonyl carbon. They are often enzymatically more stable than the corresponding esters but are more susceptible to hydrolysis than amides. Carbonates are derivatives of carboxylic acids and alcohols, and carbamates are carboxylic acid and amine derivatives. The bioconversion of many carbonate and carbamate prodrugs requires esterases for the formation of the parent drug.

4. Amides as Prodrugs:

Amides are derivatives of amine and carboxyl functionalities of a molecule. In prodrug design, amides have been used only to a limited extent owing to their relatively high enzymatic stability *in-vivo*. An amide bond is usually hydrolysed by ubiquitous carboxylesterases, peptidases or proteases. Amides are often designed for enhanced oral absorption by synthesizing substrates of specific intestinal uptake transporters.

5. Oximes as derivatives of Ketones, Amidines and Guanidines:

Oximes are derivatives of ketones, amidines and guanidines, thus providing an opportunity to modify molecules that lack hydroxyl, amine or carboxyl functionalities. They can be used to enhance the membrane permeability and absorption of a parent drug, and are hydrolyzed by the versatile microsomal cytochrome P450 (CYP450) enzymes.

3.5 PREREQUISITES OF IDEAL PRODRUG

An ideal prodrug should possess following properties:

1. Pharmacological inertness.
2. Rapid transformation, chemically or enzymatically, into the active form at the target site.
3. Non-toxic metabolic fragments followed by their rapid elimination.

3.6 OBJECTIVES OF PRODRUG DESIGN

The main objectives of a prodrug designing are

- To bring active drugs to their respective active sites.
- To provide the desired pharmacological effects while minimizing adverse metabolic and/or toxicological events.
- To improve the clinical and therapeutic effectiveness of those drugs which suffer from some undesirable properties that otherwise hinder their clinical usefulness.
- To avoid the practice of clinically co-administering two drugs in order to enhance pharmacological activity or prevent clinical side effects. Simultaneous administration does not guarantee equivalent absorption or transportation to site of action. So, mutual prodrug concept is useful when two synergistic drugs need to be administered at the same site at the same time. Mutual prodrugs are synthesized towards a pharmacological objective improving each drug's efficacy, optimizing delivery, and lowering toxicity.

3.7 CLASSIFICATION OF PRODRUGS

Depending upon constitution of the lipophilicity method of bioactivation and catalyst involved; they are classified in two groups.

(A) Carrier - linked prodrugs,

(B) Bio precursor prodrugs

(A) Carrier Linked Prodrugs:

- They are one where the active drug is covalently linked to an inert carrier. They are generally ester or amide.
- Such prodrugs have greatly modified lipophilicity due to the attached carrier. The active drug is released by hydrolytic cleavage either chemically or enzymatically.

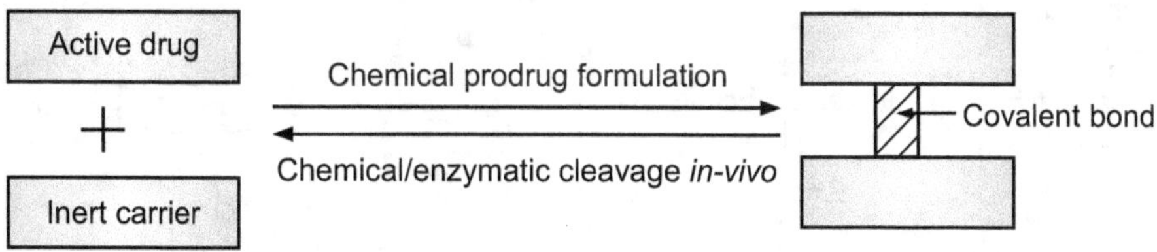

Fig. 3.3

The unique feature of this approach is that the physicochemical properties can be tailored by means of changing the structure of the promoiety.

Carrier-linked prodrugs consist of the attachment of a carrier group to the active drug to alter its physicochemical properties. The subsequent enzymatic or non-enzymatic mechanism releases the active drug moiety. Hence, the carrier-linked prodrugs have a major drawback that they are linked through covalent linkage with specialized non-toxic protective groups or carriers or promoieties in a transient manner to alter or eliminate undesirable properties in the parent molecule.

Carrier- linked prodrugs may further be classified as follows:

1. **Double prodrugs or pro-prodrugs or cascade-latentiated prodrugs**, where a prodrug is further derivatized in a fashion such that only enzymatic conversion to prodrug is possible before the later can cleave to release the active drug.

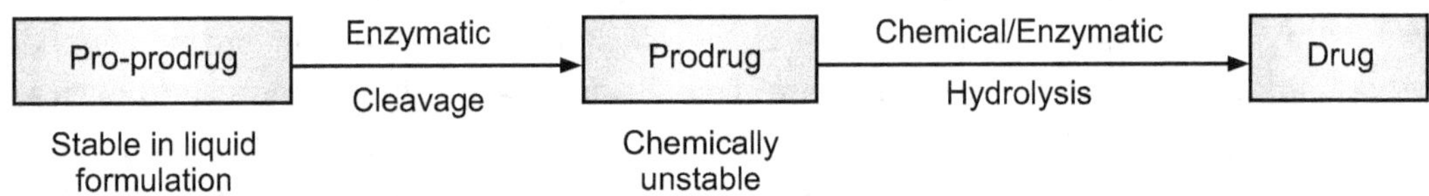

Fig. 3.4

2. **Macromolecular prodrugs,** where macromolecules like polysaccharides, dextrans, cyclodextrins, proteins, peptides and polymers are used as carriers to form the macromolecular prodrugs.
3. **Site-specific prodrugs**, where a carrier acts as a transporter of the active drug to a specific targeted site.
4. **Mutual prodrugs**, where the carrier used is another biologically active drug instead of some inert molecule. A mutual prodrug consists of two pharmacologically active agents coupled together so that each acts as a promoiety for the other agent and vice versa. The carrier selected may have the same biological action as that of the parent drug and thus might give synergistic action, or the carrier may have some additional biological action that is lacking in the parent drug, thus ensuring some additional benefit.

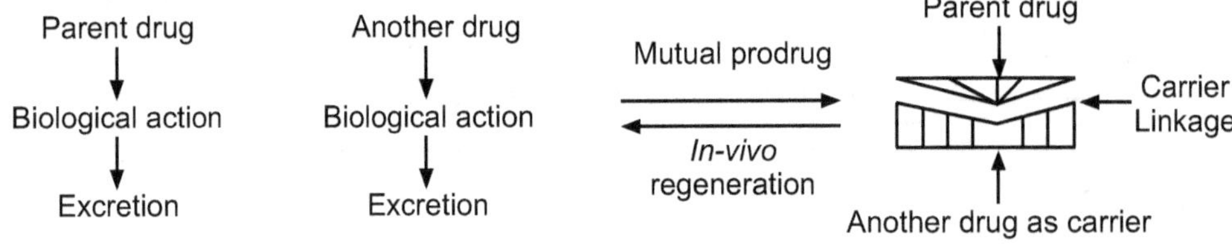

Fig. 3.5

The carrier may also be a drug that might help to target the parent drug to a specific site or organ or cells or may improve site specificity of a drug. The carrier drug may be used to overcome some side effects of the parent drugs as well.

Example: Benorylate a mutual prodrug of Aspirin and Paracetamol.

Benorylate

Acetyl salicyclic acid

+

Paracetamol

Benorylate is not hydrolyzed in the gastric juice and is more slowly absorbed than either acetyl salicylic acid or paracetamol. However, after absorption, it gets hydrolyzed quantitatively to the parent drugs. The major advantage of Benorylate as a prodrug of acetylsalicylic acid is that, it can be used to treat chronic inflammation at a decreased dosage and reduced risk of irritation to the gastric mucosa. Furthermore, it is believed that Paracetamol inhibits the erosion action of acetyl salicylic acid by stimulating the stomach prostaglandin synthetase.

Advantages of Carrier linked Prodrug:

1. It increases absorption.
2. It reduces injection site pain.
3. It eliminates unpleasant taste.
4. It decreases toxicity.
5. It decreases metabolic inactivation.
6. It increases chemical stability.

(B) Bioprecursor/Metabolic Precursor Prodrugs:

They are inert molecules obtained by chemical modification of the active drug, but do not contain a carrier. Such a moiety has almost the same lipophilicity as the parent drug and is bioactivated generally by redox biotransformation only enzymatically.

Bioprecursor don't have a temporary linkage between the active compound and carrier group but results from a molecular modification of the active compound itself. This modification generates new compound which acts as substrate for the metabolizing enzyme, a metabolite being the expected active agent.

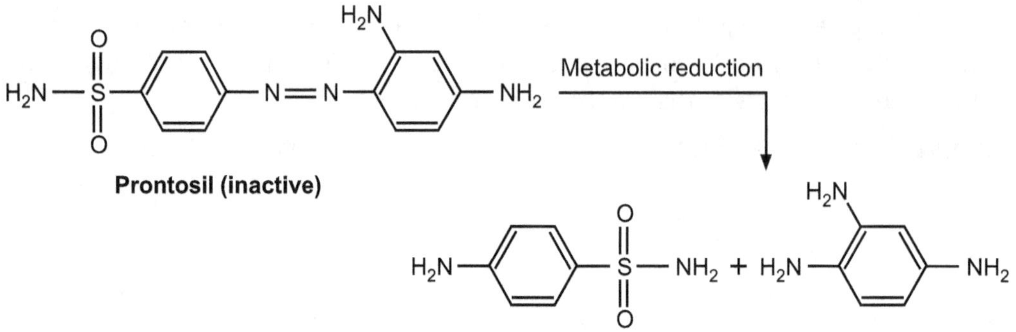

Prontosil (inactive)

Metabolic reduction

Sulphanilamide (antibacterial)

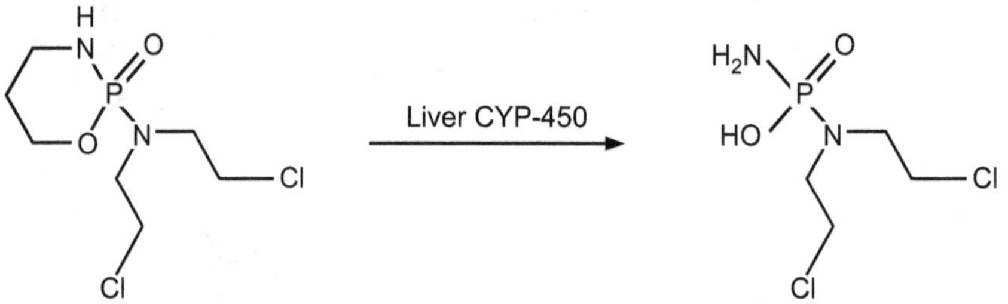

Liver CYP-450

Cyclophosphamide (inactive)   **Phosphoramide mustard (antineoplastic)**

3.8 APPLICATIONS OF PRODRUGS DESIGN

Prodrugs approach has been successfully applied to encompassing variety of drugs, various goals achieved not only for correction of pharmacokinetic behavior, but also pharmaceutical, organoleptic, physical and chemical properties of parent drug compound which enhance the stability and patient compliance improving the efficacy of therapy.

3.8.1 Pharmacokinetic Applications

Pharmacokinetic properties of drugs are important for its pharmacodynamic efficacy. Therefore drawbacks in pharmacokinetic parameters which affect the bioavailability and mean residence time of drug in body can be modulated by Prodrug approach. Following are the goals achieved by prodrug approach.

1. Prodrugs for improvement of bioavailability by alteration of drug's solubility.

2. Prodrugs for site selective drug delivery.

3. Prodrugs for longer duration of action.

4. Prodrugs for minimizing toxicity.

5. Prodrugs for protection from pre-systemic metabolism.

1. Prodrugs for Improvement of Bioavailability:

Chemical modification of drugs is used to improve physicochemical properties such as solubility, stability, and lipophilicity.

(a) Prodrugs to increase lipophilicity: Prodrugs are used to increase lipophilicity so that the drugs are available for oral administration, ocular or topical drug delivery. The main reason for designing prodrugs is to increase oral bioavailability, and the intestinal absorption, which are enhanced by masking the polar moiety of the drug.

Example: Dabigatran, a potent inhibitor of the active site of thrombin is very polar molecule, therefore its oral bioavailability is negligible. Dabigatran etexilate, the first oral alternative to warfarin, was developed as a prodrug of dabigatran. The oral bioavailability of dabigatran etexilate is 6.5%. After oral administration, dabigatran etexilate is converted to the active drug dabigatran by esterases.

Dabigatran etexilate

Esterases

Dabigatran

Lipophilic prodrugs are also used to enhance ocular absorption and transdermal absorption for certain drugs.

(b) Prodrugs to increase polarity: Prodrugs are designed to increase aqueous solubility by esterification with amino acids or phosphate group.

Example: Fosamprenavir, a protease inhibitor used as antiviral, is converted to amprenavir by alkaline phosphatase in the gut epithelium. The phosphate promoiety is linked to a free hydroxyl group which makes fosamprenavir 10-fold more water soluble than amprinavir. Because of prodrug, the dosage regimens of amprinavir get reduced into 2 times per day instead of administering the drug 8 times daily.

Fosampinavir (Prodrug)

2. **Prodrugs for Site Selective Drug Delivery:**

   Prodrugs are applied for targeting drugs to a specific organ or tissue; they are widely used in chemotherapy. Targeted prodrugs are used to increase absorption and decrease toxicity; they are targeted to an enzyme or membrane transporter.

   (a) **Tumor targeted drug delivery:** Cancer chemotherapeutics are toxic and non-selective which limits their use for cancer therapy. Their selectivity depends on the rapidly dividing cells that are more prone to toxic effects. Hence, they are toxic for rapidly proliferating normal tissue such as hair follicles, gut epithelia, bone marrow, and red blood cells. Therefore, in order to improve toxicity and efficacy, chemotherapy prodrugs were designed to target tumor cells. This targeting is achieved by binding drugs to ligands having high affinity to specific antigens, receptors, or transporters that are over expressed in tumor cells.

   One of the targeting methods is enzyme activated prodrug therapy, where the non-toxic prodrug is converted to the active drug in the tumor tissue.

   (b) **Drug-antibody conjugate:** Tumor specific mAbs bind to receptors on tumor cells and the cytotoxic drug is selectively delivered to the tumor. For example, mylotarg consists of anti-CD33 mAbs conjugated to the cytotoxic ozogamicin, which was approved by the FDA for treatment of acute myeloid leukemia.

   (c) **Antibody enzyme conjugates:**
   - **Antibody-directed enzyme prodrug therapy (ADEPT):** In this approach tumor specific antibody is delivered into tumor cells. Then the prodrug is administered systemically, and converted to the active toxic drug inside the tumor.
   - **Gene-directed enzyme prodrug therapy (GDEPT):** In this method, a gene encoding the activating enzyme is delivered to tumor cells as a first step. The second step is an administration of the inactive prodrug which is converted to the toxic drug by the tumor enzyme. Viral vectors are the most popular vectors used for gene delivery.

   (d) **Membrane transporter prodrug targeting:** Membrane transporters selectively transport peptides, amino acids, phosphates, ascorbic acid, bile acids and others. For example, dipeptides and tripeptides are transported in the intestinal epithelial cells by peptide transporters (PepT1).

Targeting specific transporters, which have an important role in drug absorption, distribution, and elimination, via a prodrug is efficient and selective strategy, in which a prodrug is selectively attached to a molecule that targets a specific membrane transporters; PepT1 is the most promising transporter due to its selectivity and high capacity.

Example: Acyclovir, an antiviral drug used to treat herpes simplex virus, by acting as a competitive substrate for DNA polymerase, has low oral bioavailability, because of its hydrophilic nature and poor permeability which limited its efficacy.

Valacyclovir   **Acyclovir**

To increase the oral bioavailability of acyclovir, L-valine (valacyclovir) prodrug was developed to target PepT transporters in the G.I. This prodrug has a high affinity for PepT transporter; therefore, it is highly absorbed through small intestine and is converted to acyclovir in the gut lumen.

3. Prodrugs for Longer Duration of Action:

Drugs with short half-life require frequent dosing, to maintain blood concentration, which leads to poor patient compliance and fluctuation in the drug concentration. The development of prodrugs with long duration of action can be used to overcome these problems.

Long acting antipsychotic therapy is important to control symptoms and prevent relapse. These long acting agents also improve patient compliance and increase efficacy.

Example: Fluphenazine decanoate, an ester prodrug of fluphenazine, is used as long acting intramuscular depot injection for the treatment of schizophrenia. This prodrug is administered once every 2 weeks.

Fluphenazine decanoate

4. Prodrugs for minimizing toxicity:

For therapeutically active drugs it is preferred to have minimum or no toxicity, therefore, prodrugs can be used to minimize toxicity of many drugs.

Example: Doxorubicin, an anthracycline antibiotic, which is highly used as anticancer drug, but its use is limited by its cardiotoxicity. Hence, there was a crucial need to design drug targeting system to increase doxorubicin availability in tumor tissue and decrease its accumulation in cardiac tissue. A galactoside prodrug that is linked to doxorubicin via a carbamate spacer was developed. This prodrug is solely activated by β-galactosidase that is highly expressed in tumor tissue; additionally, the hydrophilic nature of galactoside moiety prevents its distribution to other tissues. This prodrug is more effective and less toxic than its parent drug due to low concentration in cardiac tissue.

5. Prodrugs for Protection from Pre-systematic Metabolism:

Presystemic metabolism causes low oral bioavailability of drugs; certain sites or groups in the molecule are subjected to presystemic metabolism, therefore prodrugs can be used to block these sites and increase oral bioavailability.

Example 1: Nalbuphine is a potent analgesic drug used in moderate to severe pain; it has a low oral bioavailability of only 17% due to presystemic metabolism at the 3-hydroxyl position. Nalbuphine acetylsalicylate an ester prodrug of nalbuphine was synthesized and it has shown an increased oral bioavailability in dogs by 5-folds.

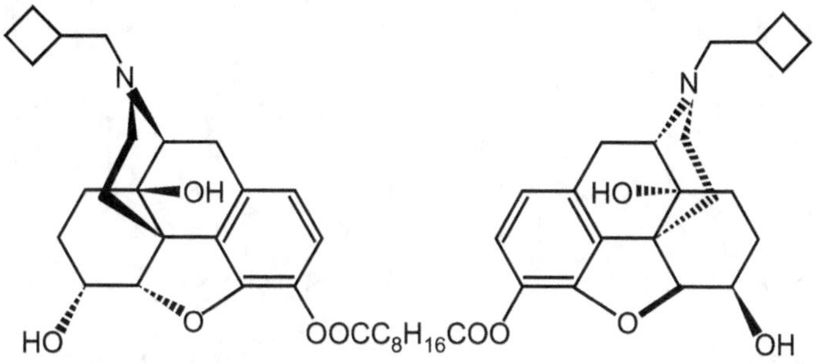

Sebacoyl dinalbuphine ester

Example 2: Estrogens such as estradiol and ethinyl estradiol have low oral bioavailability due to the conjugation at the phenolic hydroxyl position. Estrogen sulfamate prodrug was synthesized by replacing the phenolic hydroxyl group with sulfamate; this sulfamate prodrug protects estrogens from the liver first pass effect which leads to higher systemic activity of oral estrogens.

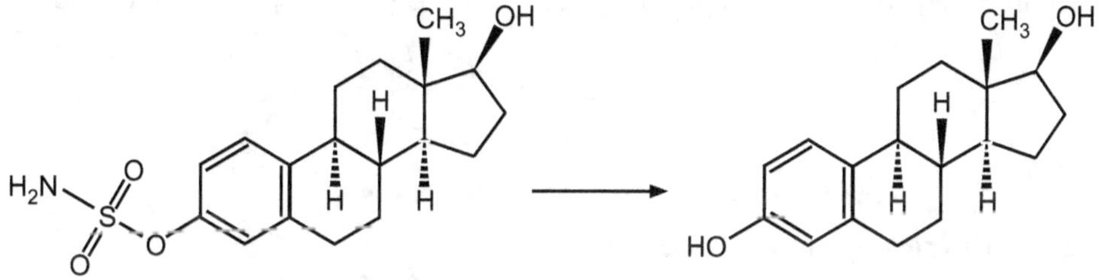

Estradiol sulfamate   **Estradiol**

3.8.2 Pharmaceutical Applications of Prodrugs

The undesirable organoleptic properties and physicochemical problems associated with drug formulation can be resolved.

1. **Taste Masking (Improvement of Taste):**

    Taste is an important factor in the development of dosage forms, and masking bitter taste of oral drugs is crucial for patient compliance especially in pediatric and geriatric patients. Drugs interact with taste buds on the tongue to give bitter taste. Many technologies were developed to prevent this interaction, including use of physical barrier, chemical or solubility modification and solid dispersion.

    Chemical modification to eliminate interaction with taste receptors can be achieved by using prodrug approach.

    Example: Paracetamol, an antipyretic and pain killer drug, has a bitter taste. It is believed that the phenolic hydroxyl group of paracetamol interacts by hydrogen bonding with bitter taste receptors. Therefore, blocking the hydroxyl group with a suitable linker could inhibit the interaction and mask the bitter taste of paracetamol.

Paracetamol   **Paracetamol prodrug**

2. **Odour Masking (Improvement of Odour):**

    Odour is an aesthetic concern for drugs with high vapor pressure or low boiling point, which makes them difficult to be formulated.

    Example: Ethyl mercaptan a tuberculostatic agent used for the treatment of leprosy has unpleasant smell because of low boiling point (25°C). The most attractive derivative prodrugs were its ethyl thiol esters; diethyl dithiolisophthalate prodrug of ethyl mercaptan was developed; this prodrug was found to be highly active and odorless.

    $C_2H_5SH \longrightarrow$

    Ethyl mercaptan   **Phthalate ester**

3. **Change of Physical Form of the Drug:**

    Some drugs which are in liquid form are unsuitable for formulation as a tablet, especially if their dose is high. The method of converting such a liquid drug into solid prodrug involves formation of symmetrical molecules having a higher tendency to crystallize.

    Example: Esterification of trichlorethanol with P-acetamidobenzoic acid ester.

    $Cl_3CCH_2OH \longrightarrow Cl_3CH_2COOC$ ——— $NHCOCH_3$

    Trichloroethanol   **P-Acetamidobenzoic acid ester**

4. **Reduction of G.I. Irritation:**

    Several drugs cause irritation and damage to the gastric mucosa through direct contact, increased stimulation of acid secretion or through interference with protective mucosal layer.

    Example: The NSAIDs, salicylates lower the gastric pH and induce or aggravate ulceration. This can be overcome by use of prodrug approach e.g. Salsalate.

5. **Minimizing Pain at Injection Site:**

    Pain at the injection site is caused by precipitation of drug that causes cell lyses and tissue injury. This problem may be related to the vehicle composition or vehicle pH needed for formulation purposes.

Example: Phenytoin injection, is approved for the treatment of status epilepticus has poor aqueous solubility and leads to soft tissue injury and pain in the site of administration, due to phenytoin precipitation. A phosphate ester prodrug of phenytoin (Fosphenytoin) was approved by the FDA in 1996. This prodrug has high aqueous solubility, no apparent pain was observed upon its use and its intramuscular bioavailability was 100%.

Fosphenytoin   Phenytoin

6. Enhancement of Solubility and Dissolution Rate (Hydrophilicity) of Drug:

Hydrophilicity or water solubility is desired where dissolution is the rate limiting step in the absorption of poorly aqueous soluble agents or when parental or ophthalmic formulation of such agents is desired. Many drugs in the pipeline in recent drug development are hydrophobic in nature (BCS Class-II) and possess poor bioavailability.

The prodrug approach is also made useful for rectification of the solubility problem and for better gastrointestinal absorption.

Example: Sulindac, a prodrug of Sulindac sulfide being more water soluble with sufficient lipophilicity, makes this drug suitable for oral administration.

Sulindac   Sulindac sulfide

7. Enhancement of Chemical Stability:

A drug may destabilize during its shelf life stability. The commonest conventional approach is to lyophilize the solution into a powder, which can be reconstituted before use. The prodrug design of such agents is a good alternative to improve stability.

Example: The aqueous solution of an antineoplastic drug (Azacytidine) is readily hydrolyzed, but the bisulfite prodrug shows stability to such degradation at acidic pH and is also more water soluble than the parent drug.

Azacytidine   **Stable bisulfite prodrug**

QUESTIONS

Multiple Choice Questions:

1. To understand the drug receptor interaction it is necessary to quantify the relation between ....
    (a) Drug and its toxicity
    (b) Drug and its absorption
    (c) Drug and its biological activity
    (d) Drug and intermediate product

2. Identify the metabolite of prontosil responsible for its antibacterial activity.
    (a) Sulphacetamide
    (b) Sulphanilamide
    (c) p-Amino benzoic acid
    (d) Probenecid

3. Which of the following strategies will increase the polarity and water solubility of a drug?
    (a) Removing polar functional groups.
    (b) Adding extra alkyl groups.
    (c) Replacing an aromatic ring with a nitrogen containing heterocyclic ring.
    (d) Replacing an alkyl group with a larger alkyl group.

4. Esters are frequently used as prodrugs. Which of the following statements is false?
    (a) Ester prodrugs are more easily absorbed from the gut than the parent drug if the parent drug is highly polar.
    (b) Esters are more susceptible to hydrolysis if the alcohol moiety has an electron donating group.
    (c) Esters can be used to mask a polar alcohol, phenol or carboxylic acid group.
    (d) It is preferable if the leaving group from ester hydrolysis is a natural chemical such as an amino acid.

5. The activation of prodrug does not occur at any time during ....
    (a) absorption
    (b) distribution
    (c) metabolism
    (d) elimination

6.	L-dopa is an example for ....
	(a)	Carrier linked prodrug				(b)	Bioprecursor
	(c)	Mutual Prodrug					(d)	None of the above

7.	Chloramphenicol succinate ester is used to increase .... of chloramphenicol.
	(a)	lipid solubility					(b)	water solubilty
	(c)	bioavailability					(d)	distribution

8.	The carrier group of carrier linked prodrugs must be ....
	(a)	pharmacologically active			(b)	biologically detachable
	(c)	reactive to the drug				(d)	chemically reactive

9.	Chloramphenicol palmitate is a prodrug of the antibiotic chloramphenicol. Which of the following statements is true?
	(a)	Chloramphenicol palmitate is more water soluble than chloramphenicol.
	(b)	Chloramphenicol palmitate is active than chloramphenicol.
	(c)	Chloramphenicol palmitate is used to achieve higher concentrations for injections.
	(d)	Chloramphenicol palmitate is used to reduce the bitter taste of chloramphenicol.

10.	Candoxatril is an ester prodrug for candoxatrilat which inhibits protease enzymes. Which of the following statements is incorrect?
	(a)	Hydrolysis of the ester reveals a carboxylic acid group on candoxatrilat.
	(b)	The parent drug can be administered orally, whereas the ester prodrug cannot.
	(c)	The bicyclic leaving group is non-toxic.
	(d)	The bicyclic system is electron withdrawing and speeds up the rate of ester hydrolysis.

11.	Which of the following statements is true with respect to phosphate prodrugs?
	(a)	Phosphate esters are more polar in nature than the parent drug.
	(b)	Phosphate esters are less water soluble than the parent drug.
	(c)	Phosphate esters are more likely to cross cell membranes than the parent drug.
	(d)	Phosphate esters are resistant to drug metabolism.

12.	Some drugs containing an ester group are inactive *in-vitro*, but are active once the drug has been absorbed *in-vivo*. What term is used for such drugs?
	(a)	Postdrugs						(b)	Predrugs
	(c)	Metabolites					(d)	Prodrugs

13.	Esters are frequently used as prodrugs. Which of the following statements is false?
	(a)	Ester prodrugs are more easily absorbed from the gut than the parent drug if the parent drug is highly polar.
	(b)	Esters are more susceptible to hydrolysis if the alcohol moiety has an electron donating group.

(c) Esters can be used to mask a polar alcohol, phenol or carboxylic acid group.

(d) It is preferable if the leaving group from ester hydrolysis is a natural chemical such as an amino acid.

14. Chloroquin is an antimalarial drug which belongs to the class of ....

    (a) 4-amino quinoline   (b) 8-amino quinoline

    (c) 9-amino quinoline   (d) Acidine

15. Which of the following statements is true with respect to phosphate prodrugs?

    (a) Phosphate esters are more polar in nature than the parent drug.

    (b) Phosphate esters are less water soluble than the parent drug.

    (c) Phosphate esters are more likely to cross cell membranes than the parent drug.

    (d) Phosphate esters are resistant to drug metabolism.

16. What is not the reason to use prodrug?

    (a) To reduce pain.
    (b) To alter absorption, distribution and metabolism.
    (c) To avoid an unpleasant taste.
    (d) To increase toxicity.

Answers :

1. (c)	2. (b)	3. (c)	4. (b)	5. (d)	6. (a)	7. (b)	8. (b)	9. (d)	10. (b)
11. (a)	12. (a)	13. (b)	14. (a)	15. (a)	16. (d)				

Answer the following Questions:

1. Define prodrugs. Explain basic concept behind designing of prodrugs.
2. Give an account of designing of prodrugs.
3. Give in detail functional groups that are amenable to prodrug design.
4. Define prodrugs. Give objective of designing of prodrugs.
5. Define prodrugs. Classify them.
6. Write a short note on Carrier linked prodrug. Give its advantages.
7. Define mutual prodrug. Explain it with suitable example.
8. Write in brief various applications of designing of prodrugs.
9. Give a detail note on pharmacokinetic application of prodrug design.
10. Give a detail account on pharmaceutical application of prodrug design.
11. Explain how prodrug design is helpful for reduction of toxicity of drug with suitable example.

■■■

Chapter ... 4

ANTIMALARIAL AGENTS

♦ LEARNING OBJECTIVES ♦

After completing this sub-unit the students should be able:

- *To learn the causes and different types of malaria*
- *To study life cycle of malaria.*
- *To study treatment to be carried out for malaria.*
- *To study different categories of drugs used in treatment of malaria.*
- *To study the synthetic pathway of some selected antimalarial drugs.*

4.1 MALARIA

Malaria, (mala-aria means bad air), is one of the most widespread diseases caused by a *Plasmodium* parasite. It is a serious, life-threatening, and sometimes fatal, disease spread by mosquitoes. The parasite is transmitted to humans through the bites of infected mosquitoes. The disease is uncommon in temperate climates. Malaria is still common in tropical and subtropical countries.

Malaria is a mosquito-borne disease and it does not spread from person to person. In rare certain circumstances only it spreads without a mosquito such as transmission from a pregnant woman to an unborn child (congenital malaria), by blood transfusions, or when intravenous-drug users share needles. Except for the above conditions, malaria is not considered as contagious.

Following the mosquito bite, there is about a 7 to 30 days period before symptoms appear (incubation period). The incubation period for *P. vivax* is usually 10-17 days, but can be much longer (about one year and rarely, as long as 30 years!). *P. falciparum* usually has a short incubation period (10-14 days). Other species of *Plasmodium* that cause malaria have incubation periods similar to *P. vivax*.

Some varieties of the malaria parasite, which typically cause milder forms of the disease, can persist for years and cause relapses. Scientists around the world are trying to develop a safe and effective vaccine for malaria. As of yet, however, there is still no malaria vaccine approved for human use.

Malaria is caused by four species of a one-cell protozoan of the *Plasmodium* genus:

1. **P. falciparum:** This species is estimated to cause approximately 50% of all malaria. It has an incubation period of 1 to 3 weeks (average, 12 days). It causes the most severe form and the most debilitating form of the disease, because patients feel ill between acute attacks. One reason why it leaves the patient so weak is that it infects up to 65% of the patient's erythrocytes.

2. **P. vivax:** This species is the second most common species, accounting for about 40% of all malaria cases. It can be very chronic, because it can re-infect liver cells. It has an incubation period of 1 to 4 weeks (average, 2 weeks). This form of malaria can cause spleen rupture and anemia. Relapses can occur due to the periodic release of dormant parasites (hypnozoites) from the liver cells.

3. **P. malariae:** It accounts only 10% of all malarial cases, relapses are very common. It has an incubation period of 2 to 4 weeks (average, 3 weeks). In addition to the usual symptoms, this form also causes nephritis. The RBC infected ion associated with P. malariae can last for many years.

4. **P. ovale:** This species is the least common. It has an incubation period of 9 to 18 days (average, 14 days). Relapses have been known to occur in individuals infected with this plasmodium. The relapse may be associated with the ability of the organism to lie dormant in hepatic tissue for extended periods of time.

4.2 TYPES OF MALARIA

1. **Uncomplicated Malaria:**

   The most common symptoms of uncomplicated malaria are:
   - fever and chills.
   - headaches.
   - nausea and vomiting and
   - general weakness and body aches.

   Other signs and symptoms may include:
   - sweating
   - chest or abdominal pain
   - cough

2. **Complicated or Severe Malaria:**

   This occurs when malaria affects different body systems. The most common symptoms of complicated malaria are:
   - Severe anemia (due to destruction of red blood cells).
   - Kidney failure.
   - Cerebral malaria - seizures, unconsciousness, abnormal behavior, or confusion.
   - Cardiovascular collapse.
   - Low blood sugar (in pregnant women after treatment with quinine).

In most cases, malaria deaths are related to one or more serious complications, including:

- **Cerebral malaria:** If parasite-filled blood cells block small blood vessels to brain (cerebral malaria), swelling of brain or brain damage may occur. Cerebral malaria may cause seizures and coma.

- **Breathing problems:** Accumulated fluid in lungs (pulmonary edema) can make it difficult to breathe.

- **Organ failure:** Malaria can cause kidneys or liver to fail, or spleen to rupture. Any of these conditions can be life-threatening.

- **Anemia:** Malaria damages red blood cells, which can result in anemia.

- **Low blood sugar:** Severe forms of malaria itself can cause low blood sugar (hypoglycemia), as can quinine - one of the most common medications used to combat malaria. Very low blood sugar can result in coma or death.

4.3 DIGNOSIS AND PREVENTION OF MALARIA

Diagnosis of Malaria:

Diagnosis of malaria depends on the demonstration of parasites in the blood, usually by microscopy. Additional laboratory findings may include mild anemia, mild decrease in blood platelets (thrombocytopenia), elevation of bilirubin, and elevation of aminotransferases.

Prevention of Malaria:

Mosquitoes are most active between dusk and dawn. To protect from mosquito bites, some precautions are needed to take, such as:

- **Covering (protecting) skin:** Wear pants and long-sleeved shirts.

- **Apply insect repellant to skin and clothing:** Sprays containing DEET (Diethyltoluamide) can be used on skin and sprays containing permethrin are safe to apply to clothing.

- **Sleep under a net:** Bed nets, particularly those treated with insecticide, help to prevent mosquito bites while sleeping.

4.4 PARASITE TRANSMISSION CYCLE

- **Uninfected mosquito:** A mosquito becomes infected by feeding on a person who has malaria.

- **Transmission of parasite:** If this mosquito bites in the future to any person, it can transmit malaria parasites to that person.

- **In the liver:** Once the parasites enter in the body of that person, they travel to liver - where some types can lie dormant for as long as a year.

- **Into the bloodstream:** When the parasites mature, they leave the liver and infect red blood cells. This is when people typically develop malaria symptoms.

- **On to the next person:** If an uninfected mosquito bites to that infected person at this point in the cycle, it will become infected with malaria parasites and can spread them to the other people it bites.

4.5 LIFE CYCLE OF MALERIA

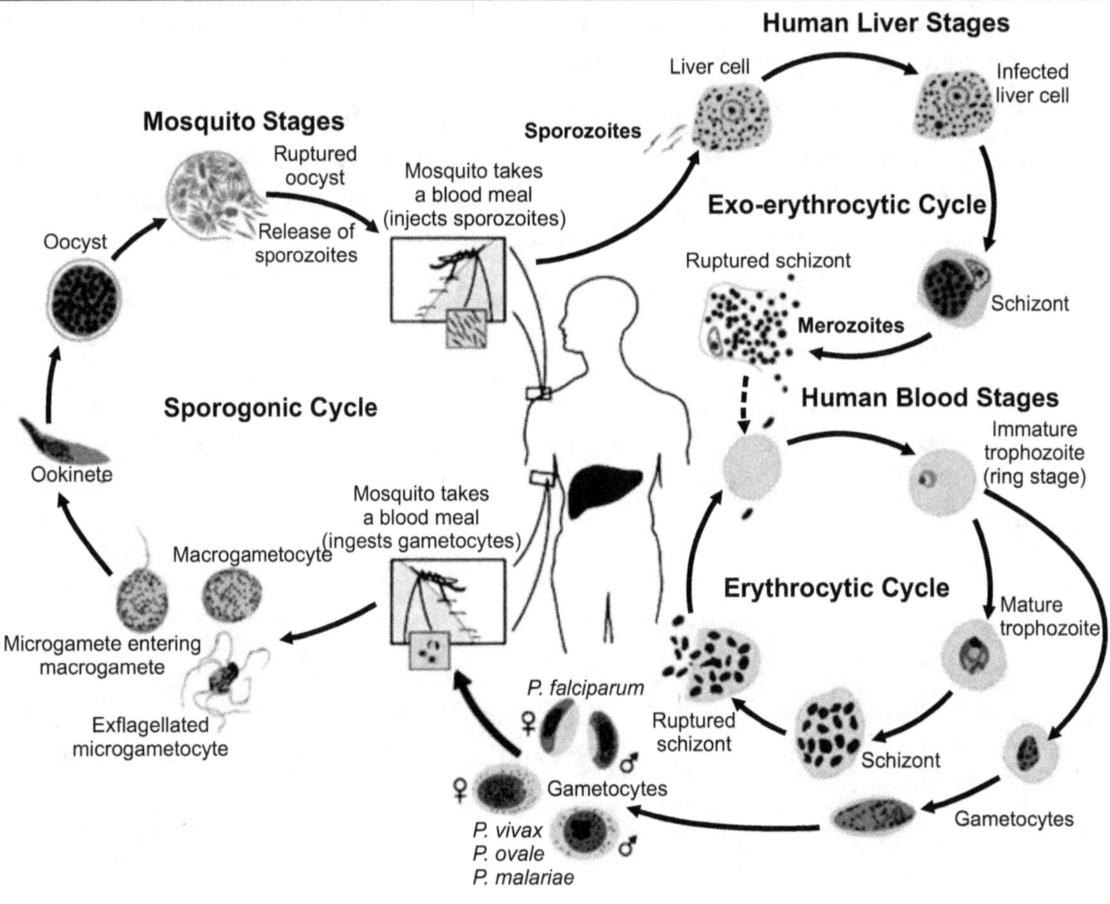

Fig. 4.1

1. Malaria infection begins when an infected female *Anopheles* mosquito bites a person, injecting *Plasmodium* parasites, in the form of sporozoites, into the bloodstream.

2. The sporozoites pass quickly into the human liver.

3. The sporozoites multiply asexually in the liver cells over the next 7 to 10 days, causing no symptoms.

4. In an animal model, the parasites, in the form of merozoites, are released from the liver cells in vesicles.

5. Merozoites pass through the heart and arrive in the lungs, where they settle within lung capillaries.

6. The vesicles eventually ruptured and released the merozoites enter in the blood phase of their development.

7. In the bloodstream, the merozoites invade red blood cells (erythrocytes) and multiply again until the cells burst.

8. Then they invade more erythrocytes. This cycle is repeated, causing fever each time parasites break free and invade blood cells.

9. Some of the infected blood cells leave the cycle of asexual multiplication. Instead of replicating, the merozoites in these cells develop into sexual forms of the parasite, called gametocytes that circulate in the blood stream.

10. When a mosquito bites an infected human, it ingests the gametocytes, which develop further into mature sex cells called gametes.

11. The fertilized female gametes develop into actively moving ookinetes that burrow through the mosquito's mid-gut wall and form oocysts on the exterior surface.

12. Inside the oocyst, thousands of active sporozoites develop. The oocyst eventually bursts, releasing sporozoites into the body cavity that travel to the mosquito's salivary glands.

13. The cycle of human infection begins again when the mosquito bites another person.

4.6 TREATMENT OF MALARIA

There are four possible sites for drug therapy:

1. Kill the sporozoites injected by the mosquito and/or prevent the sporozoites from entering the liver.

2. Kill the schizonts residing in hepatocytes and/or prevent them from becoming merozoites.

3. Kill the merozoites in the blood and/or prevent them from developing into gametocytes.

4. Kill the gametocytes before they can enter the mosquito and reproduce into zygotes. The main focus of drug therapy at this site should be on the male gametocytes. This would block the female gametocytes from mating.

Anti-malarial drugs are good examples of anti-infective agents with poor selective toxicity. Contrast them with the antibiotics tetracyclines, chloramphenicol, and aminoglycosides act against bacterial ribosomes, but not mammalian ones. Penicillins and cyclosporines inhibit bacterial cell wall crosslinking, and mammals have cell membranes, not cell walls. The fluoroquinolones inhibit bacterial gyrase, but not mammalian topoisomerases.

The biochemistry of *Plasmodium spp.* is similar to that of mammals, making it difficult to design drugs that will not affect the patient adversely. Indeed, some have indications beyond treating and preventing malaria.

4.7 CLASSIFICATION OF ANTIMALARIAL DRUGS

1. **Cinchona alkaloids:** Quinine sulphate.
2. **4-aminoquinoline:** Chloroquine, Hydroxychloroquine, Amodiaquine, Mefloquine.
3. **8-aminoquinoline:** Primaquine phosphate, Pamaquine, Pentaquine.
4. **9-Aminoacridines:** Mepacrine hydrochloride (Quinacrine hydrochloride).
5. **Guanidine analogues (Biguanides) and dihydro triazines:** Cycloguanil pamoate, Proguanil.
6. **Pyrimidine analogues (Diaminopyrimidines):** Pyrimethamine, Trimethoprim.
7. **Miscellaneous:** Artesunete, Artemether, Atovoquone.

4.8 DRUG PROFILE

4.8.1 Cinchona Alkaloids

The cinchona tree produces four alkaloids that are enantiomeric pairs, quinine and quinidine and their desmethoxy analogues cinchonidine (for quinine) and cinchonine (for quinidine). Their numbering system is based on rubane. The stereochemistry differs at positions 8 and 9, with quinine and cinchonidine being S, R and Quinidine and cinchonine being R, S.

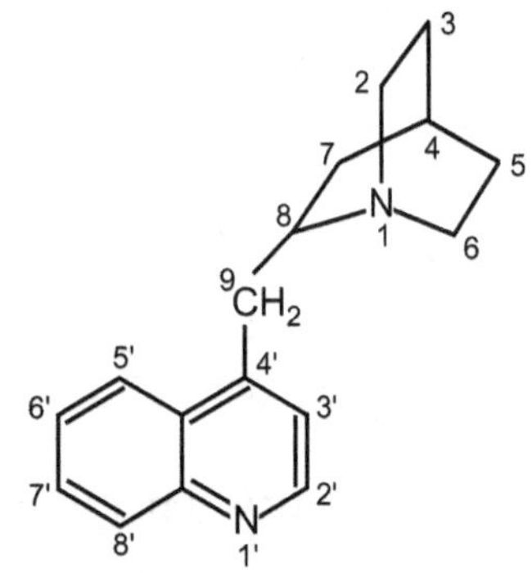

Rubane

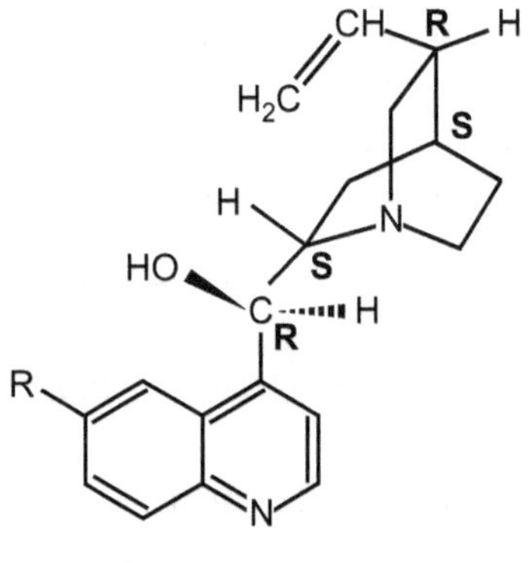

Quinine R = OCH$_3$
Cinchonidine R = H

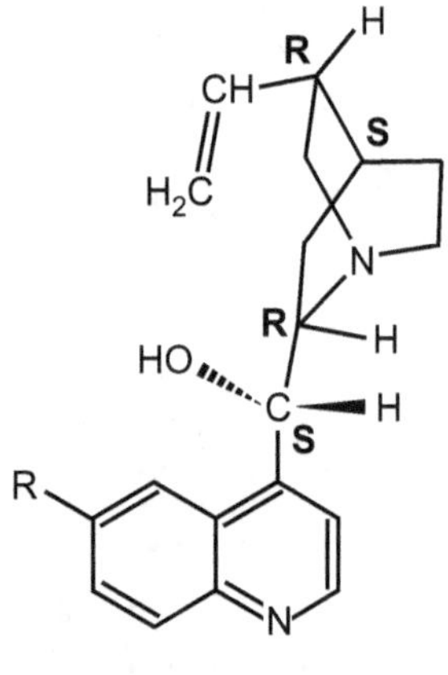

Quinidine R = OCH$_3$
Cinchonine R = H

1. **Quinine Sulphate:**

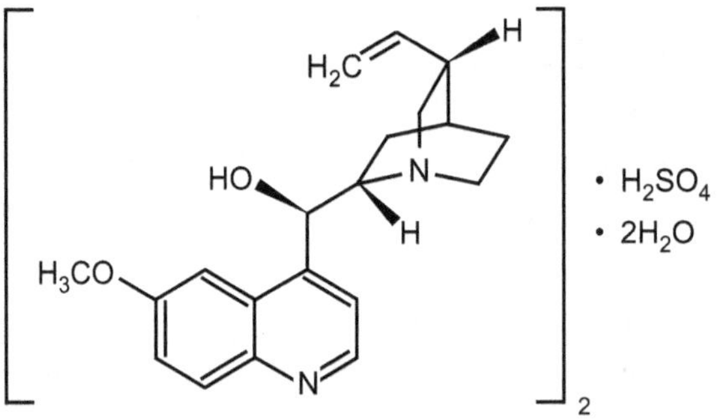

Quinine sulphate

- Quinine is an alkaloid isolated in 1820 from the bark of *Cinchona officinalis Lin.* belonging to the family *Rubiaceae* or other species of *Cinchona*.
- It is a 4-quinolinemethanol derivative bearing a substituted quinuclidine ring.
- Quinine only affects the erythrocytic form of the plasmodia.
- It is employed extensively for the suppression and control of malaria caused due to *P. vivax, P. malariae and P. ovale.* It has been found to be less effective in *P. falciparum.*

Uses:

- Quinine was the first known antimalarial.
- It is also a mild antipyretic and analgesic.
- It is also useful in some muscular disorders, especially nocturnal leg cramps and myotonia congenital.
- The 'drug' may be employed in combination with pyrimethamine and a sulphonamide, but it seems to be antagonized by chloroquine.
- It has been employed successfully to treat chloroquine-resistant strains of *P. falciparum.*

4.8.2 4-Aminoquinolines

4-aminoquinolines are the closest of the antimalarials that are based on the quinine structure. This group is substituted at the same position 4 as quinine and has an asymmetric carbon equivalent to quinine's C-9 position. Just as with quinine, both isomers are active, and the 4-aminoquinoline racemic mixtures are used.

For the newest drug in this series, mefloquine, only the R,S isomer is marketed. A significant difference from the commercial cinchona alkaloids is replacing the 6-methoxy on quinine with a 7-chloro substituent on the 4-aminoquinolines.

1. Chloroquine:

Chloroquine

- Chloroquine is a 4-aminoquinoline which is substituted at position 4 by a [5-(diethylamino)pentan-2-yl]amino group and at position 7 by chlorine.
- It is chemically, 7-Chloro-4-[[4-(diethylamino)-1-methyl] butyl] amino]-quinoline.
- It is shown to inhibit the parasitic enzyme heme polymerase that converts the toxic heme into non-toxic hemazoin, thereby resulting in the accumulation of toxic heme within the parasite.

Uses:

- Chloroquine is an aminoquinoline used for the prevention and therapy of malaria.
- It is also effective in extraintestinal amebiasis and as an anti-inflammatory agent for therapy of rheumatoid arthritis and lupus erythematosus.

2. Amodiaquine:

Amodiaquine

- Amodiaquine is an orally active 4-aminoquinoline derivative.
- It is a quinoline having a chloro group at the 7-position and an aryl amino group at the 4-position.
- It is chemically, 4-[(7-chloroquinolin-4-yl)amino]-2-(diethylaminomethyl)phenol.
- It likely is able to inhibit heme polymerase activity in the body. This results in accumulation of free heme, which is toxic to the parasites.
- As it is associated with a higher incidence of hepatitis and agranulocytosis, it is recommended for use only as treatment and not for prophylaxis against malaria.

Uses:

- Amodiaquine is an aminoquinoline used for the therapy of malaria.
- It is effective against some chloroquine-resistant strains, particularly *P. falciparum*,
- It also possesses anti-inflammatory properties.

3. Mefloquine:

Mefloquine

- Mefloquine is a quinolinemethanol derivative with antimalarial activity.
- It consists of quinoline bearing trifluoromethyl substituents at positions 2 and 8 as well as a (2-piperidinyl) hydroxymethyl substituent at position 4.
- It is chemically, [2,8-bis(trifluoromethyl)quinolin-4-yl]-piperidin-2-yl methanol
- It is a weak base, preferentially accumulates in lysosomes and disrupts lysosomal function and integrity, thereby leading to host cell death.

Uses:
- Mefloquine is a quinoline derivative used for the prevention and therapy of *P. falciparum* malaria.
- It also possesses anti-inflammatory and potential chemosensitization and radio-sensitization activities.
- It is contraindicated in patients with active depression.

4.8.3 8-Aminoquinolines

The other major group of antimalarial drugs based on the cinchona alkaloid quinoline moiety is the substituted 8-aminoquinolines. All 8-aminoquinolines can cause hemolytic anemia in erythrocytic glucose-6-phosphate dehydrogenase deficient patients.

Mechanism of Action:

Although structurally related to the cinchona alkaloids, the 8-aminoquinolines have a different mechanism of action. They appear to disrupt the parasite's mitochondria, results in disruption of several processes, including maturation into the subsequent forms. An advantage is destroying exoerythrocytic forms before the parasite can infect erythrocytes, the step in the infectious process that makes malaria so debilitating.

Structure Activity Relationship:
- 8-Aminoquinolines have a 6-methoxy moiety like quinine.
- Substituents on quinoline are located at position 8 rather than carbon-4.
- All agents in this series have 4-5 carbon alkyl linkage or bridge between the two nitrogens.
- Pamaquine and Primaquine have one asymmetric carbon.

1. Primaquine Phosphate:

Primaquine phosphate

- Primaquine phosphate is a synthetic, 8-aminoquinoline derivative with antimalarial properties.
- It is chemically, 8-[(4-Amino-1-methylbutyl) amino]-6-methoxy quinoline phosphate.
- It is active against latent tissue forms of *P. vivax* and *P. ovale*, and it is active against the hepatic stages of *P. falciparum*.
- It is also active against exoerythrocytic stages of *P. vivax* and *P. ovale* and primary exoerythrocytic stages of *P. falciparum*.
- It acts by binding to and altering the properties of protozoal DNA.

Uses:
- Primaquine is an aminoquinoline that has been used for the prevention and therapy of malaria for more than 50 years.

2. Pamaquine:

Pamaquine

- Pamaquine is an 8-aminoquinoline antimalarial drug. It was first introduced for treatment of malaria in 1926.
- It is chemically, 8-(4-Diethylamino-1-methylbutylamino)-6-methoxyquinoline.
- The mechanism of action is as under 8-aminoquinoline.

Uses:

- Pamaquine was initially employed for the treatment of malaria, but has since been superseded by primaquine phosphate.

4.8.4 9-Aminoacridines

1. Quinacrine Hydrochloride (Mepacrine Hydrochloride):

Quinacrine hydrochloride

- Quinacrine hydrochloride is the dihydrochloride salt of the 9-amino-acridine derivative.
- It is chemically, 6-Chloro-9-[[4-(diethylamino)-1-methylbutyl]amino]-2-methoxy-acridine dihydrochloride dehydrate.
- It inhibits the erythrocytic state of development of the malarial parasite.
- It is found to be more toxic and less effective than chloroquine.

Uses:

- Quinacrine hydrochloride is an acridine derivative formerly widely used as an antimalarial, but superseded by chloroquine in recent years.
- It has potential antineoplastic and antiparasitic activities.
- It is also used as an anthelmintic and in the treatment of giardiasis, amebiasis, tapeworm and pinworm infestations.

4.8.5 Guanidine Analogues (Biguanides) and Dihydro Triazines

1. Proguanil (Chlorguanide):

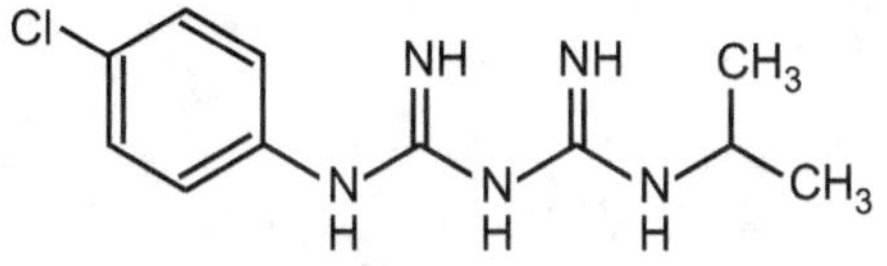

Proguanil

- Proguanil is a biguanide derivative which is active against several protozoal species.
- It is chemically, 1-(p-Chlorophenyl)-5-isopropylbiguanide.
- It is active against the pre-erythrocytic (liver) forms of malaria.
- It is also active against the erythrocytic forms, but their activity is slow.
- It acts by inhibiting the enzyme dihydrofolate reductase, which is involved in the reproduction of the malaria parasites *P. falciparum and P. vivax* within the red blood cells.

Uses:

- Proguanil is used as an antimalarial, an antiprotozoal drug.
- It is used mainly for prophylactic treatment of malaria.

2. Cycloguanil Pamoate:

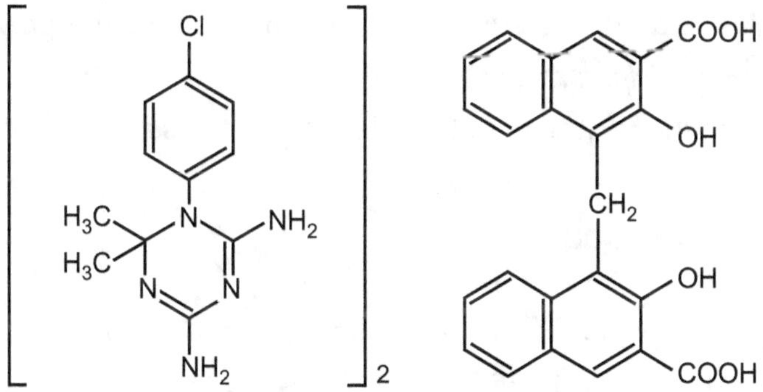

Cycloguanil Pamoate

- Cycloguanil is the active metabolite of proguanil.
- It is chemically, 4, 6-Diamino-1-(p-chlorophenyl)-1, 2-dihydro-2, 2-dimethyl-s-triazine compound (2:1) with 4, 4' methylene-bis [3-hydroxy-2-naphthoic acid].
- It acts by inhibiting the enzyme dihydrofolate reductase.

Uses:

- Cycloguanil is employed for the suppression of malaria.

4.8.6 Pyrimidine Analogues (Diaminopyrimidines)

The pyrimidine analogues have a close similarity to the pteridine moiety of dihydrofolic acid, and are directly responsible for its subsequent reduction to tetrahydrofolic acid by means of the enzyme dihydrofolate reductase.

The site of action of pyrimidine analogues are exoerythrocytic and erythrocytic forms of *P. falciparum*, together with the exoerythrocytic forms of *P. vivax*.

1. Pyrimethamine:

Pyrimethamine

- Pyrimethamine is a synthetic derivative of ethyl-pyrimidine with potent antimalarial properties.
- It is chemically, 2, 4-Diamino-5-(p-chlorophenyl)-6-ethylpyrimidine.
- It acts by inhibiting dehydrofolate reductase in plasmodia; and thereby the developing parasite cannot synthesize and use nucleic acid precursors needed for their normal growth.

Uses:

- Pyrimethamine is used as a suppressive prophylactic for the preventation of severe attacks due to *P. falciparum* and *P. vivax*.
- It is also used in the treatment of toxoplasmosis and as an immunosuppressive agent.

2. Trimethoprim:

Trimethoprim

- Trimethoprim is a synthetic derivative of trimethoxybenzyl-pyrimidine with antibacterial and antiprotozoal properties.
- It is chemically, 2, 4-Diamino-5-(3,4,5-Trimethoxybenzyl) pyrimidine.
- It is a potent inhibitor of dihydrofolate reductase.

Uses:

- Trimethoprim is employed in conjunction with sulfamethopyrazine in the treatment of chloroquine-resistant malaria.
- It has also been used in conjunction with sulphonamides in the treatment of bacterial infections (*viz., trimethoprim with sulphamethoxazole*).

4.8.7 Miscellaneous Drugs

1. Artemisinin:

Artemisinin

- The marked and pronounced antimalarial activity of 'Quinghausu' as the constituent of a traditional Chinese medicinal herb *Artemisia annuna* L., (sweet wormwood) has been known in China for over 200 years. However, the active principle was first isolated in 1972 and found to be a sesquiterpene lactone with a peroxy moiety.

- All of the drugs derived from artemisinin are active against the *Plasmodium* genera that cause malaria.

- The key structure characteristic appears to be a "trioxane" consisting of the endoperoxide and doxepin oxygens.

Mechanism of Action:

- In human's erythrocyte, it has been observed that the malaria parasite actually consumes the haeomoglobin comprising mainly of Fe^{2+} iron, thereby changing it to the corresponding toxic hematin consisting of Fe^{3+} ion, subsequently get reduced to heme with its Fe^{2+} ion.

- Later on, the resulting 'heme ion' eventually interacts with the prevailing trioxane moiety, thereby releasing the 'reactive oxygen' carbon radicals and the extremely reactive $Fe^{IV} = O$ species. It has been established that the later is proved to be lethal to the parasite.

2. Artesunate:

Artesunate

- Artesunate (water soluble) is a semi-synthetic derivative of artemisinin.
- It is the newest of the antimalarial drugs and is structurally unique.
- It is the hemisuccinate ester of the lactol resulting from the reduction of the lactone carbonyl group of artemisinin.
- The mechanism of action is same as artemisinin.

Uses:

- Artesunate is a part of the artemisinin group of drugs that treat malaria.
- It also has anti-schistosomiasis, antiviral, and potential anti-neoplastic activities.

3. Artemether:

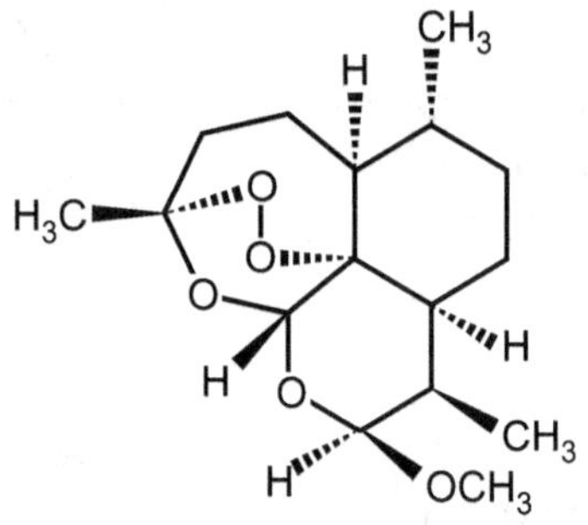

Artemether

- Artemether is an semisynthetic artemisinin derivative in which the lactone has been converted to the corresponding lactol methyl ether.
- It is active against the entire *Plasmodium* genera that cause malaria.
- The mechanism of action is same as artemisinin.
- It is administered in combination with lumefantrine for improved efficacy.
- In combination therapy it is effective against the erythrocytic stages of *Plasmodium spp.* and may be used to treat infections caused by *P. falciparum* and unidentified *Plasmodium* species.

Uses:

- Artemether is an antimalarial agent used to treat acute uncomplicated malaria.

4. Atovaquone:

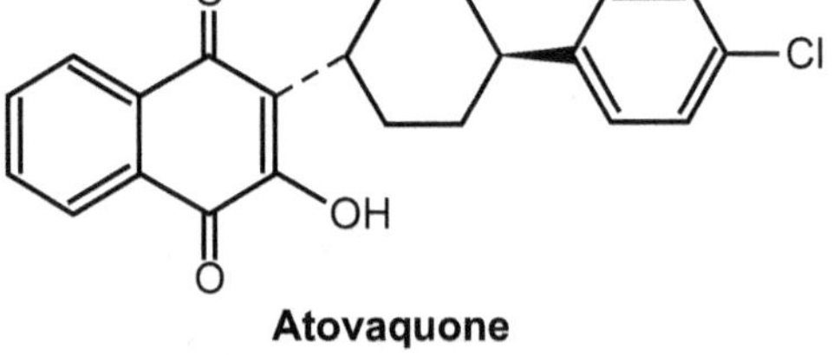

Atovaquone

- Atovaquone is a synthetic hydroxynaphthoquinone with antiprotozoal activity.
- It is chemically, 3-[4-(4-chlorophenyl)cyclohexyl]-4-hydroxynaphthalene-1,2-dione.
- Atovoquone blocks the mitochondrial electron transport at complex-III of the respiratory chain of protozoa, thereby inhibiting pyrimidine synthesis, preventing DNA synthesis and leading to protozoal death.

Uses:

- Atovaquone is used in combination with proguanil for prevention and treatment of *P. falciparum* malaria.

SYNTHESIS

1. Chloroquine:

2. Pamaquine:

QUESTIONS

Multiple Choice Questions:

1. A natural product derivative developed as an antimalarial is ....
    (a) Artemether   (b) Paludrine
    (c) Pyrimethamine   (d) Halofantrine

2. Proguanil is metabolized to a triazine derivative which is an active metabolite. Name the metabolite.
    (a) Thioguanil   (b) Diguanil
    (c) Cycloguanil   (d) P-chlorophenyl biguanide

3. Amodiaquine is derivative of ....
    (a) 3-amino quinoline   (b) 4-amino quinoline
    (c) 2-amino quinoline   (d) 5-amino quinoline

4. Pamaquine is derivative of
    (a) 4-amino quinoline   (b) 8-amino quinoline
    (c) 2-amino quinoline   (d) 5-amino quinoline

5. Cycloguanil contains the following heterocyclic ring in its structure:
    (a) Triazine   (b) Pyrazole
    (c) Furan   (d) Tetrazine

6. Pamaquine is sythesized from ....
    (a) Anisole   (b) Toluene
    (c) Phenol   (d) Cresol

7. Identify the drug which is NOT used in the treatment of malaria caused by Plasmodium falciparum:
    (a) Pyrimethamine   (b) Pamaquine
    (c) Quinine   (d) Isoniazid

8. Chloroquine is an antimalarial drug which belongs to the class of
    (a) 4-amino quinoline   (b) 8-amino quinoline
    (c) 9-amino quinoline   (d) Acidine

9. Which of the following causes 50% malaria disease?
    (a) plasmodium falciparum   (b) plasmodium vivax
    (c) plasmodium ovale   (d) plasmodium malariae

10. Which one of the following is called as an intermittent fever?
    (a) Malaria   (b) Tuberculosis
    (c) HIV   (d) Cancer

11. Which form is the starting point for the life cycle of Malaria?

    (a) Merozoites   (b) Sporozoites

    (c) Schizaonts   (d) Oocysta

12. The tetracycline used for the treatment of malaria is ....

    (a) Aureomycin   (b) Minocycline

    (c) Doxycycline   (d) Demeclocycline

13. Which metabolite of the mepacrine gives yellow colour of urine?

    (a) 9-amino mepacrine   (b) 8-amino mepacrine

    (c) 7-amino mepacrine   (d) 6-amino mepacrine

14. Quinacrine or Mepacrine is derivative of ....

    (a) 4-amino quinoline   (b) 8-amino quinoline

    (c) Acridine   (d) 5-amino quinoline

15. Which of the following statements is FALSE for artemisinin?

    (a) It is a sesquiterpene lactone endoperoxide.

    (b) It is a drug of choice in prophylaxis of malaria.

    (c) It does not cure relapsing malaria.

    (d) It is useful in treatment of cerebral falciparum malaria.

16. Treatment of Malaria is achieved with the combination of pyrimethamine with all of the following except ....

    (a) Sulphadoxine   (b) Dapsone

    (c) Trimethoprim   (d) Sulphadiazine

17. Artemisinin contains the following group in its structure :

    (a) Endoperoxide   (b) Exoperoxide

    (c) Epoxide   (d) Acid hydrazide

18. Identify the drug which is NOT used in the treatment of malaria caused by Plasmodium falciparum.

    (a) Artemisinin   (b) Primaquine

    (c) Quinine   (d) Mefloquine

Answers :

1. (a)	2. (c)	3. (b)	4. (b)	5. (a)	6. (a)	7. (d)	8. (a)	9. (a)	10. (a)
11. (b)	12. (c)	13. (a)	14. (c)	15. (b)	16. (a)	17. (a)	18. (b)		

Answer the Following Questions:

1. Write a short note on diagnosis, symptoms and treatment of malaria.
2. What are the causal organisms responsible for malaria? How do the antimalarials affect the life cycle of mosquito? Explain.
3. Give a brief note on cinchona alkaloids.
4. Classify the synthetic antimalarials based on their basic chemical nucleus. Give examples of at least one compound from each class.
5. How would you synthesize the following drugs?
    (a) Chloroquine
    (b) Pamaquine
6. Give the structure, chemical name and the uses of:
    (a) Amodiaquine
    (b) Mefloquine.
    (c) Proguanil
    (d) Quinacrine hydrochloride
7. Write a short note on various types of malaria with their symptoms.
8. Write a brief note on life cycle of malaria.
9. Write in brief classification of antimalarial drugs with suitable examples.
10. Give a comprehensive account of Artemisinin.
11. Give a brief account of the mode of action of antimalarials.
12. Give mode of action and SAR of 8-Aminoquinolines.

Unit III

chapter ... 5

ANTI-TUBERCULAR AGENTS

♦ LEARNING OBJECTIVES ♦

After completing this sub-unit the students should be able:
- *To study definition, symptoms and diagnosis of Tuberculosis.*
- *To study different classes of anti-tubercular drugs along with their Mode of Action.*
- *To study different drugs used against tuberculosis with their MOA and uses.*
- *To learn the synthetic scheme for some selected antitubercular agents.*

5.1 INTRODUCTION

Tuberculosis (TB) is an infectious disease usually caused by *Mycobacterium tuberculosis* bacteria. It is a disease that has been known from the earliest of recorded history. Koch identified the causative organism tubercle bacillus; *Mycobacterium tuberculosis*. It is estimated that, one-third to one-half of the world population is infected with *M. tuberculosis*, leading to approximately 6% of all deaths worldwide.

The bacteria usually attack the lungs, but they can also damage other parts of the body. Most infections do not have symptoms, in which case it is known as latent TB. About 10% of latent infections progress to active disease which, if left untreated, kills about half of those affected.

Tuberculosis spreads through the air when a person with active TB infection coughs, sneezes, spit or talks. People with latent TB do not spread the disease. Active infection occurs more often in people with HIV/AIDS and in those who smoke.

Symptoms of Tuberculosis:

The classic symptoms of active TB are a chronic cough with blood-containing mucus, fever, night sweats, and weight loss. It was historically called "consumption" due to the weight loss. Infection of other organs can cause a wide range of symptoms.

Diagnosis of Tuberculosis:

Diagnosis of active TB is based on chest X-rays, as well as microscopic examination and culture of body fluids. Diagnosis of latent TB relies on the tuberculin skin test (TST) or blood tests.

Mycobacterium Tuberculosis (MBT):

The main cause of TB is *Mycobacterium tuberculosis*, a small, aerobic, non-motile bacillus. The high lipid content of this pathogen accounts for many of its unique clinical characteristics. It divides every 16 to 20 hours, which is an extremely slow rate compared with other bacteria, which usually divide in less than an hour. Mycobacteria have an outer membrane lipid bilayer. If a Gram stain is performed, *MTB* either stains very weakly "Gram-positive" or does not retain dye as a result of the high lipid and mycolic acid content of its cell wall. *MTB* can withstand weak disinfectants and survive in a dry state for weeks. In nature, the bacterium can grow only within the cells of a host organism, but *MTB* can be cultured in the laboratory.

The *Mycobacterium tuberculosis* complex (MTBC) includes four other TB-causing mycobacteria: *M. bovis, M. africanum, M. canetti,* and *M. microti. M. africanum* is not widespread, but it is a significant cause of tuberculosis in parts of Africa. *M. bovis* was once a common cause of tuberculosis, but the introduction of pasteurized milk has almost completely eliminated this as a public health problem in developed countries. *M. canetti* is rare and seems to be limited to the Horn of Africa, although a few cases have been seen in African emigrants. *M. microti* is also rare and is seen almost only in immunodeficient people, although its prevalence may be significantly underestimated.

Mechanism of Action of Anti-Tubercular Drugs:

Tuberculosis drugs target various aspects of *Mycobacterium tuberculosis* biology, including inhibition of cell wall synthesis, protein synthesis, or nucleic acid synthesis. The mechanism of action is via inhibition of DNA-dependent RNA polymerase at the initiation step. Elongation is not inhibited. Rifampin binds to the β-subunit of the holoenzyme. Higher concentrations are required to inhibit mammalian mitochondrial RNA synthesis.

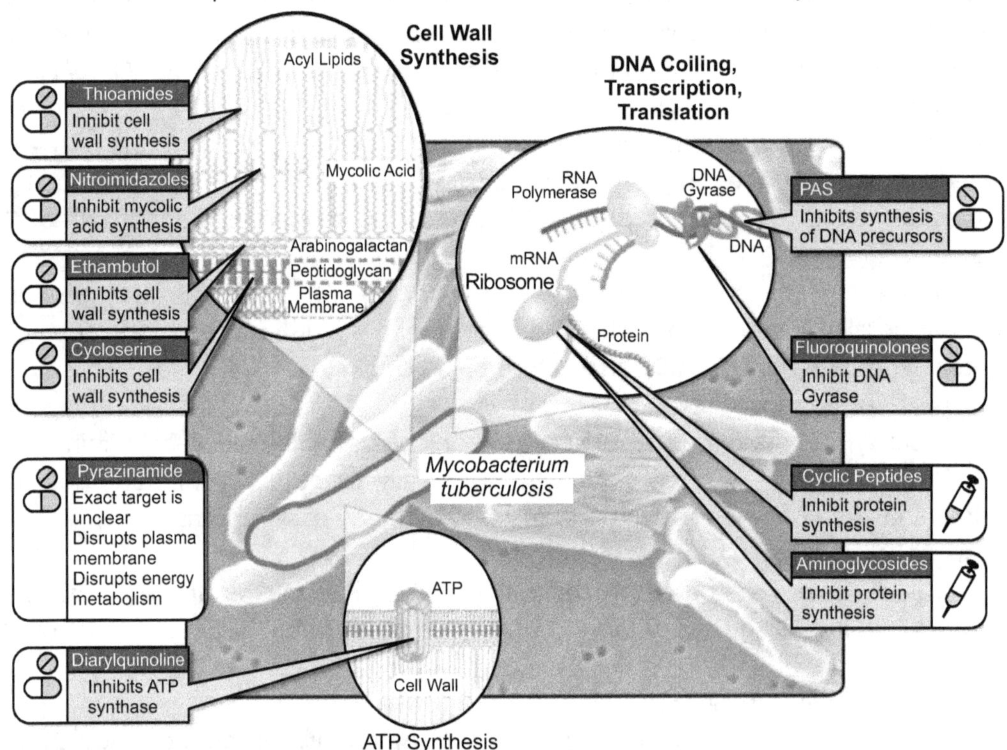

Fig. 5.1: Mechanism of action of anti-tubercular drugs

5.2 ANTI-TUBERCULAR AGENTS

The development of anti-tubercular drugs initiated with the sulphanilamide in 1938, as sulphanilamide exhibited weak bacteriostatic properties, and followed by the sulfone derivative Dapsone. Dapsone, is still considered one of the most effective drug, but due its toxicity it is not a first line agent. The discovery of the antitubercular activity of the streptomycin; an aminoglycoside antibiotic, followed by the *p*-aminosalicylic acid (PAS) and isoniazid were a significant breakthrough. Eventually, the research for better anti-tubercular agents led to the development of the synthetic drug ethambutol and, the other semisynthetic antibiotic rifampin.

The Fight Against Tubercular Infection:

The reappearance of the tuberculosis is indicated by the development of resistance to the antitubercular following a mono drug therapy and also marked by non-patient compliance. The other factor includes urban crowding, immigration, unhygienic condition, malnutrition and AIDS.

The clinical importance of combination therapy, with the use of two or more anti-tubercular drugs to reduce the emergence of strains of *M. tuberculosis* resistant to individual agents has become standard medical practice. The choice of anti-tubercular combination depends on the location of the disease (pulmonary, urogenital, gastrointestinal, or spinal cord) and also the toxicities of the individual agents.

First-line Agents for Tuberculosis:

Initially, the combination of isoniazid and ethambutol, with or without streptomycin, was the most prescribed therapy. With the discovery of the anti-tubercular properties of rifampin resulted in its replacement of the more toxic antibiotic; streptomycin. The synthetic drug pyrazinamide, because of its sterilizing ability, is also considered a first-line agent and is frequently used in place of ethambutol in combination therapy.

Second-line Agents for Tuberculosis:

It includes the antibiotics cycloserine, kanamycin, and capreomycin and the synthetic compounds ethionamide and PAS. A major advance in the treatment of tuberculosis was signalled by the introduction of the antibiotic rifampin into therapy. Clinical studies indicated that when rifampin is included in the regimen, particularly in combination with isoniazid and ethambutol (or pyrazinamide), the period required for successful therapy is shortened significantly. Previous treatment schedules without rifampin required maintenance therapy for at least 2 years, whereas those based on the isoniazid–rifampin combination achieved equal or better results in 6 to 9 months.

5.3 CLASSIFICATION OF ANTI-TUBERCULAR DRUGS

The anti-tubercular drugs can be divided into two groups:

1. **First-line:** High anti-tubercular efficacy as well as low toxicity.
   Examples: Isoniazid, Rifampicin, Pyrazinamide, Ethambutol, Streptomycin.
2. **Second-line:** Low anti-tubercular efficacy as well as high toxicity.
   Examples: Paraminosalicylic acid, Ethionamide, Cycloserine, Kanamycin, Amikacin, Ciprofloxacin, Ofloxacin, Clarithromycin, Azithromycin.

5.4 DRUG PROFILE

5.4.1 Synthetic Anti-Tubercular Agents

1. Isoniazid or Isonicotinic Acid Hydrazide (INH):

Isoniazid

- Isoniazid is a synthetic derivative of nicotinic acid with anti-mycobacterial properties.
- It is chemically, pyridine-4-carbohydrazide.
- Isoniazid is a prodrug that inhibits the formation of the mycobacterial cell wall.
- It acts by blocking the synthesis of mycolic acids, major components of the mycobacterial cell wall.
- It also interferes with mycobacterial metabolism of vitamin B6.
- It inhibits the cytochrome P450 system and hence acts as a source of free radicals.
- It is a mild monoamine oxidase inhibitor (MAO-I).
- This agent is only active against actively growing mycobacteria because, as a pro-drug, it requires activation in susceptible mycobacterial species. Resistance occurs due to decreased bacterial wall penetration.

Activation of Isoniazid:

Isoniazid must be activated by KatG, a bacterial catalase-peroxidase enzyme in *M. tuberculosis*. KatG catalyzes the formation of the isonicotinic acyl radical, which spontaneously couples with NADH to form the nicotinoyl-NAD adduct. This complex binds tightly to the enoyl-acyl carrier protein reductase InhA, thereby blocking the natural enoyl-AcpM substrate and the action of fatty acid synthase. This process inhibits the synthesis of mycolic acids, which are required components of the mycobacterial cell wall.

Uses:

- Isoniazid is bactericidal to rapidly dividing mycobacteria, but is bacteriostatic if the mycobacteria are slow-growing.
- It is often used to treat latent and active tuberculosis infections.
- It was widely used in the treatment of *M. avium* complex as part of a regimen including rifampicin and ethambutol.

2. Ethionamide:

Ethionamide

- Ethionamide is a nicotinamide derivative, with antibacterial activity.
- It is chemically, 2-ethylpyridine-4-carbothioamide.
- It is a pro-drug, requiring activation by the monooxygenase EthA.
- It acts by inhibiting the synthesis of mycolic acid, a saturated fatty acid found in the bacterial cell wall, thereby inhibiting bacterial cell wall synthesis. This eventually leads to bacterial cell wall disruption and cell lysis.

Uses:

- Ethionamide is used in combination with other anti-tuberculosis agents as part of a second-line regimen for active tuberculosis.
- It may be bacteriostatic or bactericidal in action, depending on the concentration of the drug at the site of infection and the susceptibility of the organism involved.

3. Ethambutol:

Ethambutol

- Ethambutol is an ethylenediamine derivative bacteriostatic antimycobacterial drug, effective against *M. tuberculosis* and some other mycobacteria.
- It is chemically, (2S)-2-[2-[[(2S)-1-hydroxybutan-2-yl]amino]ethylamino]butan-1-ol.
- It interferes with the biosynthesis of arabinogalactan, a major polysaccharide of the mycobacterial cell wall.
- It inhibits the polymerization of cell wall arabinan of arabinogalactan and lipoara-binomannan by blocking arabinosyl transferases and induces the accumulation of D-arabinofuranosyl-P-decaprenol, an intermediate in arabinan biosynthesis. This results in halting bacterial growth.

Uses:

- Ethambutol is an antibiotic with bacteriostatic, antimicrobial and antitubercular properties.
- It is used along with other medications to treat a number of infections including: tuberculosis, *M. avium* complex, and *M. kansasii.*

4. Pyrazinamide:

Pyrazinamide

- Pyrazinamide is a synthetic pyrazinoic acid amide derivative with bactericidal property.
- It is chemically, pyrazine-2-carboxamide.
- It is particularly active against slowly multiplying intracellular bacilli (unaffected by other drugs) by an unknown mechanism of action.
- Its bactericidal action is dependent upon the presence of bacterial pyrazinamidase, which removes the amide group to produce active pyrazinoic acid.

Uses:

- Pyrazinamide is only used in combination with other drugs such as isoniazid and rifampicin in the treatment of *M. tuberculosis.*
- It is an important component of multidrug therapy for tuberculosis.

5. Paraminosalicylic Acid:

Paraminosalicylic acid

- Paraminosalicylic (PAS) acid is an aminobenzoic acid that is salicylic acid substituted by an amino group at position 4.
- It is chemically, 4-amino-2-hydroxybenzoic acid.
- It exerts its bacteriostatic activity against *Mycobacterium tuberculosis* by competing with PABA for enzymes involved in folate synthesis, thereby suppressing growth and reproduction of *M. tuberculosis*, eventually leading to cell death.

Uses:

- Paramino salicylic acid is used in the treatment of tuberculosis infections.
- It has also been used in the treatment of inflammatory bowel disease.

5.4.2 Anti-Tubercular Antibiotics

1. Rifampicin:

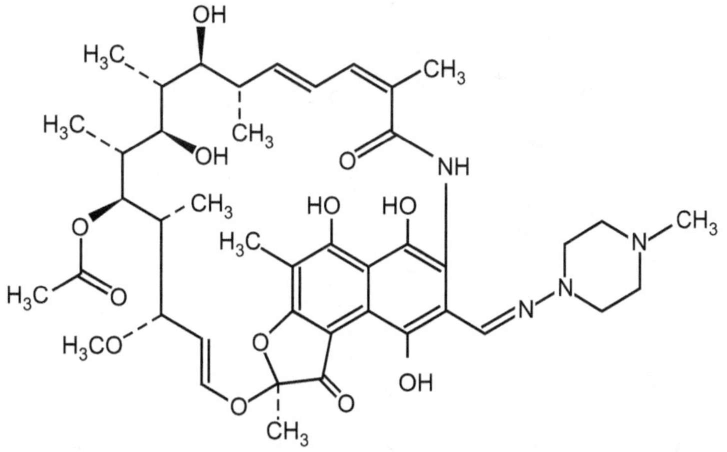

Rifampicin

- Rifampicin (Rifamycin) is a semi-synthetic antibiotic derived from *Amycolatopsis rifamycinica*.

- It is a broad-spectrum antibiotic and most widely used to treat TB.

- It inhibits DNA-dependent RNA polymerase in susceptible bacteria.

- It is N-iminopiperazine, a N-methylpiperazine, a hydrazone, a cyclic ketal, a semi-synthetic derivative and a member of rifamycins. It is a tautomer of a rifampicin zwitterion.

Uses:

- Rifampicin is used for the treatment of tuberculosis in combination with other antibiotics, such as pyrazinamide, isoniazid, and ethambutol.

- It is also used as preventive treatment against *Neisseria meningitidis* (meningococcal) infections.

- It is also recommended as an alternative treatment for infections by the tick-borne pathogens *Borrelia burgdorferi* and *Anaplasma phagocytophilum* when treatment with doxycycline is contraindicated, such as in pregnant women or in patients with a history of allergy to tetracycline antibiotics.

- It is used to treat infections by *Listeria* species, *Neisseria gonorrhoeae*, *Haemophilus influenzae*, and *Legionella pneumophila*.

- It is also used as a leprostatic drug, an *Escherichia coli* metabolite, a protein synthesis inhibitor, a neuroprotective agent, an angiogenesis inhibitor, a pregnane X receptor agonist and an antineoplastic agent.

2. Rifabutin:

Rifabutin

- Rifabutin is a rifamycin antibiotic that is similar in structure and activity to rifampin with potent antimycobacterial properties.

- It inhibits bacterial DNA-dependent RNA polymerase, thereby suppressing the initiation of RNA formation and leading to inhibition of RNA synthesis and transcription.

- It is associated with transient and asymptomatic elevations in serum amino-transferase and is a likely cause of clinically apparent, acute liver disease.

Uses:

- Rifabutin is now recommended as first-line treatment for tuberculosis.
- Rifabutin is used in the treatment of *M. avium* complex disease, a bacterial infection most commonly encountered in people with late-stage AIDS.
- It is also useful in the treatment of *Chlamydophila pneumoniae* infection.

3. Cycloserine:

Cycloserine

- Cycloserine is an analogue of the amino acid D-alanine with broad-spectrum antibiotic.

- It is chemically, (4R)-4-amino-1,2-oxazolidin-3-one.

- It interrupts peptidoglycan synthesis by inhibiting the enzymes L-alanine racemase and D-alanine ligase thereby impairing peptidoglycan formation necessary for bacterial cell wall synthesis.

Uses:

- It is used in the treatment of tuberculosis, cycloserine is classified as a second-line drug, i.e. its use is only considered if one or more first-line drugs cannot be used. Hence, cycloserine is restricted for use only against multiple drug-resistant and extensively drug-resistant strains of *M. tuberculosis*.

4. Streptomycin:

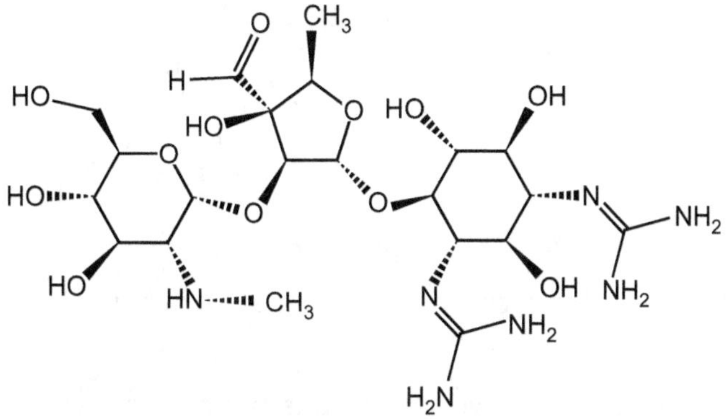

Streptomycin

- Streptomycin was the first antibiotic cure for tuberculosis.

- In 1952 Waksman was the recipient of the Nobel Prize in Physiology or Medicine in recognition "for his discovery of streptomycin, the first antibiotic active against tuberculosis.

- It is an antibiotic that inhibits both Gram-positive and Gram-negative bacteria, and is therefore a useful broad-spectrum antibiotic.

- It is a protein synthesis inhibitor. It binds to the small 16S rRNA of the 30S subunit of the bacterial ribosome, interfering with the binding of formyl-methionyl-tRNA to the 30S subunit. This leads to codon misreading, eventual inhibition of protein synthesis and ultimately death of microbial cells.

Uses:

- Streptomycin is used in the treatment of tuberculosis in combination with other antibiotics. For active tuberculosis it is often given together with isoniazid, rifampicin, and pyrazinamide.

- It is used in infective endocarditis caused by enterococcus when the organism is not sensitive to gentamicin.

- It is used in the treatment of Plague (*Yersinia pestis*).

- In veterinary medicines, streptomycin is the first-line antibiotic for use against Gram-negative bacteria in large animals (horses, cattle, sheep, etc.). It is commonly combined with procaine penicillin for intramuscular injection.

5. Capreomycin Sulphate:

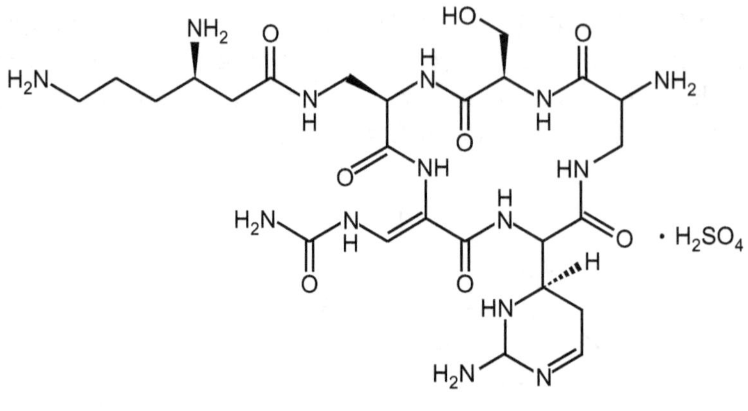

Capreomycin sulphate

- Capreomycin is a macrocyclic polypeptide antibiotic isolated from *Streptomyces capreolus*.

- Like Streptomycin and Kanamycin, it inhibits protein synthesis through modification of ribosomal structures at the 16S rRNA.

- Recent studies using site-directed mutagenesis have identified the binding site of capreomycin on 16S rRNA helix 44.

Uses:

- It is a second-line agent used in the treatment of tuberculosis in combination with other antibiotics.

SYNTHESIS

1. Isoniazid:

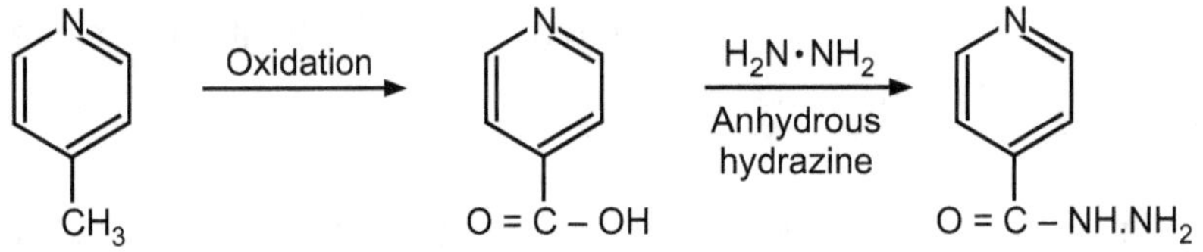

4-Methyl-pyridine → (Oxidation) → **Isonicotinic acid** → ($H_2N \cdot NH_2$, Anhydrous hydrazine) → **Isoniazid**

2. Paraminosalicylic acid:

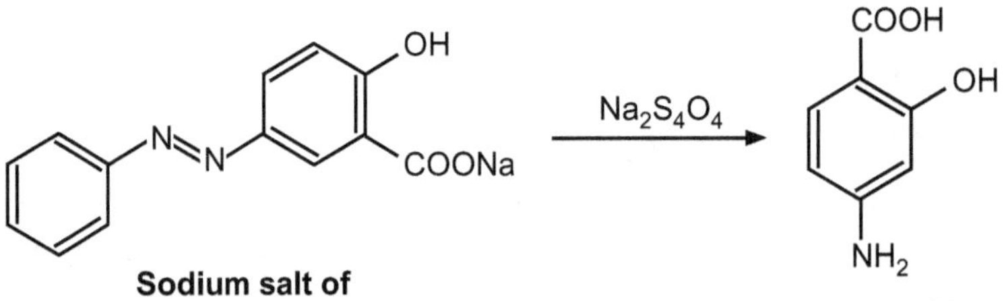

Sodium salt of 5-(phenylazo) salicylic acid → ($Na_2S_4O_4$) → **Paraminosalicylic acid**

QUESTIONS

Multiple Choice Questions:

1. Streptomycin is a …………
   (a) Di-acidic base possessing an aldehydic carbonyl group
   (b) Tri-acidic base possessing an aldehydic carbonyl group
   (c) Neutral compound possessing a ketonic group
   (d) Acidic compound possessing a carboxylic group

2. The first hydrolytic product of streptomycin with methanolic acid is …………
   (a) Streptidine + Streptose + N-methyl glucosamine
   (b) Streptidine + Methyl strepto-biosaminide dimethyl acetal
   (c) Streptamine + Streptose + N-methyl glucosamine
   (d) Streptamine + Streptose dimethyl acetal + N-methyl glucosamine

3. Streptomycin is obtained from …………
   (a) *Streptomyces griseus*   (b) *Streptomyces fradiae*
   (c) *Streptomyces alboniger*   (d) *Streptomyces rimosus*

4. ………… is the test organism used for the assay of streptomycin as per IP.
   (a) Bacillus pumilus   (b) Bacillus subtilis
   (c) Micrococcus luteus   (d) Mycobacterium smegmatis

5. An adverse effect of Streptomycin is …………
   (a) Ototoxicity   (b) Nepherotoxicity
   (c) Intestinal haemorrhage   (d) Constipation

6. Which one of the following is not a synthetic drug?
   (a) Isoniazid   (b) Rifampin
   (c) Pyrazinamide   (d) Ethionamide

7. The mechanism of PAS is :
   (a) It inhibits mycolic acid synthesis.
   (b) It inhibits folic acid synthesis.
   (c) It inhibits DNA-dependent RNA polymerase.
   (d) It makes the tuberculosis organism susceptible to reactive oxygen.

8. Which one of the following is not a first-line drug for treating antituberculosis?
   (a) Isoniazid   (b) Rifampin
   (c) Cycloserine   (d) Pyrazinamide

9. Ethambutol molecule has …………
   (a) two chiral centers and 3 stereoisomers
   (b) two chiral centers and 4 stereoisomers
   (c) two chiral centers and 2 stereoisomers
   (d) one chiral center and 2 stereoisomers

10. INH is used as …………
    (a) Antipellagra   (b) Bactericidal
    (c) Antitubercular   (d) Respiratory stimulant
11. The drug useful to treat multi-drug resistant tuberculosis is …………
    (a) Isoniazid   (b) Ethionamide
    (c) Rifampin   (d) Pyrazinamide
12. Isoniazid is synthesized from …………
    (a) alpha picoline   (b) beta picoline
    (c) Gamma picoline   (d) Hydrazine
13. The antitubercular activity of isoniazid is :
    (a) It inhibits mycolic acid synthesis.
    (b) It inhibits folic acid synthesis.
    (c) It inhibits DNA-dependent RNA polymerase.
    (d) It makes the tuberculosis organism susceptible to reactive oxygen.
14. Rifampicin acts by the following mechanism of action :
    (a) It inhibits mycolic acid synthesis.
    (b) It inhibits folic acid synthesis.
    (c) It inhibits DNA-dependent RNA polymerase.
    (d) It makes the tuberculosis organism susceptible to reactive oxygen.

Answers :

1. (b)	2. (a)	3. (a)	4. (b)	5. (a)	6. (b)	7. (b)	8. (c)	9. (b)	10. (c)
11. (b)	12. (c)	13. (a)	14. (d)						

Answer the Following Questions:

1. Write a note on causative organism of tuberculosis.
2. Write a note on mechanism of action of anti-tubercular drugs.
3. Classify antitubercular drugs with suitable examples.
4. Give a brief note on combinational therapy for the treatment of tuberculosis.
5. Explain Antitubercular antibiotics.
6. Draw structure, chemical name and uses of Isoniazid, Ethionamide, Ethambutol.
7. Give schematic route for synthesis of Isoniazid and para amino salicylic acid.

■■■

chapter ... 6

URINARY TRACT ANTI-INFECTIVE AGENTS

♦ LEARNING OBJECTIVES ♦

After completing this sub-unit the students should be able:

- *To study symptoms and diagnosis of urinary tract infection.*
- *To learn detail classification of anti-UTI agents.*
- *To study Quinolones, its classification, SAR and spectrum activity.*
- *To study different classes of anti-UTI agents with their MOA and uses.*
- *To study the synthetic scheme of some selective anti-UTI agents.*

6.1 INTRODUCTION

A urinary tract infection (UTI) is an infection that affects part of the urinary tract. The urinary tract is made up of kidneys, ureters, bladder, and urethra. UTI are caused by bacteria, but some are caused by fungi and in rare cases by viruses. UTI are more common in women than men (8 : 1).

Urinary tract infection is known as lower UTI/bladder infection/cystitis, when it affects the lower urinary tract i.e. the urethra and bladder part and it is most common UTI whereas, it is known as kidney infection/pyelonephritis, when it affects the upper urinary tract i.e., the ureters and kidneys.

Upper UTI are rarer than lower UTI. Upper UTI are also more severe and life threatening if bacteria move from the infected kidney into the blood and this condition is called urosepsis, can cause low blood pressure, shock, and even death. Lower UTI are usually treated with oral antibiotics; whereas, upper UTI are treated via intravenous antibiotics. UTI can be prevented by hydration (eight glasses of water daily) and don't hold urine for long periods of time.

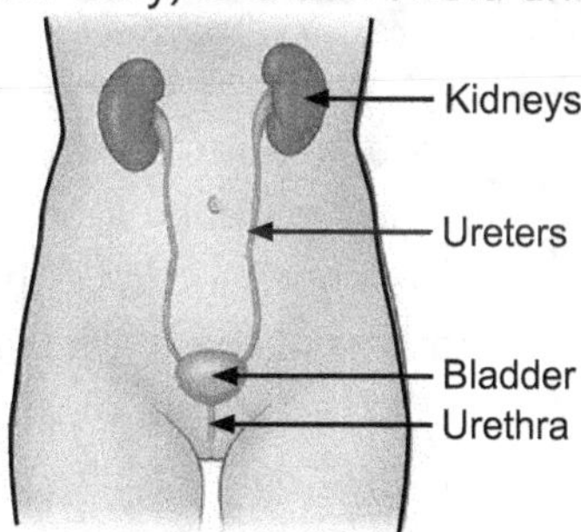

Fig. 6.1

Symptoms of Urinary Tract Infection:

Symptoms from a lower urinary tract infection include:

- Burning sensation and pain with urination.
- Increased frequency of urination without passing much urine or feeling the need to urinate despite having an empty bladder.
- Increased urgency of urination.
- Bloody urine or cloudy urine.
- Urine that has a strong odour.
- Pelvic pain in women and rectal pain in men.

Symptoms of a kidney infection include:

- Fever and flank pain usually in addition to the symptoms of a lower UTI.

Symptoms of an upper UTI include:

- Pain and tenderness in the upper back and sides, chills, fever, nausea and vomiting.

Diagnosis:

Diagnosis is symptoms - based and in complicated cases a urine culture may be useful. Rarely the urine may appear bloody. In the very old and the very young, symptoms may be vague or non-specific. The most common cause of infection is *Escherichia coli* (80–85%), though other bacteria or fungi may rarely be the cause.

If the urine contains significant bacteria, but there are no symptoms, the condition is known as asymptomatic bacteriuria. If a urinary tract infection involves the upper tract, and the person has diabetes mellitus, is pregnant, is male, or immuno-compromised, it is considered complicated. Otherwise if a woman is healthy and premenopausal, it is considered uncomplicated. In children when a urinary tract infection is associated with a fever, it is deemed to be an upper urinary tract infection.

Risk factors include female anatomy, sexual intercourse, diabetes, obesity, and family history. Although sexual intercourse is a risk factor, UTIs are not classified as sexually transmitted infections (STIs). Kidney infection, if it occurs, usually follows a bladder infection, but may also result from a blood-borne infection.

6.2 ANTI-INFECTIVE AGENTS EMPLOYED FOR URINARY TRACT INFECTION

Chemical classes of synthetic antibacterial agents include the sulfonamides, certain nitro heterocyclic compounds (nitrofurans), and the quinolones. These antibacterial agents find importance for the treatment of local, systemic, and/or urinary tract infections. Antibacterial agents that achieve adequate concentrations in the urine are effective for eradicating urinary tract infections with good oral absorption, activity against common Gram-negative urinary pathogens, and comparatively higher urinary (compared with plasma and tissue) concentrations.

6.3 CLASSIFICATION OF URINARY TRACT ANTI-INFECTIVE AGENTS

A series of synthetic antibacterial agents is patterned after nalidixic acid (a naphthyridine derivative) introduced in 1963. Isosteric heterocyclic groupings in this class include:

(a) Quinolones: Norfloxacin, Ciprofloxacin, Ofloxacin, Lomefloxacin, Sparfloxacin, Gatifloxacin, Moxifloxacin.

(b) Naphthyridines: Nalidixic acid, Enoxacin.

(c) Miscellaneous: Furazolidine, Nitrofurantoin, Methanamine.

6.4 QUINOLONES

A quinolone antibiotic is a member of a large group of broad-spectrum bacteriocidals that share a bicyclic core structure related to the substance 4-quinolone. They are used in human and veterinary medicine to treat bacterial infections, as well as in animal husbandry. The majority of quinolones in clinical use belong to the second generation class of "fluoroquinolones", which have a true quinoline framework, maintain the C-3 carboxylic acid group, and add a fluorine atom to the all carbon containing ring, typically at the C-6 or C-7 positions. They are effective against both Gram-negative and Gram-positive bacteria.

Mechanism of Action of Quinolones:

Quinolones exert their antibacterial effect by preventing bacterial DNA from unwinding and duplicating. Specifically, they inhibit the ligase activity of the type-II topoisomerases, gyrase, and topoisomerase-IV, which cut DNA to introduce supercoiling and with their ligase activity disrupted, release DNA with single and double strand breaks that lead to cell death. High activity against the eukaryotic type-II enzyme is exhibited by drugs containing aromatic substituents at their C-7 positions.

First and second generation fluoroquinolones selectively inhibit the topoisomerase-II ligase, leads to DNA fragmentation via the nucleasic activity of the intact enzyme. Third and fourth generation fluoroquinolones are more selective for the topoisomerase-IV ligase, thus have enhanced Gram-positive bacteria coverage.

The first generation of the quinolones began following introduction of the related, but structurally distinct naphthyridine-family, nalidixic acid in 1962 for treatment of UTIs in humans. Nalidixic acid was discovered by George Lesher and coworkers in a chemical distillate during an attempt at synthesis of the chloroquinoline antimalarial agent.

Naphthyridone and quinolone classes of antibiotics prevent bacterial DNA replication by inhibition of DNA unwinding events, and can be both bacteriostatic and bacteriocidal.

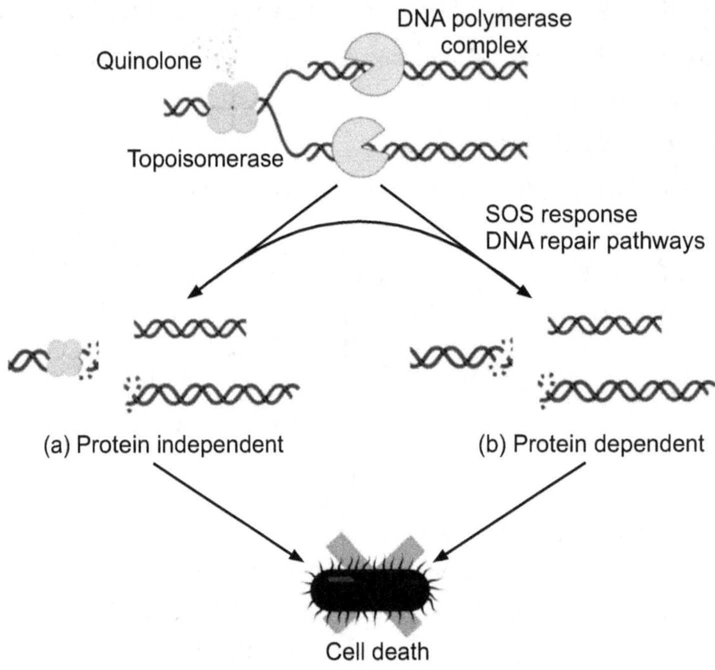

Fig. 6.2: Mechanism of action of Quinolones

6.4.1 Classification of Quinolones

Quinolones can be classified into generations based on their antibacterial spectra. The earlier-generation agents are, in general, more narrow-spectrum than the later ones, but no standard is employed to determine which drug belongs to which generation. The only universal standard applied is the grouping of the non-fluorinated drugs found within this class (quinolones) within the first-generation heading. The first generation is rarely used.

1. **First-generation:**

   Examples: Flumequine (Veterinary use), Oxolinic acid, Rosoxacin.

   A structurally related first-generation drugs, but formally not 4-quinolones, include:

   Examples: Cinoxacin, Nalidixic acid, Piromidic acid, Pipemidic acid.

2. **Second-generation:**

   Examples: Ciprofloxacin, Fleroxacin, Lomefloxacin, Nadifloxacin, Norfloxacin, Ofloxacin, Pefloxacin, Rufloxacin.

   A structurally related second-generation drugs, but formally not a 4-quinolone, include:

   Example: Enoxacin.

3.   **Third-generation:**

   Examples: Balofloxacin, Grepafloxacin, Levofloxacin, Pazufloxacin, Sparfloxacin, Temafloxacin.

   A structurally related third-generation drugs, but formally not a 4-quinolone, include:

   Example: Tosufloxacin

4.   **Fourth-generation:**

   Fourth-generation fluoroquinolones act at DNA gyrase and topoisomerase-IV. This dual action slows development of resistance.

   Example: Clinafloxacin, Gatifloxacin, Moxifloxacin, Sitafloxacin, Prulifloxacin, Besifloxacin, Delafloxacin.

5.   **Veterinary used Quinolones**

   Quinolones have been widely used in animal husbandry, and several agents have veterinary-specific applications.

   Examples: Danofloxacin, Difloxacin, Enrofloxacin, Ibafloxacin, Marbofloxacin, Orbifloxacin, Sarafloxacin.

6.4.2 Structure Activity Relationship of Quinolones

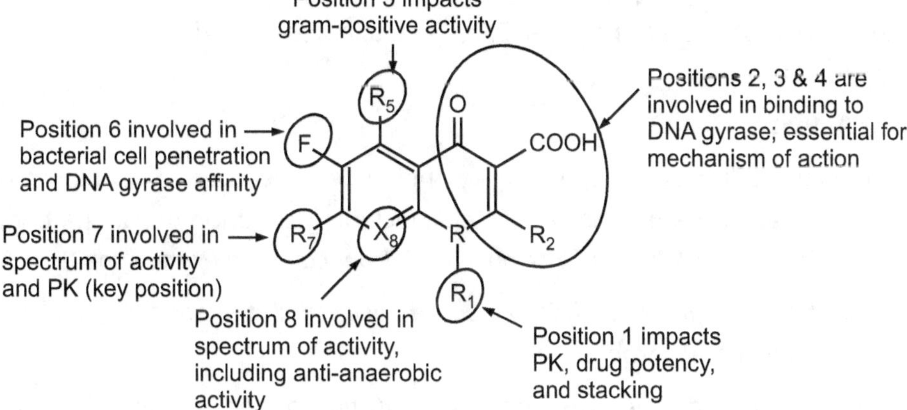

Fig. 6.3

1.   The structure activity studies have shown that the 1,4-dihydro-4-oxo-3-pyridine carboxylic acid moiety is essential for antibacterial activity.

2.   The pyridine system must be annulated with an aromatic ring.

3.   Isosteric replacements of nitrogen for carbon atoms at positions 2 (cinnolines), 5 (1,5-naphthyridines), 6 (1,6-naphthyridines), and 8 (1,8-naphthyridines) are consistent with retention of antibacterial activity.

Cinnolines   **1,5-Naphthyridines**   **1,6-Naphthyridines**   **1,8-Naphthyridines**

4. Introduction of substituents at position 2 greatly reduces or abolishes activity.

5. Substituents at positions 5, 6, 7 (especially), and 8 of the annulated ring results in better active compounds.

    (a) Piperazinyl and 3-aminopyrrolidinyl substitutions at position 7 of the quinolone class have been shown enhanced activity against *P. aeruginosa*.

    (b) Fluorine atom substitution at position 6 results in significantly enhanced antibacterial activity.

6. Alkyl substitution at the 1-position is essential for activity, with lower alkyl (methyl, ethyl, cyclopropyl) compounds generally having progressively greater potency.

7. Aryl substitution at the 1-position is also consistent with antibacterial activity, with 2,4-difluorophenyl group providing optimal potency.

8. Ring condensations at the 1,8-, 5,6-, 6,7- and 7,8- positions also lead to active compounds.

Spectrum of Activity:

- The effective antibacterial spectrum of the earliest members of the quinolone class were confined to Gram-negative bacteria, including common urinary pathogens such as *Escherichia coli, Klebsiella, Enterobacter, Citrobacter*, and *Proteus spp.*

- Strains of *P. aeruginosa, Neisseria gonorrhoeae*, exhibited resistant, and the Gram-positive cocci and anaerobes.

- Newer members of the class possessing 6-fluoro and 7-piperazinyl substituent exhibit an extended spectrum of activity that includes effectiveness against additional Gram-negative pathogens (e.g., *P. aeruginosa, H. influenzae, N. gonorrhoeae*), Gram-positive cocci (e.g., *S. aureus*).

- The quinolones generally exhibit poor activity against most anaerobic bacteria.

- Bacterial strains that have developed resistance to the antibacterial antibiotics, such as penicillin-resistant *gonococci*, methicillin-resistant *S. aureus*, and amino glycoside resistant *P. aeruginosa* are susceptible to the quinolones.

- Due to the chelating properties of the quinolones, they are incompatible with antacids, hematinics, and mineral supplements containing divalent or trivalent metals.

6.5 DRUG PROFILE

1. Nalidixic Acid:

Nalidixic acid

- Nalidixic acid is the first of the synthetic quinolone antibiotics.
- It is chemically 1-ethyl-7-methyl-4-oxo-1,8-naphthyridine-3-carboxylic acid.
- Its ring structure is a 1,8-naphthyridine nucleus that contains two nitrogen atoms.
- It is effective primarily against Gram-negative bacteria, with minor anti-Gram-positive activity.
- In lower concentrations, it acts in a bacteriostatic manner; that is, it inhibits growth and reproduction. In higher concentrations, it is bactericidal, meaning that it kills bacteria instead of merely inhibiting their growth.
- It is effective inhibitor of cellular deoxyribonucleic acid synthesis, is added to conjugating bacteria at any time during mating, it stops genetic transfer provided the donor bacterium is sensitive to the drug.
- It selectively and reversibly blocks DNA replication in susceptible bacteria.
- Nalidixic acid and related antibiotics inhibit a subunit of DNA gyrase and topoisomerase-IV and induce formation of cleavage complexes.

Uses:

- Nalidixic acid is used for treating urinary tract infections caused by certain bacteria.
- It is used for treating urinary tract infections, caused, for example, by *Escherichia coli*, *Proteus, Shigella, Enterobacter*, and *Klebsiella*.

2. Norfloxacin:

Norfloxacin

- Norfloxacin is a broad-spectrum antibiotic that is active against both Gram-positive and Gram-negative bacteria.

- It is chemically, 1-ethyl-6-fluoro-4-oxo-7-piperazin-1-ylquinoline-3-carboxylic acid.

- It functions by inhibiting DNA gyrase, a type-II topoisomerase, and topoisomerase-IV, enzymes necessary to separate bacterial DNA, thereby inhibiting cell division.

- It does not bind to DNA gyrase, but does bind to the substrate DNA.

- The cytotoxicity of fluoroquinolones is likely a 2-step process involving,

    (i) Conversion of the topoisomerase-quinolone-DNA complex to an irreversible form, and

    (ii) Generation of a double-strand break by denaturation of the topoisomerase.

Uses:

- Norfloxacin is used in uncomplicated urinary tract infections (including cystitis) and complicated urinary tract infections.

- It is also used in uncomplicated urethral and cervical gonorrhoea and in prostatitis due to *Escherichia coli*.

3. Enoxacin:

Enoxacin

- Enoxacin is an oral broad-spectrum antibacterial agent belonging to a 1,8-naphthyridine derivative, used in the treatment of urinary tract infections and gonorrhoea.

- It is chemically, 1-ethyl-6-fluoro-4-oxo-7-piperazin-1-yl-1,8-naphthyridine-3-carboxylic acid.

- It acts by inhibiting bacterial DNA gyrase and topoisomerases-IV. The inhibition of these enzymes prevents bacterial DNA replication, transcription, repair and recombination.

Uses:

- Enoxacin can be used to treat a wide variety of infections, particularly gastroenteritis including infectious diarrhoea, respiratory tract infections, gonorrhoea and urinary tract infections.

4. Ciprofloxacin:

Ciprofloxacin

- Ciprofloxacin is a broad-spectrum antibiotic of the fluoroquinolone class.

- It is chemically, 1-cyclopropyl-6-fluoro-4-oxo-7-piperazin-1-yl quinoline-3-carboxylic acid.

- It binds to and inhibits bacterial DNA gyrase, an enzyme essential for DNA replication.

- It is active against some Gram-positive and many Gram-negative bacteria.

- It has a role as an anti-infective agent, a topoisomerases-IV inhibitor, an antibacterial drug, a DNA synthesis inhibitor, an antimicrobial agent, an environmental contaminant and a xenobiotic.

Uses:

- Ciprofloxacin is a second-generation fluoroquinolone antibiotic that is widely used in the therapy of mild-to-moderate urinary and respiratory tract infections caused by susceptible organisms.

- It is also used to treat a wide variety of other infections, including infections of bones and joints, endocarditis, gastroenteritis, malignant otitis externa, cellulitis, prostatitis and anthrax.

5. Ofloxacin:

Ofloxacin

- Ofloxacin is a synthetic fluorinated carboxyquinolone, is an anti-infective agent and an antibacterial drug.

- It is a racemate, and it is chemically, (±)-9-fluoro-2,3-dihydro-3-methyl-10-(4-methyl-1-piperazinyl)-7-oxo-7H-pyrido[1,2,3-de]-1,4-benzoxazine-6-carboxylic acid.

- Ofloxacin is an oxazinoquinolone carrying carboxy, fluoro, methyl and 4-methylpiperazino substituents.
- It has a role as a DNA synthesis inhibitor. It inhibits the supercoiling activity of bacterial DNA gyrase, halting DNA replication.

Uses:

Ofloxacin is used in the treatment of bacterial infections such as:

- Community-acquired pneumonia,
- Uncomplicated skin and skin structure infections,
- Non-gonococcal urethritis, cervicitis, prostatitis, epididymitis and uncomplicated cystitis,
- Mixed Infections of the urethra and cervix,
- Acute pelvic inflammatory disease,
- Complicated urinary tract infections,
- Acute, uncomplicated urethral and cervical gonorrhoea.

6. Lomefloxacin:

Lomefloxacin

- Lomefloxacin is a synthetic broad-spectrum fluoroquinolone with antibacterial activity.
- It is chemically, 1-ethyl-6,8-difluoro-7-(3-methylpiperazin-1-yl)-4-oxoquinoline-3-carboxylic acid.
- It is a difluorinated quinolone with a longer elimination half-life (7 –8 hours).
- It inhibits DNA gyrase, a type-II topoisomerase involved in the induction or relaxation of supercoiling during DNA replication. This inhibition leads to a decrease in DNA synthesis during bacterial replication, resulting in cell growth inhibition and eventually cell lysis.

Uses:

- Lomefloxacin is used to treat bacterial infections including bronchitis and urinary tract infections.
- It is also used to prevent urinary tract infections prior to surgery.
- It has a role as an antimicrobial agent, a photosensitizing agent trand an antitubercular agent.

7. Sparfloxacin:

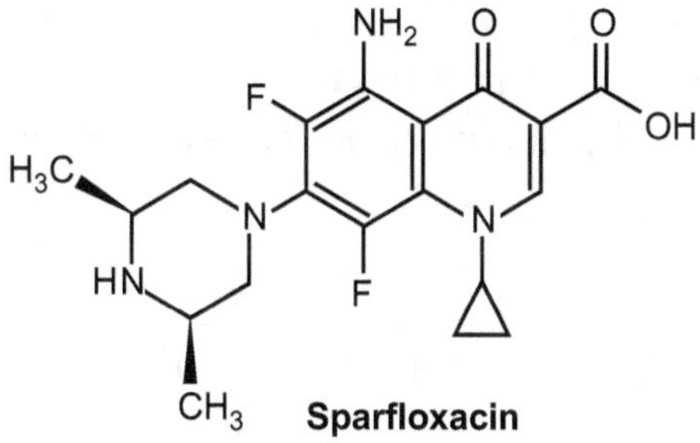

Sparfloxacin

- Sparfloxacin is a fluoroquinolone antibiotic used in the treatment of bacterial infections.

- It is chemically, 5-amino-1-cyclopropyl-7-[(3R,5S)-3,5-dimethylpiperazin-1-yl]-6,8-difluoro-4-oxoquinoline-3-carboxylic acid.

- It exerts its antibacterial activity by inhibiting DNA gyrase, a bacterial topoisomerase. DNA gyrase is an essential enzyme which controls DNA topology and assists in DNA replication, repair, deactivation, and transcription.

Uses:

- Sparfloxacin is a compound indicated for treating community-acquired lower respiratory tract infections (acute sinusitis, exacerbations of chronic bronchitis caused by susceptible bacteria, community-acquired pneumonia).

8. Gatifloxacin:

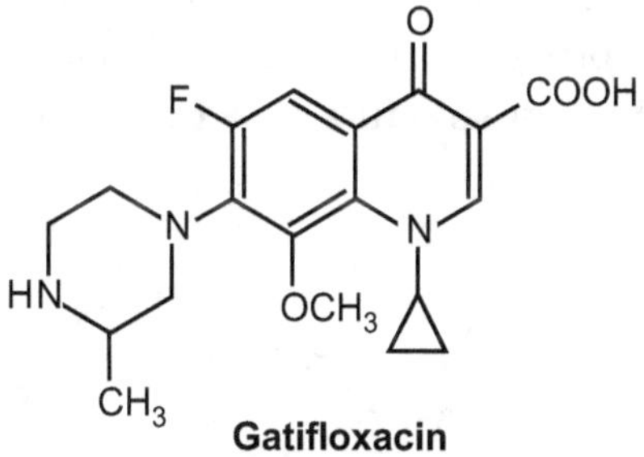

Gatifloxacin

- Gatifloxacin is an antibiotic of the fourth-generation fluoroquinolone family with anti-infective activity.

- It is a synthetic 8-methoxyfluoroquinolone with antibacterial activity against a wide range of Gram-negative and Gram-positive microorganisms.

- It is chemically, (±)-1-Cyclopropyl-6-fluoro-1,4-dihydro-8-methoxy-7(3-methyl-1-piperazinyl)-4-oxo-3-quinoline carboxylic acid.

- It exerts its effect through inhibition of DNA gyrase, an enzyme involved in DNA replication, transcription and repair, and inhibition of topoisomerase-IV, an enzyme involved in partitioning of chromosomal DNA during bacterial cell division.

Uses:

- Gatifloxacin ophthalmic solution is used to treat bacterial conjunctivitis (pinkeye; infection of the membrane that covers the outside of the eyeballs and the inside of the eyelids) in adults and children 1 year of age and older.

9. Moxifloxacin:

Moxifloxacin

- Moxifloxacin is a fluoroquinolone antibiotic with antibacterial activity.
- It is chemically, 1-Cyclopropyl-6-fluoro-7-((4aS,7aS)-hexahydro-1H-pyrrolo [3,4-b]pyridin-6(2H)-yl)-8-methoxy-4-oxo-1,4-dihydroquinoline-3-carboxylic acid.
- Moxifloxacin binds to and inhibits the bacterial enzymes DNA gyrase (topoisomerase-II) and topoisomerase-IV, resulting in inhibition of DNA replication and repair and cell death in sensitive bacterial species.

Uses:

- Moxifloxacin is used to treat a number of infections, including: respiratory tract infections, cellulitis, anthrax, intra-abdominal infections, endocarditis, meningitis, and tuberculosis.
- It is also used for the treatment of acute bacterial sinusitis, acute bacterial exacerbation of chronic bronchitis, community acquired pneumonia, complicated and uncomplicated skin and skin structure infections, and complicated intra-abdominal infections.

10. Furazolidone:

Furazolidone

- Furazolidone, is a nitrofuran derivative with antiprotozoal and antibacterial activity.
- It is chemically, 3-[(5-nitrofuran-2-yl)methylideneamino]-1,3-oxazolidin-2-one.
- It binds bacterial DNA which leads to the gradual inhibition of monoamine oxidase.

Uses:

- Furazolidone is a nitrofuran antimicrobial agent used in the treatment of diarrhoea or enteritis caused by bacteria or protozoan infections.
- It is also active in treating typhoid fever, cholera and salmonella infections.

11. Nitrofurantoin:

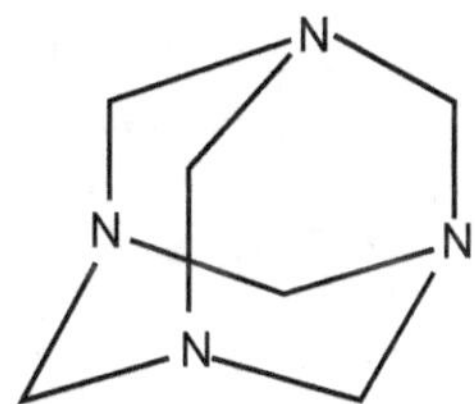

Nitrofurantoin

- Nitrofurantoin is a synthetic derivative of imidazolidinedione.
- It is chemically, 1-[[[5-nitro-2-furanyl]methylene]amino]-2,4- imidazolidinedione.
- It inhibits bacterial DNA, RNA, and cell wall protein synthesis.
- It is activated by bacterial flavoproteins to intermediates that inactivate bacterial ribosomal proteins.
- It is one of the most common causes of drug induced liver disease and can cause either an acute or a chronic hepatitis-like syndrome that can be severe and lead to liver failure or cirrhosis.

Uses:

- Nitrofurantoin is an oral antibiotic widely used either short term to treat acute urinary tract infections or long term as chronic prophylaxis against recurrent infections.

12. Methenamine:

Methenamine

- Methenamine or Hexamethylenetetramine, also known as hexamine or urotropin, is a heterocyclic organic compound with the formula $(CH_2)_6N_4$.
- It is chemically, 1,3,5,7-tetrazatricyclo[3.3.1.1^{3,7}]decane.
- It has a cage-like structure similar to adamantane.
- It is a heterocyclic organic compound with antibiotic activity.
- In the body methenamine is converted to formaldehyde, a non-specific bactericidal agent.

Uses:

- Methenamine is typically used long-term to treat chronic urinary tract infections and to prevent the recurrence of infections.

SYNTHESIS

1. Ciprofloxacin:

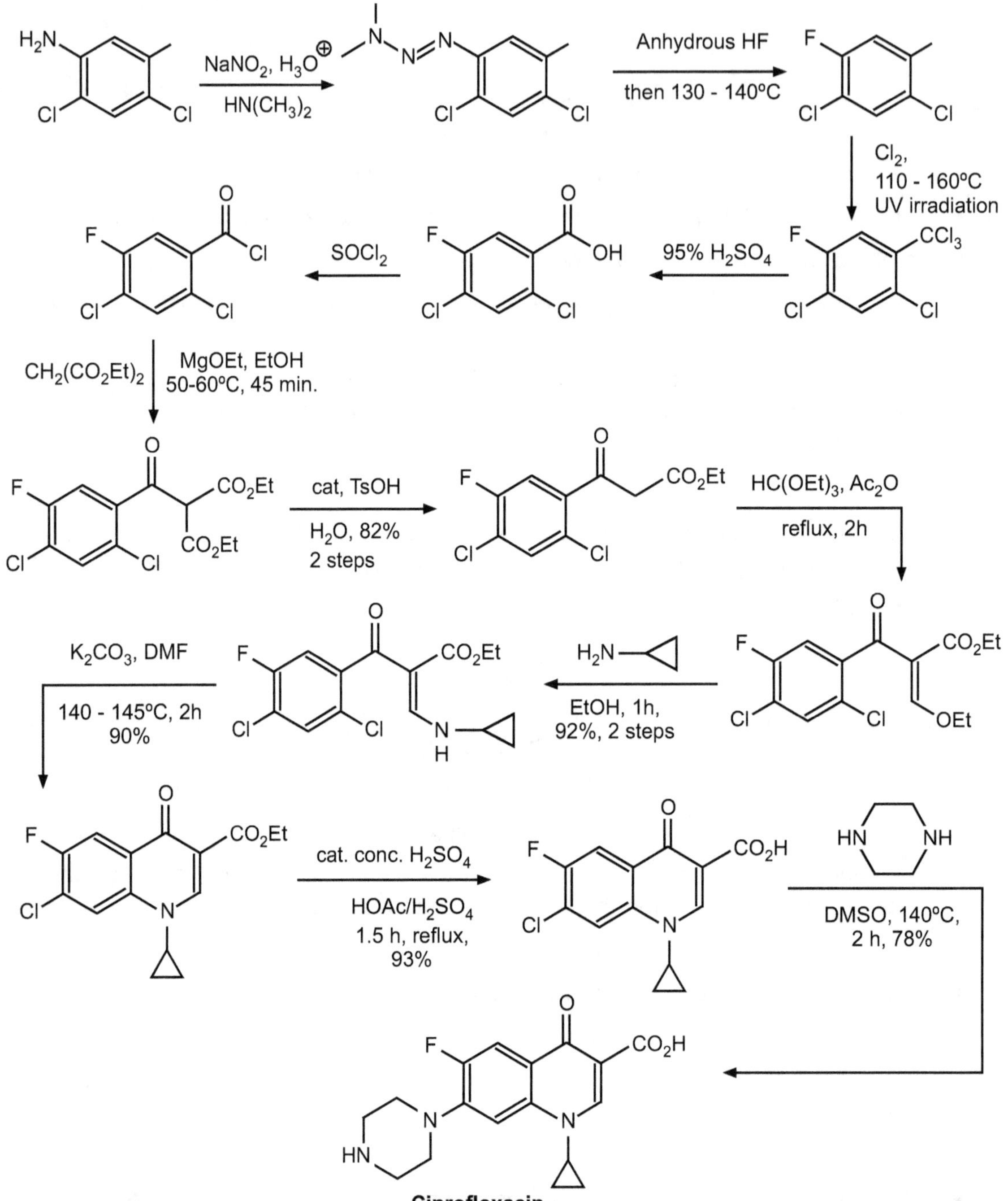

2. Nitrofurantoin:

$H_2N - NH_2$ + Cl—CH₂—CO_2H → H_2N—N(H)—CH₂—CO_2H → (KNCO) → Semicarbazidoacetic acid

Hydrazine   **Chloroacetic acid**   **Hydrazinoacetic acid**   **Semicarbazidoacetic acid**

O_2N-furan-CH(OAc)₂

Nitrofurantoin   **1-aminoidantoin**

QUESTIONS

Multiple Choice Questions:

1. Which one of the following is not a side-effect of fluoroquinolones?

   (a) Phototoxicity   (b) Ototoxicity

   (c) Convulsion   (d) Arthralgia

2. Fluoroquinolones are indicated for all of the following except …………

   (a) Urinary tract infection   (b) Tuberculosis

   (c) Bone infection   (d) Bronchial asthma

3. The N-1 position of ciprofloxacin contains …………

   (a) Cyclopropyl   (b) Methyl

   (c) Ethyl   (d) Piperazine

4. Which of the following is a synthetic antibacterial agent?

   (a) Aminoacridines   (b) Aminoglycosides

   (c) Fluoroquinolones   (d) Tetracyclines

5. The C-6 position of Norfloxacin contains …………

   (a) Piperazine   (b) 4-Methylpiperazine

   (c) 3,5-dimethylpiperazine   (d) Fluoride

6. Following are fluoroquinolone derivatives except …………

   (a) Norfloxacin   (b) Ciprofloxacin

   (c) Ofloxacin   (d) Cinoxacin

---

7. The C-7 position of gatifloxacin contains

    (a) Piperazine   (b) 4-Methylpiperazine
    (c) 3,5-dimethylpiperazine   (d) 3-Methylpiperazine

Answers :

1. (b)	2. (d)	3. (a)	4. (c)	5. (d)	6. (d)	7. (c)

Answer the Following Questions:

1. Give Symptoms of Urinary tract infection.
2. Explain anti-infective agents employed for urinary tract infection.
3. What are quinolones? Explain how they are useful in treatment of urinary tract infection.
4. Explain quinolone therapy as anti-infective agents employed for urinary tract infection.
5. Write mechanism of action of quinolones as anti-infective agents employed for urinary tract infection.
6. What are quinolones? Give detail classification with suitable examples.
7. Give detail account of SAR of quinolones.
8. Give synthetic route of Ciprofloxacin and Nitrofurantoin.

■■■

Chapter ... 7

ANTIVIRAL AGENTS

♦ LEARNING OBJECTIVES ♦

After completing this sub-unit the students should be able:

- *To learn definition, different classes, replication and transformation of viruses.*
- *To study diseases caused by viruses.*
- *To learn in brief various classes of antiviral agents.*
- *To study various antiviral agents along with their MOA and uses.*
- *To learn the synthetic scheme for some selected antiviral agents.*

7.1 INTRODUCTION

Antiviral drugs are the agents that are used in the treatment of an infectious diseases caused by a virus. Viruses are responsible for infectious diseases such as HIV/AIDS, influenza, herpes simplex type-I (cold sores of the mouth) and type-II (genital herpes), herpes zoster (shingles), viral hepatitis, encephalitis, infectious mononucleosis, and the common cold.

Viruses consist of nucleic acid (either DNA or RNA) and aprotein coat. Because viruses do not have the enzymes that are needed to manufacture cellular components, they are obligate parasites, which means they must enter a cell for replication to occur. The nucleic acid of the virus instructs the host cell to produce viral components, which leads to an infection. In some cases, as in herpes infections, the viral nucleic acid may remain in the host cell without causing replication of the virus and damage to the host (viral latency). In other cases, the production of virus by the host cell may cause the death of the cell. A major problem in treating some viral diseases is that latent viruses can become activated.

7.2 CLASSIFICATION OF VIRUSES

Viruses are classified on the basis of several features:
- Nucleic acid content (DNA or RNA)
- Viral morphology (helical, icosahedral)
- Site of replication in cell (cytoplasm or nucleus)
- Coating (enveloped or non-enveloped)
- Serological typing (antigenic signatures)
- Cell types infected (B-Lymphocytes, T-Lymphocytes, Monocytes)

The Baltimore classification in 1971 places viruses into one of seven groups depending on a combination of their nucleic acid (DNA or RNA), strandedness (single-stranded or double-stranded), sense, and method of replication. Named after David Baltimore, a Nobel Prize-winning biologist, these groups are designated by Roman numerals.

Viruses can be placed in one of the seven following groups:

(i) **dsDNA viruses** e.g. Adenoviruses, Herpesviruses, Poxviruses.

(ii) **ssDNA viruses** (+ strand or "sense") DNA : e.g. Parvoviruses.

(iii) **dsRNA viruses** : e.g. Reoviruses.

(iv) **(+) ssRNA viruses** (+ strand or sense) RNA : e.g. Picornaviruses, Togaviruses.

(v) **(−) ssRNA viruses** (−strand or antisense) RNA : e.g. Orthomyxoviruses, Rhabdoviruses.

(vi) **ss RNA-RT viruses** (+ strand or sense) RNA with DNA intermediate in life-cycle e.g. Retroviruses.

(vii) **dsDNA-RT viruses** DNA with RNA intermediate in life-cycle : e.g. Hepadnaviruses.

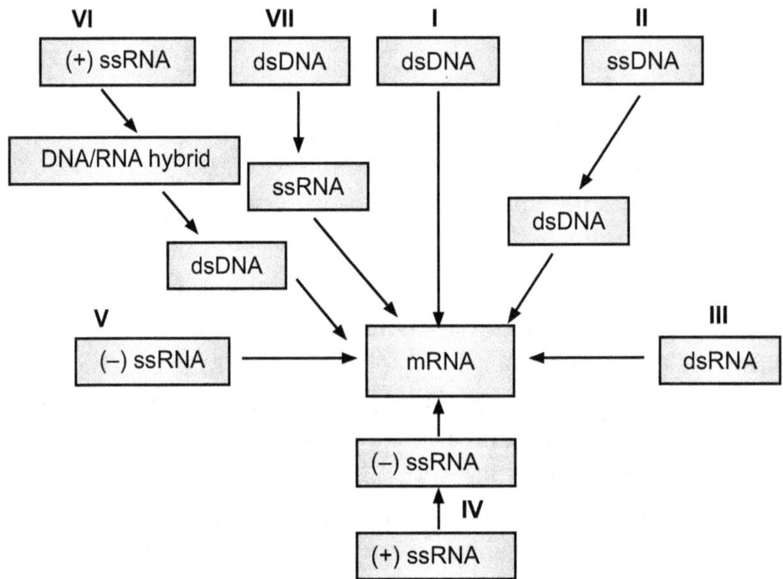

Fig. 7.1: The Baltimore classification of viruses

DNA Viruses:

- **Group I** viruses possess double-stranded DNA. Viruses that cause chickenpox and herpes are found here.
- **Group II** viruses possess single-stranded DNA.

RNA Viruses:

- **Group III** viruses possess double-stranded RNA genomes, e.g. rotavirus.
- **Group IV** viruses possess positive-sense single-stranded RNA genomes. Many well known viruses are found in this group, including the picornaviruses (which is a family

of viruses that includes well-known viruses like hepatitis-A virus, enteroviruses, rhinoviruses, poliovirus, and foot-and-mouth virus), SARS virus, hepatitis-C virus, yellow fever virus, and rubella virus.

- **Group V** viruses possess negative-sense single-stranded RNA genomes. The deadly Ebola and Marburg viruses are well known members of this group, along with influenza virus, measles, mumps and rabies.

Reverse transcribing viruses:

- **Group VI** viruses possess single-stranded RNA viruses that replicate through a DNA intermediate. The retroviruses are included in this group, of which HIV is a member.
- **Group VII** viruses possess double-stranded DNA genomes and replicate using reverse transcriptase. The hepatitis-B virus can be found in this group.

Replication and Transformation of viruses:

Viruses, in general, utilize only the enzyme-system of the host-cell for two purposes, namely: first, to synthesize DNA; and secondly, to replicate virus, thereby enabling it to perform their usual metabolic activities. They may carry out either the transformation or the replication processes of the cell at the same time. By virtue of the fact that viruses are obligate intra-cellular parasites, therefore, their replication phenomenon solely depends on the host's cellular processes.

7.3 VIRUS REPLICATION

A virus must use cell processes to replicate. The viral replication cycle can produce dramatic biochemical and structural changes in the host cell, which may cause cell damage. These changes, called cytopathic (causing cell damage) effects, can change cell functions or even destroy the cell. Some infected cells, such as those infected by the common cold virus known as rhinovirus, die through lysis (bursting) or apoptosis (programmed cell death or "cell suicide"), releasing all progeny virions at once. The symptoms of viral diseases result from the immune response to the virus, which attempts to control and eliminate the virus from the body, and from cell damage caused by the virus.

Many viruses, such as HIV (Human Immunodeficiency Virus), leave the infected cells of the immune system by a process known as budding, where virions leave the cell individually. During the budding process, the cell does not undergo lysis and is not immediately killed. However, the damage to the cells that the virus infects may make it impossible for the cells to function normally, even though the cells remain alive for a period of time. Most productive viral infections follow similar steps in the virus replication cycle: attachment, penetration, uncoating, replication, assembly, and release. The host cell is destroyed at the end of the replication cycle. It's important to remember that this doesn't always happen: sometimes the host cell lives on and continues to replicate the virus.

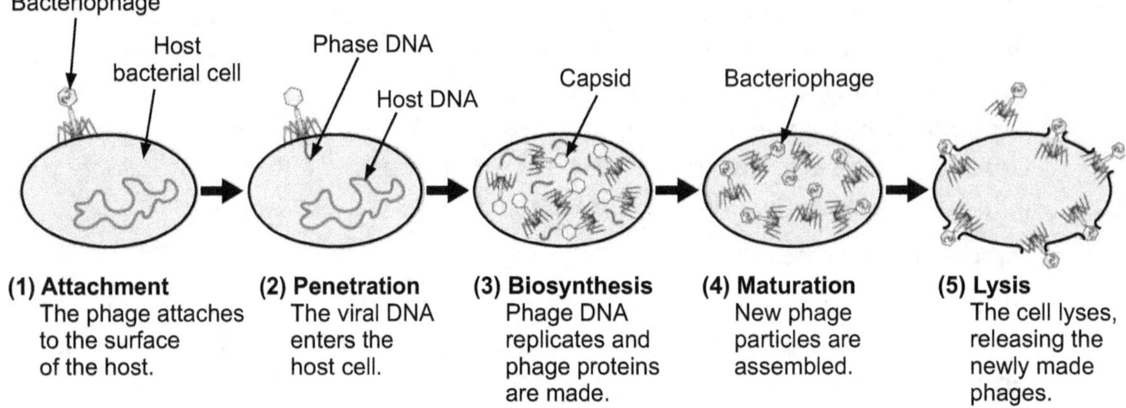

Fig. 7.2: Virus replication

7.4 DISEASES CAUSED BY VIRUSES

A number of diseases are caused by different types of viruses:

1. **Herpes simplex viruses:** Eye infections, skin diseases, encephalitis and genital infections.
2. **Influenza viruses :** Influenza A, B and C.
3. **Rabies viruses:** Rabies, encephalitis.
4. **Polio viruses:** Poliomyelitis.
5. **Parainfluenza virus :** Parainfluenza.
6. **Variola virus :** Smallpox.
7. **Vaccinia virus :** Cowpox.
8. **Varicella-zoster virus:** Chickenpox and herpes zoster.
9. **Rhino viruses:** Respiratory diseases, common cold.

7.5 ANTIVIRAL DRUGS

Antiviral drugs are a class of medication used specifically for treating viral infections rather than any other microbial infections. Most antivirals are used for specific viral infections, while a broad-spectrum antiviral is effective against a wide range of viruses. Unlike most antibiotics, antiviral drugs do not destroy their target pathogen; instead they inhibit their development.

Antiviral drugs are one class of antimicrobials, a larger group which also includes antibiotic (also termed antibacterial), antifungal and antiparasitic drugs, harmless to the host, and therefore can be used to treat infections. They should be distinguished from viricides, which are not medication, but deactivate or destroy virus particles, either inside or outside the body. Natural antivirals are produced by some plants such as Eucalyptus and Australian tea trees.

Many factors account for the difficulty in developing antiviral agents. The structure of each virus differs, and specific therapy is often unsuccessful because of periodic changes in the antigenic proteins of the virus (antigenic proteins provoke an immune response in the host). The need for a host cell to support the multiplication of the virus makes treatment difficult because the agent must be able to inhibit the virus without seriously affecting the host cells.

An antiviral agent must act at one of the five basic steps in the viral replication cycle in order to inhibit the virus:

- Attachment and penetration of the virus into the host cell.
- Uncoiling of virus (e.g., removal of the protein surface and release of the viral DNA or RNA).
- Synthesis of new viral components by the host cell as directed by the virus DNA.
- Assembly of the components into new virus.
- Release of the virus from the host cell.

7.6 CLASSIFICATION OF ANTIVIRAL DRUGS

(A) Anti-Influenza Viral Drugs:
Examples: Amantadine, Rimantadine, Oseltamivir, Zanamivir.

(B) Anti-Herpes Viral Drugs :
Examples: Idoxuridine, Acyclovir, Valacyclovir, Famcyclovir, Gancyclovir, Foscarnet.

(C) Anti-Retro Viral Drugs:

(a) Nucleoside reverse transcriptase inhibitors (NRTIs):
Examples: Zidovudine, Didanosine, Zalcitabine, Stavudine, Lamivudine, Abacavir, Tenofovir.

(b) Non-nucleoside reverse transcriptase inhibitors (NNRTIs):
Examples: Nevirapine, Efavirenz, Loviride, Delavirdine.

(c) Protease inhibitors:
Examples: Amprenavir, Lopinavir.

(D) Non-selective Anti-viral Drugs:
Examples: Ribavirin, Adefovirdipivoxil, interferon-α.

7.7 DRUG PROFILE

7.7.1 Anti-influenza Viral Drugs

1. Amantadine Hydrochloride:

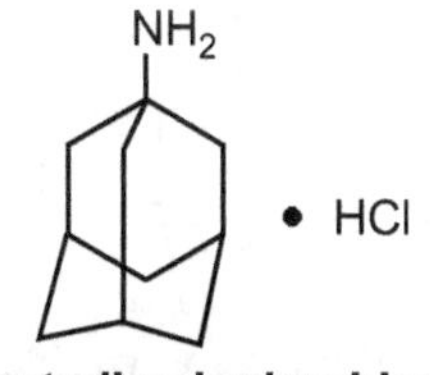

Amantadine hydrochloride

- Amantadine hydrochloride is a synthetic tricyclic amine with antiviral, antiparkinsonian, and antihyperalgesic activities.

- It is chemically, adamantan-1-amine; hydrochloride.

- It exerts its antiviral effect (against the influenza-A virus) by interfering with the function of the transmembrane domain of the viral M2 protein, thereby preventing the release of infectious viral nucleic acids into host cells.

- It also prevents virus assembly during virus replication.

Uses:

- Amantadine hydrochloride is used in the prophylactic or symptomatic treatment of influenza-A.

- It is also used as an antiparkinsonian agent, to treat extrapyramidal reactions, and for postherpetic neuralgia.

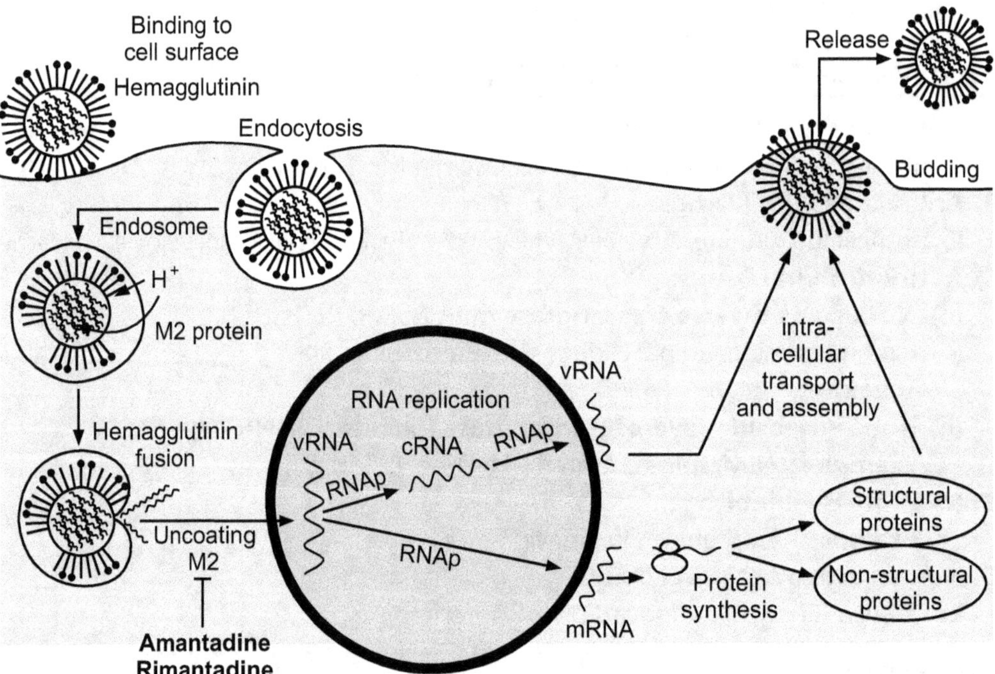

Fig. 7.3: Mechanism of action of Amantadine and Rimantadine

2. Rimantadine Hydrochloride:

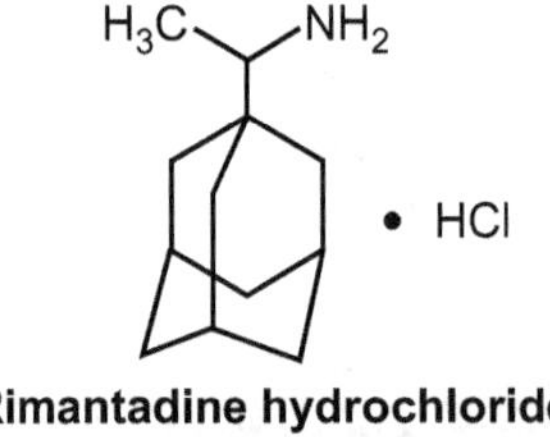

Rimantadine hydrochloride

- Rimantadine hydrochloride is a cyclic amine and alpha-methyl derivative of amantadine with antiviral activity.
- It is chemically, 1-(1-adamantyl)ethanamine; hydrochloride.
- It is a closely-related adamantane derivative with similar biological properties and exerts its antiviral effect as that of amantadine.

Uses:

- Rimantadine hydrochloride is used in the prophylactic or symptomatic treatment of influenza-A.
- It is also used as an antiparkinsonian agent, to treat extrapyramidal reactions, and for postherpetic neuralgia.

7.7.2 Anti-Herpes Viral Drugs

1. Idoxuridine:

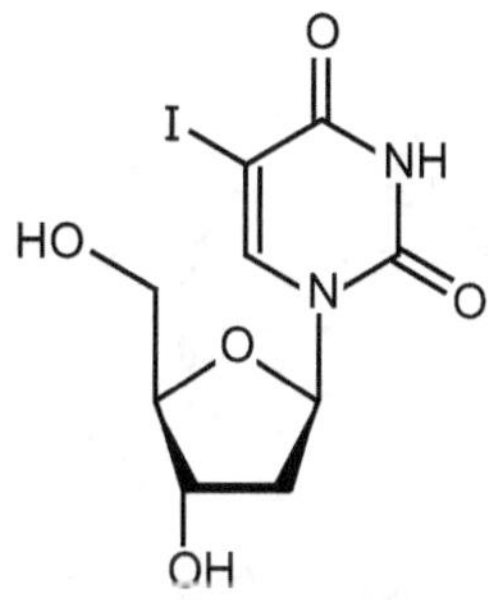

Idoxuridine

- Idoxuridine is an iodinated analogue of deoxyuridine.
- It is chemically 5-Iodo-2'-deoxyuridine.
- It has antiviral activity against herpes simplex virus (HSV) and potential radio-sensitizing activities.
- It incorporates into DNA and sensitizes cells to ionizing radiation by increasing DNA strand breaks.
- Idoxuridine is converted to its mono-, di-, and triphosphate forms, incorporated into DNA and disrupts viral replication.

Uses:

- Idoxuridine is solely employed for the topical therapy of herpes simplex keratitis of the eye.
- It has also been administered intravenously for the treatment of herpetic encephalitis.

2. Acyclovir:

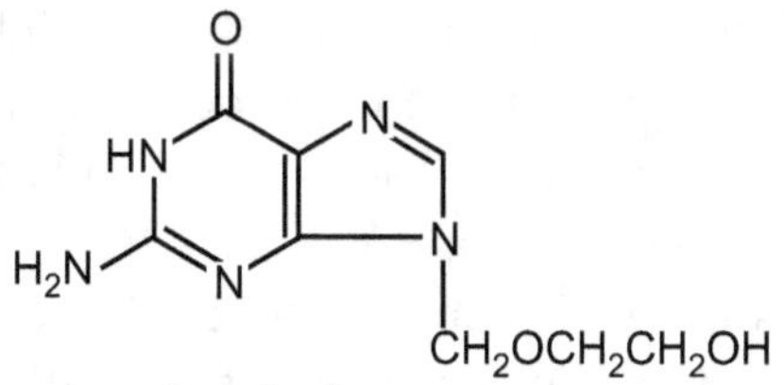

Acyclovir

- Acyclovir is a synthetic analog of the purine nucleoside, guanosine.
- It is the most effective of a series of acyclic nucleosides that possess antiviral activity.
- It is chemically, 2-amino-9-(2-hydroxyethoxymethyl)-1H-purin-6-one.
- After conversion *in-vivo* to the active metabolite acyclovir triphosphate by viral thymidine kinase, acyclovir competitively inhibits viral DNA polymerase by incorporating into the growing viral DNA chain and terminating further polymerization.

Uses:

- Acyclovir is active against herpes simplex viruses type 1 and 2, varicella-zoster virus and other viruses of the herpes virus family.
- It treats cold sores around the mouth (caused by herpes simplex), shingles (caused by herpes zoster), and chickenpox.
- This is also used to treat outbreaks of genital herpes.

3. Gancyclovir:

Gancyclovir

- Gancyclovir is a synthetic guanine derivative with antiviral activity.
- It is chemically, 2-amino-9-(1,3-dihydroxypropan-2-yl-oxymethyl)-1H-purin-6-one.
- An active metabolite of gancyclovir, gancyclovir-5-triphosphate inhibits viral DNA synthesis by competitive inhibition of viral DNA polymerases and incorporation into viral DNA, resulting in eventual termination of viral DNA elongation.

Uses:

- Gancyclovir is an antiviral drug used to treat or prevent AIDS-related cytomegalovirus infections.
- It is also used in cytomegalovirus pneumonitis in bone marrow transplant recipients and immunosuppressed patients.
- It has also been found to be an effective treatment for herpes simplex virus epithelial keratitis.

7.7.3 Anti-Retro Viral Drugs

The Nucleoside Reverse Transcriptase Inhibitors (NRTIs) inhibit reverse transcription by causing chain termination after they have been incorporated into viral DNA. For these drugs to be active they need to be phosphorylated intracellularly. NRTIs interrupt the HIV replication cycle via competitive inhibition of HIV reverse transcriptase and termination of the DNA chain. NRTIs are structurally similar to the DNA nucleoside bases and become incorporated into the proviral DNA chain, resulting in termination of proviral DNA formation.

1. Zidovudine:

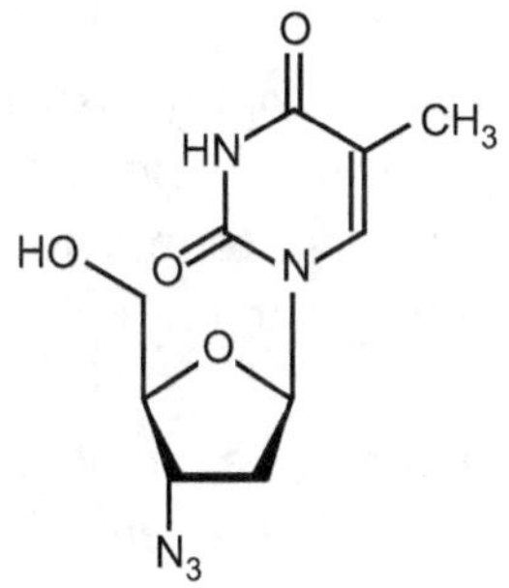

Zidovudine

- Zidovudine is a synthetic dideoxynucleoside.
- It is also known as azidothymidine (AZT).
- It is chemically, 1-[(2*R*,4*S*,5*S*)-4-azido-5-(hydroxymethyl)oxolan-2-yl]-5-methyl-pyrimidine-2,4-dione.
- It acts after intracellular phosphorylation to its active metabolite, by inhibiting DNA polymerase, resulting in the inhibition of DNA replication and cell death.
- It works by selectively inhibiting HIV's reverse transcriptase, the enzyme that the virus uses to make a DNA copy of its RNA.
- It is a principal part of the clinical pathway for both pre-exposure prophylaxis and post-exposure treatment of mother-to-child transmission of HIV during pregnancy, labor, and delivery and has been proven to be integral to uninfected siblings' perinatal and neonatal development.

Uses:

- Zidovudine is used in HIV treatment with other antiretroviral therapies and is used to prevent the likelihood of HIV resistance.
- It is used in combination with other agents in the therapy and prophylaxis of the human immunodeficiency virus (HIV) infection and the acquired immunodeficiency syndrome (AIDS).
- Without AZT, as many as 10 to 15% of fetuses with HIV-infected mothers will themselves become infected. AZT has been shown to reduce this risk to as little as 8% when given in a three-part regimen post-conception, delivery, and six weeks post-delivery.

2. Didanosine:

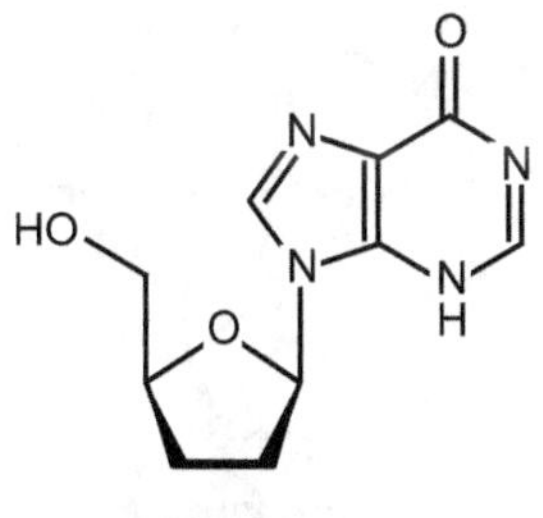

Didanosine

- Didanosine is a purine nucleoside analogue and reverse transcriptase inhibitor.
- It is a nucleoside analogue of adenosine.
- It is chemically, 9-[(2R,5S)-5-(hydroxymethyl)oxolan-2-yl]-1H-purin-6-one.
- It is phosphorylated to the active metabolite of dideoxyadenosine triphosphate, by cellular enzymes, and acts as a chain terminator by incorporation and inhibits viral reverse transcriptase by competing with natural dATP.

Uses:

- Didanosine is an antiviral drug, used as a medication to treat HIV/AIDS.
- It is used in combination with other agents in the therapy of human immuno-deficiency virus (HIV) infection and the acquired immunodeficiency syndromes (AIDS).

3. Zalcitabine:

Zalcitabine

- Zalcitabine is a pyrimidine 2',3'-dideoxyribonucleoside compound having cytosine as the nucleobase.
- It is chemically, 4-amino-1-[(2R,5S)-5-(hydroxymethyl)oxolan-2-yl]pyrimidin-2-one.
- Active metabolite of zalcitabine obtained after intracellular phosphorylation, preferentially inhibits the γ-form of DNA polymerase present in tumor cell mitochondria, resulting in the inhibition of tumor cell mitochondrial DNA replication and tumor cell death.

Uses:

- Zalcitabine has a role as an antiviral drug, an antimetabolite and a HIV-1 reverse transcriptase inhibitor.
- It is used in combination with antiretroviral agents for the treatment of HIV infection.

4. Lamivudine:

Lamivudine

- Lamivudine is a monothioacetal that consists of cytosine having a (2R,5S)-2-(hydroxymethyl)-1,3-oxathiolan-5-yl moiety attached at position 1.
- It is chemically, 4-amino-1-[(2R,5S)-2-(hydroxymethyl)-1,3-oxathiolan-5-yl]pyrimidin-2-one.
- It acts by inhibiting both type-1 and type-2 of HIV reverse transcriptase and also the reverse transcriptase of hepatitis-B virus.
- It is phosphorylated to active metabolites that compete for incorporation into viral DNA.
- Active metabolites inhibit the HIV reverse transcriptase enzyme competitively and act as a chain terminator of DNA synthesis.

Uses:

- Lamivudine is used as an antiviral in the treatment of AIDS and hepatitis-B.
- It has been used for treatment of chronic hepatitis-B at a lower dose than for treatment of HIV/AIDS.

5. Loviride:

Loviride

- Loviride is a non-nucleoside reverse transcriptase inhibitor (NNRTI) that entered phase-III clinical trials in the late 1990s, but failed to gain marketing approval because of poor potency.
- It is chemically, 2-(2-acetyl-5-methylanilino)-2-(2,6-dichlorophenyl)acetamide.

Uses:

- Loviride is an antiviral drug that is active against HIV.

6. Delavirdine:

Delavirdine

- Delavirdine is a synthetic, non-nucleoside reverse transcriptase inhibitor.

- It is chemically, N-[2-[4-[3-(propan-2-yl-amino) pyridin-2-yl] piperazine-1-carbonyl]-1H-indol-5-yl]methane sulphonamide.

- It has a role as a HIV-1 reverse transcriptase inhibitor and an antiviral drug.

- It binds directly to viral reverse transcriptase (RT) and blocks the RNA-dependent and DNA-dependent DNA polymerase activities by disrupting the enzyme's catalytic site.

- It is an inhibitor of the cytochrome P450 system, delavirdine may result in increased serum levels of co-administered protease inhibitors metabolized by the cytochrome P450 system.

Uses:

- Delavirdine is used in combination with other anti-retroviral drugs.

- It has been shown to reduce HIV viral load and increase CD_4 leukocyte counts in patients.

- It is used in the treatment of HIV-1 infection in combination with appropriate antiretroviral agents.

7. Saquinavir:

Saquinavir

- Saquinavir is quinolines and L-asparagine derivative with HIV-1 protease inhibitor activity.

- Proteases are enzymes that cleave protein molecules into smaller fragments. HIV protease is vital for both viral replication within the cell and release of mature viral particles from an infected cell.

- It binds to the active site of the viral protease and prevents cleavage of viral polyproteins, preventing maturation of the virus.

- It inhibits both HIV-1 and HIV-2 proteases.

Uses:

- Saquinavir is used together with other medications to treat or prevent HIV/AIDS.

8. Indinavir:

Indinavir

- Indinavir is a N-(2-hydroxyethyl)piperazine, a piperazinecarboxamide and a dicarboxylic acid diamide.
- It is an antiretroviral protease inhibitor.
- It can cause transient and usually asymptomatic elevations in serum aminotransferase levels and mild elevations in indirect bilirubin concentration.

Uses:

- Indinavir is used in the therapy and prevention of human immunodeficiency virus (HIV) infection and the acquired immunodeficiency syndrome (AIDS).

9. Ritonavir:

Ritonavir

- Ritonavir is an L-valine derivative that is an antiretroviral drug from the protease inhibitor class.
- It has a role as an antiviral drug, a HIV protease inhibitor, an environmental contaminant and a xenobiotic.
- It is a member of 1,3-thiazoles, a L-valine derivative, a carbamate ester, a member of ureas and a carboxamide.

Uses:

- Ritonavir is used in the treatment of human immunodeficiency virus (HIV) infection and the acquired immunodeficiency syndrome (AIDS).
- It is often used as a fixed-dose combination with another protease inhibitor, lopinavir.
- It is also used in combination with dasabuvir sodium hydrate, ombitasvir and paritaprevir for the treatment of chronic hepatitis-C virus genotype-1 infection as well as cirrhosis of the liver.

7.7.4 Non-selective Antiviral Drugs

1. Ribavirin:

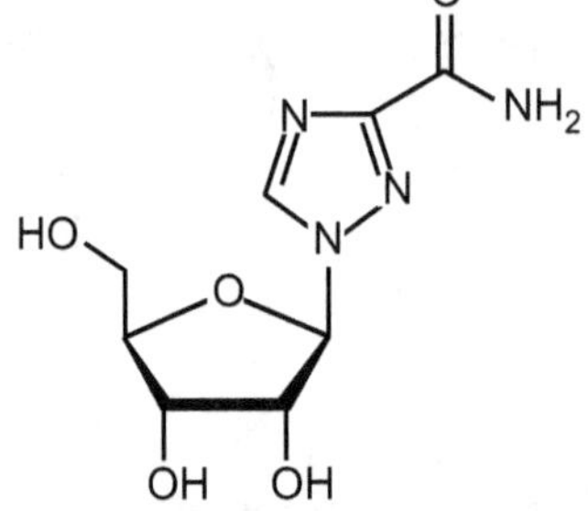

Ribavirin

- Ribavirin is a 1-ribosyltriazole that is the 1-ribofuranosyl derivative of 1,2,4-triazole-3-carboxamide.
- It is a nucleoside inhibitor, used to stop viral RNA synthesis and viral mRNA capping.
- It is a prodrug, which when metabolized, resembles purine RNA nucleotides, which interferes with RNA metabolism required for viral replication.

Uses:

- Ribavirin is used to treat hepatitis-C and viral hemorrhagic fevers.
- It is also used in the treatment of influenza types A and B, oral treatment of hepatitis, genital herpes, and lassa fever (hemorrhagic fever).

SYNTHESIS

1. Acyclovir:

Synthesis-1:

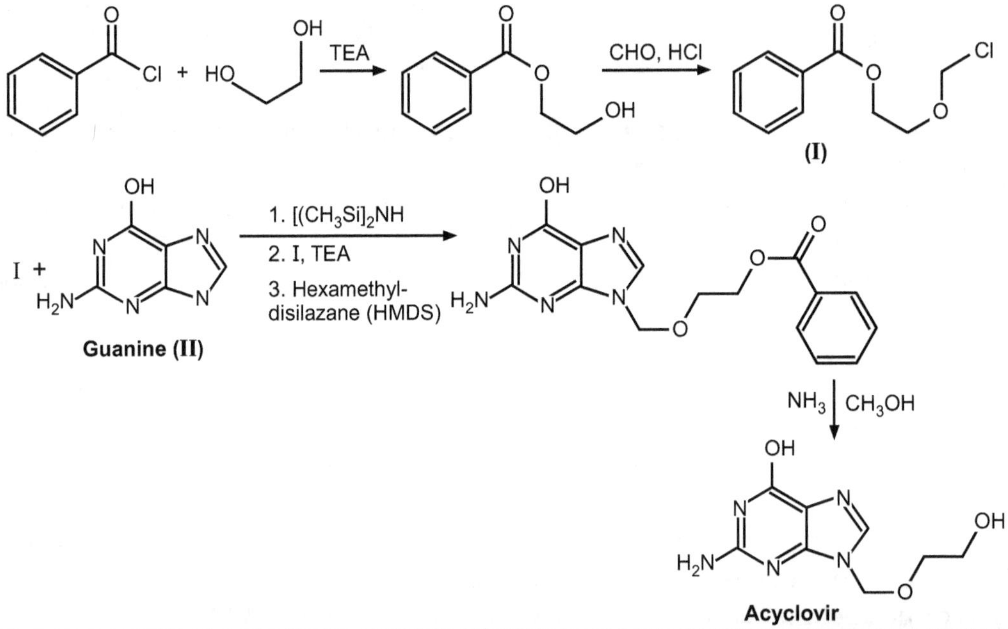

Guanine (II)

Acyclovir

Synthesis-2:

QUESTIONS

Multiple Choice Questions:

1. What are the two main targets currently used in anti-HIV therapy?
   (a) Reverse transcriptase and protease
   (b) Reverse transcriptase and integrase
   (c) Protease and integrase
   (d) The viral glycoproteins gp120 and gp41

2. Which one of the following does not possess purine nucleus?
   (a) Gancyclovir   (b) Ribavirin
   (c) Adefovir   (d) Didanosine

3. Which one of the following drugs is most effective in preventing transmission of HIV virus from the mother to the foetus?
   (a) Lamivudine   (b) Zidovudine
   (c) Indinavir   (d) Ribavirin

4. Which of the following enzymes is responsible for processing HIV proteins during the production of new viruses?
   (a) Integrase   (b) Protease
   (c) Reverse transcriptase   (d) DNA polymerase

5. Which one of the following does not possess purine nucleus?
   (a) Gancyclovir   (b) Acyclovir
   (c) Vidarabine   (d) Idoxuridine

6. Which of the following protease inhibitors was developed by a hybridization strategy?
   (a) Ritonavir   (b) Indinavir
   (c) Saquinavir   (d) Amprenavir

Answers :

1. (a)	2. (b)	3. (b)	4. (b)	5. (d)	6. (b)

Answer the Following Questions:

1. What are the various diseases caused by different types of viruses?
2. Give brief account of replication and transformation in viruses.
3. Classify the 'antiviral drugs' on the basis of their mode of action with suitable examples.
4. How would you synthesize Acyclovir?
5. Define virus and give in detail Baltimore classification.
6. Write a note on Replication and Transformation of viruses.
7. What do you know about virus replication? Explain in detail.
8. Give an account of various diseases caused by viruses.
9. Define antiviral drugs with suitable examples from each class.
10. Write chemical names, uses and mode of action of Amantadine, Zidovudine, Didanosine and Indinavir.
11. Write a brief note on anti-retro viral drugs.

| Unit IV |

Chapter ... 8

ANTIFUNGAL AGENTS

♦ LEARNING OBJECTIVES ♦

After completing this sub-unit the students should be able:
- *To learn the morphology of fungi and fungal infections.*
- *To study various diseases caused by fungi.*
- *To study detail classification of antifungal agents.*
- *To study antifungal drugs in detail with their MOA and uses.*
- *To learn the synthetic scheme of some selected antifungal drugs.*

8.1 INTRODUCTION

Fungi belong to a diverse group of organisms that includes yeasts, moulds and dermatophytes. They are classified in a separate kingdom from animals, plants and bacteria, and physiologically have most in common with animals. Most fungi live harmlessly in the environment, especially in soil and decaying matter, but approximately 200 species can cause disease in the human host.

Fungal infections are not usually serious in otherwise fit, healthy adults, but they can be embarrassing and distressing. Very ill and immune-compromised patients are at risk of serious fungal infections, especially if they have had multiple courses of antibiotics and have undergone invasive procedures. Exogenous infection (cross-infection) caused by fungi can occur from one patient to another at home and in healthcare settings.

More than 300,000 species of fungi have been identified, but most live harmlessly in the environment where they play an important role in breaking down and recycling organic material from dead animals and plants. Only a few species are pathogenic (able to cause disease).

Some fungi, for example yeasts, assume a very simple structure and exist as single cells. More complex forms display filamentous branching structures called hyphae. These can become highly interwoven to form a mesh called a mycelium.

A fungal infection is called a mycosis, whereas mycology is the study of fungi. Fungal infections affecting the skin are sometimes referred to as dermatophytic infections.

8.2 FUNGAL DISEASES

The fungal kingdom includes yeasts, molds, rusts and mushrooms. Most fungi are saprophytic, which means that they live on dead organic matter in the soil or on decaying leaves or wood. A few of these fungi can cause opportunistic infections if they are introduced into a human through wounds or by inhalation. Some of these infections can be fatal. There are relatively few obligate animal parasites (i.e., microorganisms that can only live on mammalian hosts) among the fungi, although *Candida albicans* is commonly found as part of the normal flora of the gastrointestinal tract and vagina. The obligatory parasites are limited to dermatophytes that have evolved to live on/ in the keratin-containing hair and skin of mammals, where they cause diseases such as ringworm and athletes foot.

All fungi produce spores, which may be transported by direct contact or through the air. Although most topical fungal infections are readily treated, the incidence of life threatening systemic fungal infections, including those caused by yeasts such as *Candida albicans* and molds such as *Aspergillus fumigans* are increasing, and mortality remains high.

8.3 CLASSIFICATION OF ANTIBIOTICS

(a) **Antifungal antibiotics:** Amphotericin-B, Nystatin, Natamycin, Griseofulvin.

(b) **Synthetic Antifungal agents:** Clotrimazole, Econazole, Butoconazole, Oxiconazole, Tioconazole, Miconazole, Ketoconazole, Terconazole, Itraconazole, Fluconazole, Naftifine hydrochloride, Tolnaftate.

8.3.1 Antifungal Antibiotics

The antifungal antibiotics make up an important group of antifungal agents. All of the antibiotics are marked by their complexity.

There are two classes of antifungal antibiotics:

(a) **Polyenes:** Amphotericin-B, Nystatin, Natamycin.

(b) **Griseofulvin**

(a) Polyene Antibiotics:

A number of structurally complex antifungal antibiotics have been isolated from soil bacteria of the genus *Streptomyces*. The compounds are similar, in that they contain a system of conjugated double bonds in macrocyclic lactone rings. They contain the conjugated *–ene* system of double bonds. Hence, they are called the polyene antibiotics.

The common features of the polyene antibiotics are:

(i)   A series of hydroxyl groups on the acid-derived portion of the ring and

(ii) A glycosidically linked deoxyaminohexose called mycosamine.

The number of double bonds in the macrocyclic ring differs also,

(i)   Natamycin, the smallest macrocycle, is a pentene,

(ii) Nystatin is a hexaene, and

(iii) Amphotericin-B is a heptaene.

Mechanism of Action of Polyene Antibiotics:

Polyene antibiotics contain three-dimensional shape, a barrel-like non-polar structure capped by a polar group (the sugar). They penetrate the fungal cell membrane, acting as 'false membrane components," and bind closely with ergosterol, causing membrane disruption, cessation of membrane enzyme activity, and loss of cellular constituents, especially K^+ ions.

The drug is fungistatic at low concentrations and fungicidal at high concentrations. This suggests that at low concentrations the polyenes bind to a membrane-bound enzyme component, such as an ATPase.

Uses of Polyene Antibiotics:

The polyenes have no activity against bacteria, rickeitsia, or viruses, but they are highly potent; broad-spectrum antifungal agents.

(i)   Polyene antibiotics have activity against certain protozoa, such as Leishmania spp.

(ii) They are effective against pathogenic yeasts, molds, and dermalophytes.

(iii) In low concentrations polyenes antibiotics, *in-vitro* inhibit various species such as *Candida, Cryptococcus, Aspergilllus and Cephalosporium.*

Amphotericin-B is the only polyene useful for the treatment of serious systemic infections. The other polyenes are indicated only as topical agents for superficial fungal infections.

8.3.2 Drug Profile for Antifungal Antibiotics

1. Amphotericin-B:

Amphotericin-B

- Amphotericin-B is a polyene antifungal antibiotic isolated in 1956 and purified from the fermentation beer of a soil culture of the actinomycete *Streptomyces nodosus*.
- As the name implies, Amphotericin-B is an amphoteric substance, with a primary amino group attached to the mycosamine ring and a carboxyl group on the macrocycle.

- It acts by binding to ergosterol, an essential component of the fungal cell membrane, thereby causing depolarization of the membrane and altering cell membrane permeability. This leads to leakage of important intracellular components, cell rupture, and eventually cell death.

Uses:

- Parenteral Amphotericin-B has broad spectrum of activity and is indicated for the treatment of severe, potentially life-threatening fungal infections.
- Limited use of amphotericin-B is because of high risk of adverse reactions.
    - Nearly 80% of patients treated with amphotericin-B develop nephrotoxicity.
    - Fever headache, anorexia, gastrointestinal distress, muscle and joint pain are common.
    - Pain at the site of injection and thrombophlebitis are frequent complications of intravenous administration.

2. Nystatin:

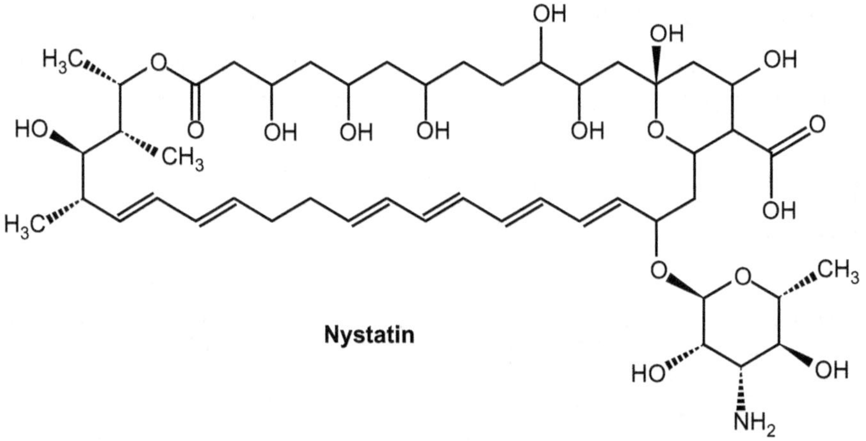

Nystatin

- Nystatin is a polyene antifungal antibiotic. It can be used as topical and oral antifungal agent.
- It is isolated in 1951 from a strain of the actinomycete *Streptomyces noursei.*
- The aglycone portion of nystatin is called as Nystatinolide, whereas glycone part is called as mycosamine.
- It has activity against many species of yeast and *candida albicans.*

Uses:

- Nystatin is used for the treatment of local and gastrointestinal monilial infections caused by *Candida albicans* and other *Candida* species.
- Nystatin is used largely to treat skin and oropharyngeal candidiasis.

3. Natamycin:

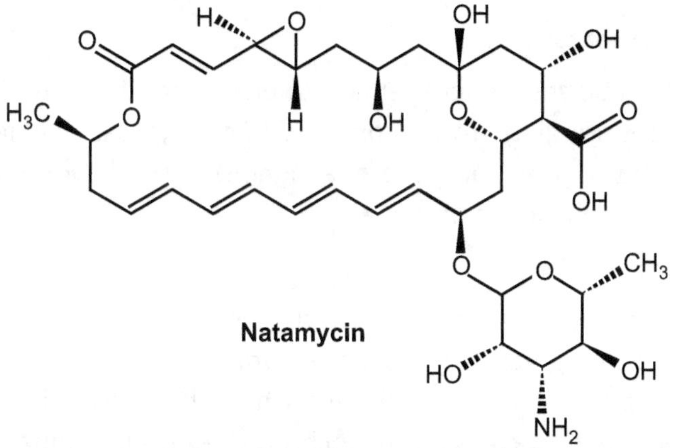

Natamycin

- Natamycin is a polyene antibiotic obtained from cultures of *Streptomyces natalensis*.
- It exerts its antifungal effects by binding to sterols in the fungal cell membrane thereby increasing membrane permeability. This leads to a leakage and loss of essential cellular constituents.
- It is a smaller polyene and it is fungistatic and fungicidal within the same concentration range.

Uses:

- Natamycin is used for a variety of fungal infections, mainly topically.
- It possesses *in vitro* activity against a number of yeasts and filamentous fungi, including *Candida, Aspergillas, Cephalosporium, Penicillium,* and *Fusarium* spp.
- 5% ophthalmic suspensions are used for the treatment of fungal conjunctivitis, blepharitis, and keratitis.

4. Griseofulvin:

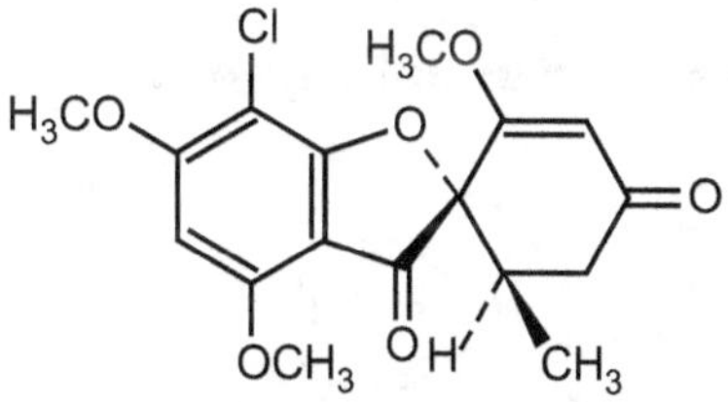

Griseofulvin

- Griseofulvin is an antibiotic obtained from the fungus *Penicillium griseofulvum*.
- It is chemically, (2S,5'R)-7-chloro-3',4,6-trimethoxy-5'-methylspiro[1-benzofuran-2,4'-cyclohex-2-ene]-1',3-dione.
- Griseofulvin binds to tubulin, disrupting microtubule function and inhibiting mitosis.

Uses:

- Griseofulvin is a fungistatic agent used to treat superficial fungal skin infections such as tinea capitis and pedis.
- It is used for the treatment of refractory ringworm infections of the body, hair, nails, and feet caused by species of dermatophytic fungi.

8.3.3 Synthetic Antifungal Agents

(a) Azole Antifungal Agents:

The azoles are synthetic antifungal agents with unique mechanism of action. They can be used to treat infections ranging from simple dermatophytoses to life threatening, deep systemic fungal infections. They are effective against most fungi that cause superficial infections of the skin and mucous membranes.

Mechanism of Action:

The fungicidal effect of azoles is because of damage to the cell membrane; with the loss of essential cellular components such as potassium ions and amino acids, whereas the fungistatic effects of azoles at low concentration have been associated with inhibition of membrane-bound enzymes such as a cytochrome P_{450} class enzyme, lanosterol and 14α-demethylase.

Structure Activity Relationship:

1. The basic structural requirement for members of the azole class is a weakly basic imidazole or 1,2,4-triazole ring bonded by a nitrogen-carbon linkage to the rest of the structure.
2. The most potent antifungal azoles possess two or three aromatic rings, at least one of which is halogen substituted (e.g., 2,4-dichlorophenyl. 4-chlorophenyl, or 2,4-difluorophenyl) and other non-polar functional groups.
3. Only 2, and/or 2,4 halogen (fluorine) or sulphonic acid substitution yields effective azole compounds.
4. Substitution at other positions of the ring yields inactive compounds.
5. The non-polar functionality confers high lipophilicity to the antifungal azoles.

8.3.4 Drug Profile for Azole Antifungal Agents

1. Clotrimazole:

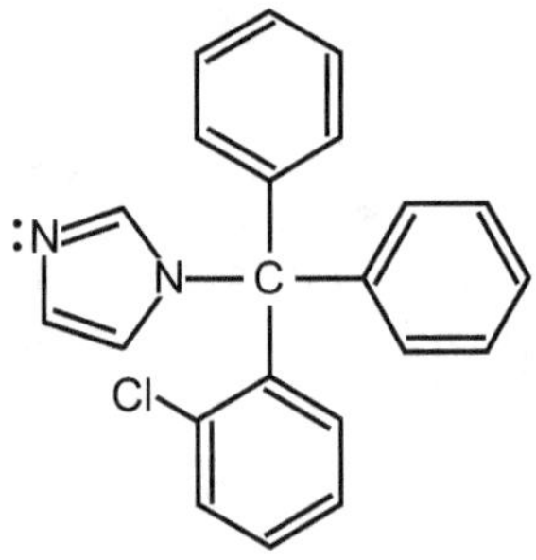

Clotrimazole

- Clotrimazole is a synthetic, imidazole derivative with broad-spectrum, antifungal activity.
- It is chemically, 1-[(2-chlorophenyl)-diphenylmethyl]imidazole.

- It acts by inhibiting 14α-demethylase, a microsomal cytochrome P_{450}-dependent enzyme, which catalyzes conversion of lanosterol to ergosterol, an essential component of the fungal cell wall, thus increases cellular permeability thereby resulting in leakage of cellular contents and eventually inhibits fungal cell growth, causes cell lysis.

Uses:

- Clotrimazole is a broad spectrum antifungal drug used topically for the treatment of tinea infections and oral candidiasis.

2. Econazole:

Econazole

- Econazole is an imidazole antifungal agent.
- It is chemically, 1-[2-[(4-chlorophenyl)methoxy]-2-(2,4-dichlorophenyl)ethyl] imidazole.
- Mechanism of action is same as that of Clotrimazole.

Uses:

- Econazole is used topically in dermatomycoses.
- 1% cream is used for the topical treatment of local tinea infections and cutaneous candidiasis.
- It also has some action against Gram-positive bacteria.

3. Butoconazole:

Butoconazole

- Butoconazole is a synthetic imidazole derivative with fungistatic properties.
- It is chemically, 1-[4-(4-chlorophenyl)-2-(2,6-dichlorophenyl)sulfanylbutyl]imidazole.
- Mechanism of action is same as that of Clotrimazole.

Uses:

- Butoconazole is active against many dermatophytes and yeasts.
- It is used as its nitrate salt in gynaecology for treatment of vulvovaginal infections caused by *Candida* species, particularly *Candida albicans*.
- It also contains antibacterial effects against some Gram-positive organisms.

4. Oxiconazole:

Oxiconazole

- Oxiconazole is a broad spectrum imidazole derivative with antifungal activity.
- It is chemically, (Z)-1-(2,4-dichlorophenyl)-N-[(2,4-dichlorophenyl)methoxy]-2-imidazol-1-yl-ethanimine.
- Mechanism of action is same as that of Clotrimazole.

Uses:

- Oxiconazole is used in cream, lotion and powder for the topical treatment of fungal skin infections such as tinea pedis, tinea corporis, and tinea capitis.

5. Tioconazole:

Tioconazole

- Tioconazole is a synthetic imidazole derivative with fungicidal activity.
- It is chemically, 1-[2-[(2-chlorothiophen-3-yl)methoxy]-2-(2,4-dichlorophenyl) ethyl]-imidazole.
- Mechanism of action is same as that of Clotrimazole.

Uses:

- Tioconazole is active against pathogenic *Candida* and used for the treatment of vulvovaginal candidiasis.
- It is more effective against *Torulopsis glabrata* than other azoles.
- Topical formulations are used for ringworm, jock itch, athlete's foot, and tinea versicolor or "sun fungus".

6. Miconazole:

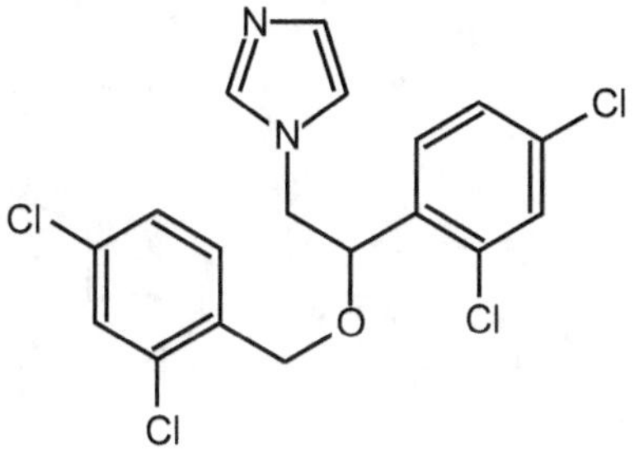

Miconazole

- Miconazole is a synthetic derivative of imidazole with an antifungal activity.
- It chemically, 1-[2-(2,4-dichlorophenyl)-2-[(2,4-dichlorophenyl)methoxy]ethyl]-imidazole.
- Mechanism of action is same as that of Clotrimazole.

Uses:

- Miconazole is used in the treatment of candidal skin infections.
- It is intended for the treatment of serious systemic fungal infections, such as candidiasis, coccidioidomycosis and cryptococcosis.
- It is also used for the treatment of chronic mucocutaneous candidiasis and vaginal candidiasis.

7. Ketoconazole:

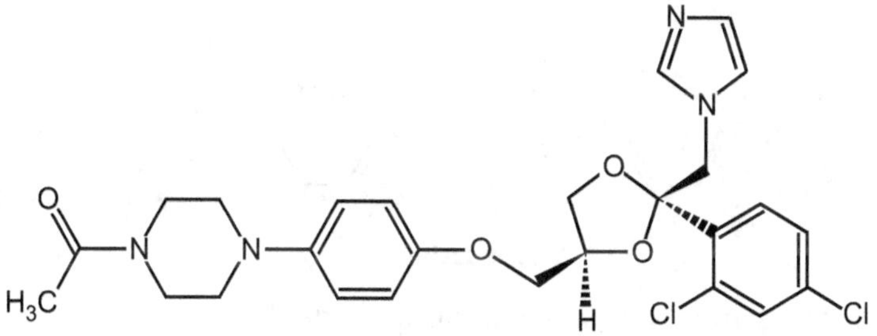

Ketoconazole

- Ketoconazole is a synthetic derivative of phenylpiperazine with broad antifungal properties.
- It is chemically, 1-[4-[4-[[(2S,4R)-2-(2,4-dichlorophenyl)-2-(imidazol-1-yl-methyl)-1,3-dioxolan-4-yl]methoxy]phenyl]piperazin-1-yl]ethanone.
- Mechanism of action is same as that of Clotrimazole.

Uses:

- Ketoconazole is a fungicidal agent with a very broad spectrum of activity against many fungal species and it is used for treatment of superficial and systemic fungal infections.
- It is also used topically in a 2% concentration in a cream and in a shampoo for the management of cutaneous *candidiasis* and *tinea* infections.

8. Terconazole:

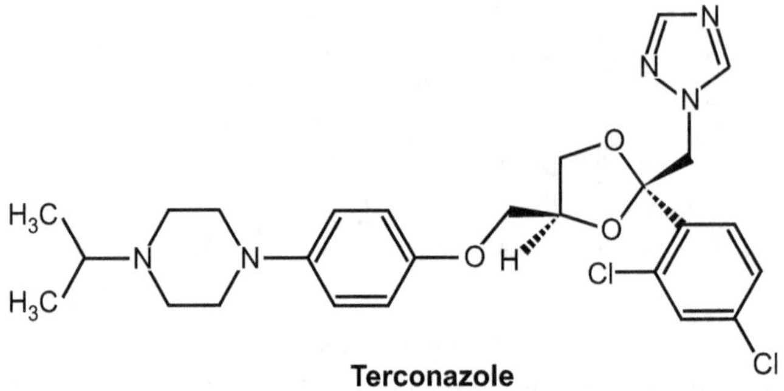

Terconazole

- Terconazole is a synthetic triazole derivative structurally related to fluconazole.
- It is chemically, 1-[4-[[(2*R*,4*S*)-2-(2,4-dichlorophenyl)-2-(1,2,4-triazol-1-yl-methyl)-1,3-dioxolan-4-yl]methoxy]phenyl]-4-propan-2-yl-piperazine.
- Mechanism of action is same as that of Clotrimazole.

Uses:

- Terconazole is an anti-fungal drug that is mainly used to treat vaginal yeast infections (or vaginal candidiasis).

9. Itraconazole:

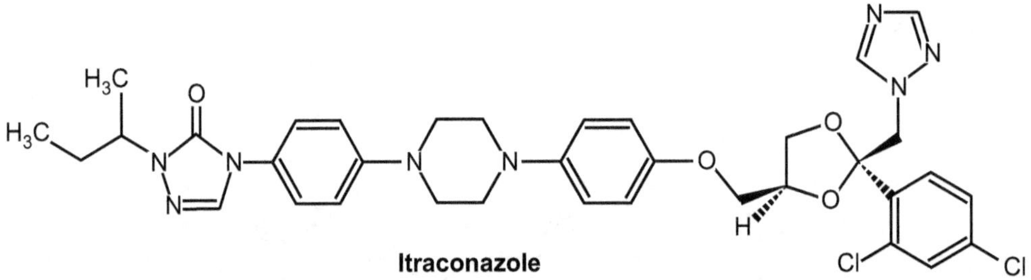

Itraconazole

- Itraconazole is a synthetic triazole antifungal agent.
- It is chemically, 2-butan-2-yl-4-[4-[4-[4-[[2-(2,4-dichlorophenyl)-2-(1,2,4-triazol-1-yl-methyl)-1,3-dioxolan-4-yl]methoxy]phenyl]piperazin-1-yl]phenyl]-1,2,4-triazol-3-one.
- It is a unique member of the azole class that contains two triazole moieties in its structure, a weakly basic 1,2,4-triazole and a nonbasic 1,2,4-triazole-3-one.
- Mechanism of action is same as that of Clotrimazole.
- Because of its low toxicity profile, this agent can be used for long-term maintenance treatment of chronic fungal infections.

Uses:

- Itraconazole is an orally active, broad-spectrum antifungal agent that has become an important alternative to ketoconazole.
- It is used in the treatment of systemic and superficial fungal infections.

10. Fluconazole:

Fluconazole

- Fluconazole is a synthetic triazole with antifungal activity.
- It is chemically, 2-(2,4-difluorophenyl)-1,3-bis(1,2,4-triazol-1-yl)propan-2-ol.
- Mechanism of action is same as that of Clotrimazole.

Uses:

- Fluconazole is an antifungal drug used for the treatment of mucosal candidiasis and for systemic infections including systemic candidiasis, coccidioidomycosis, and cryptococcosis.
- Fluconazole is recommended for the treatment and prophylaxis of disseminated and deep organ candidiasis.
- It is also used to control esophageal and oropharyngeal candidiasis.
- Because of its efficient penetration into CSF, fluconazole is an agent of choice for the treatment of cryptococcal meningitis and for prophylaxis against cryptococcosis in AIDS patients.
- It lends itself to one-dose therapies for vaginal candidiasis.

8.3.5 Drug Profile for Allylamines and Related Compounds

1. Naftifine Hydrochloride:

Naftifine hydrochloride

- Naftifine hydrochloride is an allylamine derivate with synthetic broad-spectrum antifungal activity.
- It is chemically, (E)-N-methyl-N-(naphthalen-1-yl-methyl)-3-phenylprop-2-en-1-amine; hydrochloride.

- It acts selectively by inhibiting the enzyme squalene 2,3-epoxidase, thereby inhibiting the biosynthesis of sterol. This results in a decreased amount of sterols, especially ergosterol which is the primary fungal membrane sterol, and a corresponding accumulation of squalene in fungal cells.

Uses:

- 1% concentration of Naftifine hydrochloride in a cream and in a gel is used for the treatment of ringworm, athlete's foot, and jock itch.
- It has shown efficacy for treatment of ringworm of the beard, ringworm of scalp, and tinea versicolor.

2. Tolnaftate:

Tolnaftate

- Tolnaftate is a thiocarbamate derivative with either fungicidal or fungistatic property.
- Tolnaftate is classified with the allylamine antimycotics.
- It is a selective, reversible and non-competitive inhibitor of membrane-bound squalene-2,3- epoxidase, an enzyme involved in the biosynthesis of ergosterol. Inhibition leads to the accumulation of squalene and a deficiency in ergosterol, an essential component of fungal cell walls, thereby increasing membrane permeability, disrupting cellular organization and causing cell death.

Uses:

- Tolnaftate is a thioester of β-naphthol, is fungicidal against dermatophytes, such as *Trichophyton, Microsporum,* and *Epidermophyton* spp., that cause superficial tinea infections.
- It is used in treatment of ringworm, jock itch, and athlete's foot.
- It is formulated into preparations intended to be used with artificial fingernails to counteract the increased chance of ringworm of the nail beds.

SYNTHESIS

1. Miconazole:

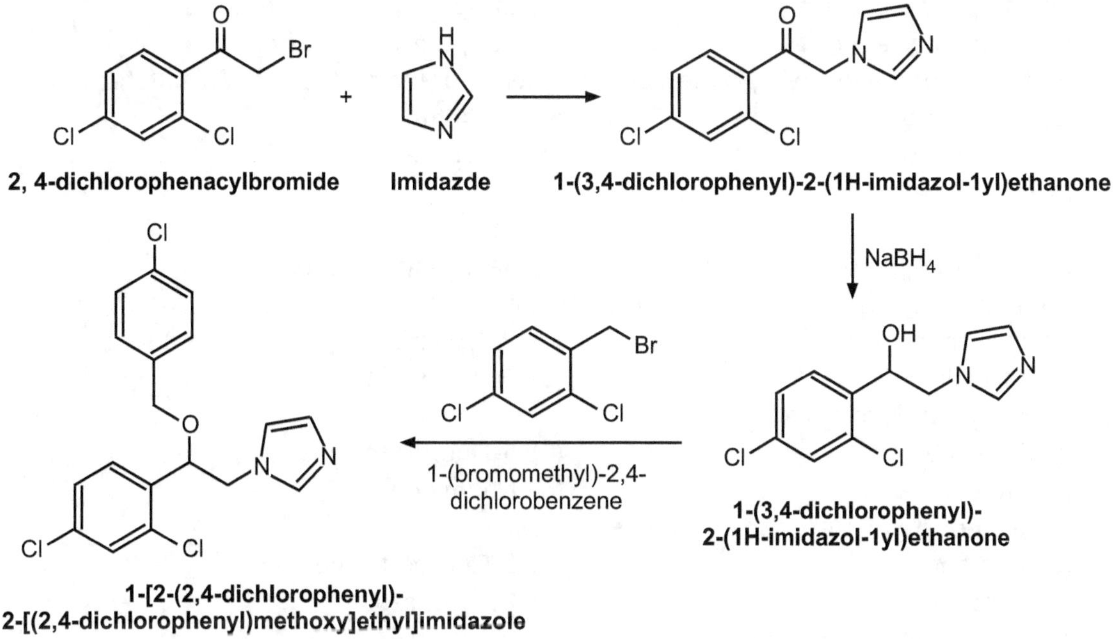

2, 4-dichlorophenacylbromide   +   **Imidazde**   →   **1-(3,4-dichlorophenyl)-2-(1H-imidazol-1yl)ethanone**

$NaBH_4$

1-(bromomethyl)-2,4-dichlorobenzene

1-(3,4-dichlorophenyl)-2-(1H-imidazol-1yl)ethanone

1-[2-(2,4-dichlorophenyl)-2-[(2,4-dichlorophenyl)methoxy]ethyl]imidazole

2. Tolnaftate:

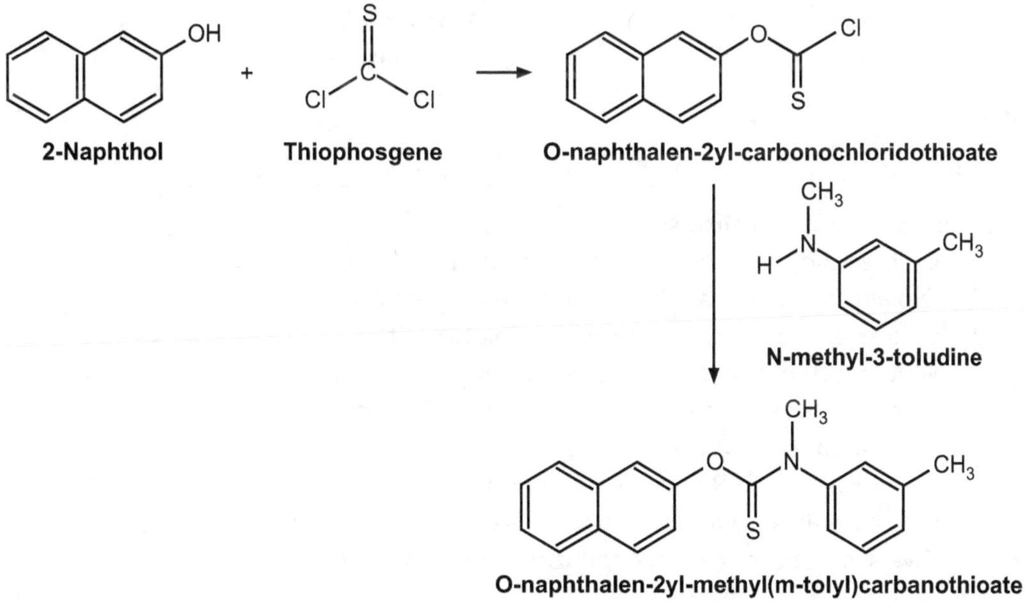

2-Naphthol   +   **Thiophosgene**   →   **O-naphthalen-2yl-carbonochloridothioate**

N-methyl-3-toludine

O-naphthalen-2yl-methyl(m-tolyl)carbanothioate

QUESTIONS

Multiple Choice Questions:

1. Nystatin is isolated from ....
   - (a) Streptomyces griesus
   - (b) Streptomyces mediterrannei
   - (c) Streptomyces nodosus
   - (d) Streptomyces noursei
2. Which one of the following is the starting material for the synthesis of Tolnaftate?
   - (a) 1-naphthol
   - (b) 2-naphthol
   - (c) 3-naphthol
   - (d) All of these
3. Mycoses is caused by .... species.
   - (a) Trichophyton
   - (b) Microsporum
   - (c) Epidermophyton
   - (d) Saprophytic yeasts
4. Amphotericin B is a .... type of antibiotic
   - (a) One amino acid
   - (b) Polypeptide
   - (c) Macrolide
   - (d) Polyene
5. Antifungal antibiotic is ....
   - (a) Naftifine
   - (b) 5-Fluorocytosine
   - (c) Nystatin
   - (d) Nafimidone
6. Inhibitor of sterol-14-α-demethylase is ....
   - (a) Naftifine
   - (b) 5-Fluorocytosine
   - (c) Ciclopirox
   - (d) Ketoconazole
7. The antifungal with bis-triazole nucleus is ....
   - (a) Ketoconazole
   - (b) Butaconazole
   - (c) Fluconazole
   - (d) Clotrimazole
8. 1,2,4-triazolone is present in ....
   - (a) Ketoconazole
   - (b) Fluconazole
   - (c) Itraconazole
   - (d) Tioconazole

Answers :

1. (d)	2. (b)	3. (d)	4. (d)	5. (c)	6. (d)	7. (b)	8. (c)

Answer the Following Questions:

1. Define fungy. Give detail account of fungal infections.
2. Explain in brief the antibiotics used in fungal infections.
3. Given detail account of polyene antibiotics with suitable examples.
4. Write mechanism of action and uses of polyene antibiotics.
5. Give structure, chemical name and uses of Griseofulvin.
6. Write a note on synthetic antifungal agents.
7. Give MOA and SAR of azole antifungal agents.
8. Give a detail account of Ketoconazole.
9. Give synthetic route for Miconazole and Tolnaftate.

■■■

Chapter ... 9

ANTI-PROTOZOAL AGENTS

♦ LEARNING OBJECTIVES ♦

After completing this sub-unit the students should be able:

- *To learn various protozoal diseases.*
- *To study the correct approaches to protozoal therapy.*
- *To study various drugs used against protozoal diseases.*
- *To study synthetic scheme of some selected antiprotozoal agents.*

9.1 INTRODUCTION

Protozoal diseases are categorized as malaria, amebiasis, giardiasis, trichomoniasis, toxoplasmosis, and as a direct consequence of the AIDS epidemic, *Pneumocystis carinii* pneumonia (PCP). Amebiasis is a disease of the large intestine caused by *Entamoeba histolytica which* can invade the wall of the colon or other parts of the body (e.g. liver, lungs, or skin). The disease occurs mainly in the tropics, but it also is seen in temperate climates in which sanitation is poor. The prevalence of amebiasis has been estimated to be as high as 20% of the population. Amebiasis may be carried without significant symptoms or may lead to severe, life-threatening dysentery.

The organism exists in one of two forms, the motile trophozoite form or the dormant cyst form. The trophozoite form is found in the intestine or wall of the colon and may be expelled from the body with the stools. The cyst form is encased by a chitinous wall that protects the organism from the environment, including chlorine used in water purification; thus, the organism may be transmitted through contaminated water and foods.

It is the cyst form that is responsible for transmission of the disease. The cyst is spread by direct person-to-person contact and is commonly associated with living conditions in which poor personal hygiene, poor sanitation, poverty, and ignorance exist. The hosts may be rendered susceptible to infection by pre-existing conditions, such as protein malnutrition, pregnancy, HIV infection, or high carbohydrate intake. Under these conditions, the organism is capable of invading body tissue.

Symptomes of Amebiasis:

Symptoms of amebiasis may range from intermittent diarrhea (foul-smelling loose/watery stools) to tenderness and enlargement of the liver (with the extra-intestinal form) to acute amoebic dysentery. Many patients may experience no symptoms, and the organism remains in the bowels as a commensal organism.

Approaches to Protozoal Therapy:

The most appropriate approach for treatment of this type of protozoal infection is through prevention. Because the infection usually occurs by consumption of contaminated drinking water and food, avoidance is the key to prevention. Drinking bottled water, or boiling or disinfecting the water, will reduce the risk. Improvement in personal hygiene and general sanitation also are beneficial.

Amebicides that are effective against both intestinal and extra-intestinal forms of the disease are limited to the nitroimidazole derivative metronidazole, and group of amebicides that are effective only against intestinal forms of the disease includes the aminoglycoside antibiotic paromomycin, the 8-hydroxyquinoline derivative iodoquinol, the arsenical compound carbarasone, and diloxanide.

9.2 DRUG PROFILE

1. **Metronidazole:**

Metronidazole

- Metronidazole is a synthetic 5-nitroimidazole derivative with antiprotozoal and antibacterial activities.
- It is a prodrug and is selective for anaerobic bacteria.
- It is chemically, 2-(2-methyl-5-nitroimidazol-1-yl)ethanol.
- It acts due to their ability to reduce the nitro group intra-cellularly to give nitroso-containing intermediates. These can covalently bind to DNA, disrupting its helical structure, and inhibiting bacterial nucleic acid synthesis, ultimately resulting in bacterial cell death.

Uses:

- Metronidazole has activity against anaerobic bacteria and protozoa.
- The drug possesses useful amebicidal activity and effective against both intestinal and hepatic amebiasis.
- It has also been found of use in treatment of such other protozoal diseases as giardiasis and balantidiasis.

2. **Tinidazole:**

Tinidazole

- Tinidazole is a 5-nitroimidazole derivative with antiprotozoal property.
- It is chemically, 1-(2-ethylsulfonylethyl)-2-methyl-5-nitroimidazole.
- It acts in similar way as that of metrinidazole.

Uses:

- Tinidazole is an orally available, broad spectrum antimicrobial agent used in the treatment of bacterial, protozoal and parasitic infections.

3. **Ornidazole:**

Ornidazole

- Ornidazole is a 5-nitroimidazole derivative with antiprotozoal property.
- It is chemically, 1-chloro-3-(2-methyl-5-nitroimidazol-1-yl)propan-2-ol.
- It acts in similar way as that of metrinidazole.

Uses:

- Ornidazole is used in the treatment of susceptible protozoal infections and for the treatment of anaerobic bacterial infections.
- It has a role as an antiprotozoal drug, an anti-infective agent and an antibacterial drug.

4. **Diloxanide:**

Diloxanide

- Diloxanide is prescribed in furoate salt for the treatment of asymptomatic amebiasis, but is ineffective as a single agent for the extraintestinal form of the disease.
- It is chemically, 2,2-dichloro-N-(4-hydroxyphenyl)-N-methylacetamide.

Uses:

- Diloxanide is an anti-protozoal drug used in the treatment of *Entamoeba histolytica*.
- It is also effective against acute intestinal amebiasis or hepatic abscesses.

5. **Iodoquinol:**

Iodoquinol

- Iodoquinol is a 8-hydroxyquinoline derivative with broad spectrum amebicidal activity.
- It is chemically, 5,7-diiodoquinolin-8-ol.
- The antifungal and antibacterial properties of 8-hydroxyquinoline are believed to result from the ability to chelate metal ions.

Uses:

- Iodoquinol is used in the treatment of amoebiasis.
- It is recommended for acute and chronic intestinal amebiasis, but is not effective in extra-intestinal disease.
- Because a relatively high incidence of topic neuropathy has occurred with its use, iodoquinol should not be used routinely for traveler's diarrhea.

6. Pentamidine Isethionate:

Pentamidine isethionate

- Pentamidine isethionate is a synthetic amidine derivative.
- It is chemically, 4-[5-(4-carbamimidoylphenoxy)pentoxy]benzenecarboximidamide;2-hydroxy- ethanesulfonic acid.
- It interacts with the minor groove of AT-rich DNA regions of the pathogen genome, interfering with DNA replication and function.

Uses:

- Pentamidine isethionate is an antiprotozoal and antifungal agent.
- It is also effective in the treatment of trypanosomiasis, leishmaniasis, and *Pneumocystis carinii* pneumonia in HIV-infected patients.

7. Atovaquone:

Atovaquone

- Atovaquone is a synthetic hydroxynaphthoquinone with antiprotozoal activity.
- It is chemically, 3-[4-(4-chlorophenyl)cyclohexyl]-4-hydroxynaphthalene-1,2-dione.
- It acts by blocking the mitochondrial electron transport at complex-III of the respiratory chain of protozoa, thereby inhibiting pyrimidine synthesis, preventing DNA synthesis and leading to protozoal death.

Uses:

- Atovaquone is an antiprotozoal and antifungal agent.
- It is used for the prevention and treatment of *Pneumocystis carinii* pneumonia.
- In combination with proguanil, it is used for prevention and treatment of *P. falciparum* malaria.

8. Eflornithine:

$$NH_2-CH_2-CH_2-CH_2-\underset{\underset{NH_2}{|}}{\overset{\overset{CHF_2}{|}}{C}}-COOH$$

Eflornithine

- Eflornithine is a difluoromethylated ornithine compound.
- It is chemically, 2,5-diamino-2-(difluoromethyl)pentanoic acid.
- Difluoromethylornithin, an amino acid derivative, is an enzyme activated inhibitor of ornithine decarboxylase, a pyridoxal phosphate-dependent enzyme responsible for catalyzing the rate-limiting step in the biosynthesis of the diamine putrescine and the polyamines spermine and spermidine. Polyamines are essential for the regulation of DNA synthesis and cell proliferation in animal tissues and microorganisms.

Uses:

- Eflornithine is used in the treatment of facial hirsutism (excessive hair growth).
- It also has antineoplastic activity.
- It is used for the treatment of West African sleeping sickness, caused by *Trypanosoma brucei*.
- It is a myelosuppressive drug that causes high incidences of anemia, leukopenia, and thrombocytopenia.

SYNTHESIS

1. Metronidazole:

2-methyl-imidazole $\xrightarrow{HNO_3}$ **2-methyl-5-nitroimidazole** $\xrightarrow[\text{2-chloroethanol}]{}$ **Metronidazole**

QUESTIONS

Multiple Choice Questions:

1. The side chain structure of Tinidazole is ....

   (a) $- CH_2 - CH_2 - SO_2 - C_2H_5$ (b) $- O - CH_2 - CH(OH) - CH_2 - NH - CH(CH_3)_2$

   (c) $- CH_2 - CH_2 - CH_2 - N(CH_3)_2$ (d) $- NH - CH(CH_3) - (CH_2)_3 - NH_2$

2. African sleeping sickness is caused by ....

   (a) T. Vaginalis   (b) T. Plasma condii

   (c) T. Cruzi   (d) T. gambiense

3. In Metronidazole which group alters energy yielding pathway?

   (a) OH   (b) CH_3CH_2OH

   (c) NO_2 (d) All of these

   Answers :

1. (a)	2. (c)	3. (b)

Answer the Following Questions:

1. Explain different protozoal diseases.

2. What is Amebiasis? Give its symptoms.

3. Explain different approaches to Protozoal Therapy.

4. Give synthetic route for Metronidazole.

5. Give chemical names, MOA and uses of :

   (a) Tinidazole

   (b) Ornidazole

   (c) Diloxanide

   (d) Iodoquinol

■■■

chapter ... 10

ANTHELMINTICS

♦ LEARNING OBJECTIVES ♦

After completing this sub-unit the students should be able:

- *To study different types of Helminths and infection caused by them.*
- *To study the detail classification of anthelmintics.*
- *To study the anthelmintic drugs in detail with their MOA and uses.*
- *To study the synthetic scheme of some selected anthelmintics.*

10.1 INTRODUCTION

Anthelmintics or anti-helminthics are a group of anti-parasitic drugs that expel parasitic worms (helminths) and other internal parasites from the body by either stunning or killing them without causing significant damage to the host. This includes both flat worms, e.g. flukes and tapeworms and round worms, i.e., nematodes. Parasitic worms also infect livestock and crops, affecting food production with a resultant economic impact. Also of importance is the infection of domestic pets. They are of huge importance for human tropical medicine and for veterinary medicine. They may also be called vermifuges (those that stun) or vermicides (those that kill).

Anthelmintics are used to treat people who are infected by helminths, a condition called helminthiasis. These drugs are also used to treat infected animals.

10.2 HELMINTHS

Helminths are parasitic worms that feed on a living host to gain nourishment and protection, while causing poor nutrient absorption, weakness and disease in the host. These worms and larvae live in the small bowel and are referred to as intestinal parasites.

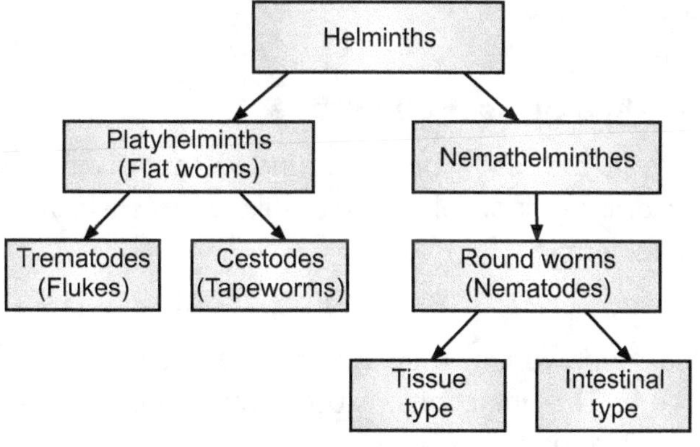

Fig. 10.1

10.2.1 Platyhelminths

They are group of soft bodied flattened invertebrates. These are found in the oceans, fresh water, and moist terrestrial habitats. The diseases caused by platyhelminths include chistosomiasis, neurocysticercosis, bladder cancer etc.

(a) Cestodes:

Cestodes (Tapeworms) are flat segmented worms that live in the intestines of some animals. Animals can be infected by these parasites when grazing in the fields. Taeniasis, seizures, anaemia and neurological problems can be caused by tapeworms.

Different types of Cestodes (Tapeworms) are,

1. *Tenia saginata* (Beef tapeworm)
2. *Tenia solium* (Pork tapeworm),
3. *Cysticercosis* (Pork tapeworm larval stage)
4. *Hymenolepis nana* (Dwarf tapeworm)
5. *Diphyllobothrium latum* (Fish tapeworm)

(b) Trematodes (Flukes):

Trematodes (Flukes), also called blood flukes belong to the invertebrate class Trematodes. They are present in almost all vertebrate classes, but most commonly fish, turtles, humans etc. Three species mainly attack humans:

(i)   Urinary blood fluke,
(ii) Intestinal blood fluke and
(iii) Oriental blood fluke

Different types of Trematodes (Flukes) are,

1. *Schistosoma mansoni*
2. *Schistosoma hematobium*
3. *Schistosoma Japonicum*
4. *Paragonimus species*
5. *Fasciolopsis buski*
6. *Fasciola hepatica*
7. *Clonorchis sinensis*

10.2.2 Nemathelminthes or Aschelminthes

They are commonly called thread worm or round worm. It is a phylum of unsegmented, triploblastic, pseudocoelomic, cylindrical or thread-like worms which are covered by a body wall having cuticle and epidermis.

Nematodes:

They are also called roundworms. They are present in every ecosystem like fresh water, soil, tropical regions etc. The infections caused by these parasites include ascariasis, trichuriasis, enterobiasis, filariasis etc.

Different types of Nematodes (Roundworms) are:

(i) Intestinal Round Worms:
1. *Ascaris lumbricoides* (common round worm)
2. *Enterobius vermicularis* (pinworm)
3. *Trichuris trichiura* (whipworm)
4. *Strongyloides stercoralis* (threadworm)
5. *Ancylostoma duodenale* and *Necator americanus* (hookworm)

(ii) Tissue Round Worms:
1. *Trichinella spiralis* (Trichinosis)
2. *Dracunculus medinensis* (guineaworm)

(iii) Filariae (Other round worms include):
1. *Wuchereria bancrofti* (filariasis)
2. *Loa loa* (loiasis)
3. *Onchocerca volvulus* (onchocerciasis) River blindness.
4. *Brugia malayi* and *Brugia timori*

10.3 CLASSIFICATION OF ANTHELMINTICS

1. **Piperazine:** Diethylcarbamazine (DEC), Piperazine Citrate
2. **Dyes:** Pyrvinium pamoate
3. **Vinyl pyrimidines:** Pyrantel pamoate
4. **Benzimidazoles:** Albendazole, Mebendazole, Thiabendazole
5. **Heterocyclics (Quinolines and Isoquinolines):** Oxaminoquine, Praziquantel
6. **Natural products:** Ivermectin , Avermectin
7. **Phenol derivatives:** Niclosamide, Bithionol
8. **Nitro derivative:** Niridazole
9. **Imidazothiazole:** Levamisole
10. **Antimonial compounds:** Antimony potassium tartrate
11. **Organophosphorus:** Metrifonate

10.4 DRUG PROFILE

10.4.1 Piperazines

1. Diethylcarbamazine Citrate:

Diethylcarbamazine citrate

- Diethylcarbamazine citrate is microfilaricidal and acts via alteration of organelle membranes of the microfilariae promoting cell death.
- It is an inhibitor of arachidonic acid metabolism in microfilariae. This makes the microfilariae more susceptible to innate immune attack.
- It is chemically, N,N-diethyl-4-methylpiperazine-1-carboxamide;2-hydroxypropane-1,2,3-tricarboxylic acid.

Uses:

- Diethylcarbamazine citrate is the first drug for filariasis caused by the nematodes *Wuchereria bancrofti*.

10.4.2 Benzimidazoles

1. Thiabendazole:

Thiabendazole

- Thiabendazole is a benzimidazole derivative with anthelminthic property.
- It is chemically, 4-(1H-benzimidazol-2-yl)-1,3-thiazole.
- Thiabendazole inhibits the helminth-specific mitochondrial enzyme fumarate reductase, thereby inhibiting the citric acid cycle, mitochondrial respiration and subsequent production of ATP, ultimately leading to helminth's death.
- It may also lead to inhibition of microtubule polymerization by binding to β-tubulin and has an overt ovicidal effect with regard to some trichostrongylids.

Uses:

- Thiabendazole is active against a variety of nematodes and is the drug of choice for strongyloidiasis.
- It is a fungicide and parasiticide.
- It is a chelating agent, which means that it is used medicinally to bind metals in cases of metal poisoning, such as lead poisoning, mercury poisoning or antimony poisoning.
- It also suppresses egg and/or larval production and may inhibit the subsequent development of those eggs or larvae which are passed in the feces.
- It is also used as a postharvest treatment for bananas, plantains and oranges.

2. Mebendazole:

Mebendazole

- Mebendazole is a synthetic benzimidazole derivate and anthelmintic agent.
- It is chemically, methyl N-(6-benzoyl-1H-benzimidazol-2-yl)carbamate.

- It works by selectively inhibiting the synthesis of microtubules via binding to colchicine binding site of β-tubulin, thereby blocking polymeration of tubulin dimers in intestinal cells of parasites.
- Disruption of cytoplasmic microtubules leads to block the uptake of glucose and other nutrients, resulting in the gradual immobilization and eventual death of the helminths.

Uses:

- Mebendazole is a broad-spectrum antihelmintic agent used commonly for roundworm (pinworm and hookworm) infections.
- It is also effective and indicated for the treatment of whipworm, threadworm, pinworm, and the intestinal form of trichinosis prior to its spread into the tissues beyond the digestive tract.

3. Albendazole:

Albendazole

- Albendazole is a broad-spectrum, synthetic benzimidazole-derivative anthelmintic.
- It is chemically, methyl N-(6-propylsulfanyl-1H-benzimidazol-2-yl)carbamate.
- It interferes with the reproduction and survival of helminths by inhibiting the formation of microtubules from tubulin. This leads to an impaired uptake of glucose, a depletion of glycogen stores, and results in the worm's death.

Uses:

- Albendazole is used in the treatment of echinococcosis, a parasitic worm that causes cysts in liver and lung.
- It is used in the treatment of dog and pork tapeworm-causing diseases, including hydatid disease and neurocysticercosis.
- It is also used to treat a variety of other roundworm infections.

4. Niclosamide:

Niclosamide

- Niclosamide is an orally bioavailable chlorinated salicylanilide, with anthelmintic activity.
- It is chemically, 5-chloro-N-(2-chloro-4-nitrophenyl)-2-hydroxybenzamide.

- It acts by inducing degradation of the androgen receptor through the proteasome-mediated pathway.

Uses:

- Niclosamide is used for the treatment of most tapeworm infections.

5. Oxamniquine:

Oxamniquine

- Oxamniquine is an anthelmintic with schistosomicidal activity against *Schistosoma mansoni,* but not against other Schistosoma spp.
- It is chemically [7-nitro-2-[((propan-2-yl-amino)methyl]-1,2,3,4-tetrahydroquinolin-6-yl]methanol.
- It causes worms to shift from the mesenteric veins to the liver where the male worms are retained; the female worms return to the mesentery, but can no longer release eggs.

Uses:

- Oxamniquine is used for treatment of schistosomiasis.

6. Praziquantal:

Praziquantal

- Praziquantal is a pyrazinoisoquinoline derivative with anthelminthic property.
- It is chemically, 2-(cyclohexanecarbonyl)-3,6,7,11b-tetrahydro-1H-pyrazino[2,1-a] isoquinolin -4-one.
- It increases the permeability of the tegument of susceptible worms, resulting in an influx and increase in intra-tegumental calcium leading to rapid contractions and paralysis of the worm's musculature through a subsequent increase in levels of calcium in the sarcoplasmic reticulum.
- In addition, vacuolization of the tegumental syncytium and blebbing results in tegument disintegration, leads to antigen exposure and elicit host defense responses to the worm. The result is the formation of granulomas and phagocytosis.

Uses:

- Praziquantel is an antihelmintic agent with activity against a broad spectrum of trematodes and cestodes.
- It is also used predominantly in the therapy of schistosomiasis, liver flukes, and cysticercosis.

7. Ivermectin:

Ivermectin

- Ivermectin is a macrocyclic lactone derived from *Streptomyces avermitilis* with antiparasitic activity.
- It exerts its anthelmintic effect via activating glutamate-gated chloride channels expressed on nematode neurons and pharyngeal muscle cells.
- Ivermectin-activated channels open very slowly, but essentially irreversibly. As a result, neurons or muscle cells remain at either hyperpolarisation or depolarization state, thereby resulting in paralysis and death of the parasites.
- Ivermectin does not readily pass the mammal blood-brain barrier to the central nervous system where glutamate-gated chloride channels locate, hence the hosts are relatively resistant to the effects of this agent.

Uses:

- Ivermectin is used to treat many types of parasite infestations. This includes head lice, scabies, river blindness (onchocerciasis), strongyloidiasis, trichuriasis, and lymphatic filariasis.

SYNTHESIS

1. Diethylcarbamazine Citrate:

Diethylcarbamoyl chloride   **1-methyl-piperazine**   **Diethylcarbamazine**

2. Mebendazole:

4-Chloro-3-nitro benzophenone + NH_4OH → (Sulpholane; CH_3OH; 125°C for 24 Hrs.) → 4-Amino-3-nitro-benzophenone

4-Amino-3-nitro-benzophenone + HCl + H_2 [Pd-on-Charcoal] as catalyst → Diaminobenzophenone hydrochloride · HCl

Diaminobenzophenone hydrochloride + H_3CS—(S-Methyl thiourea, NH_2, NH) / $HClCOOCH_3$ Methyl chloroformate (0 – 5°C) → Mebendazole

Mebendazole structure: $—NH—\overset{O}{\overset{\|}{C}}—OCH_3$

QUESTIONS

Multiple Choice Questions:

1. The essential structural unit for the anthelmintic activity of mebendazole is ....
   (a) Benzyl group   (b) Benzimidazole
   (c) Methylcarbamate   (d) Imidazole
2. The essential structural unit for the anthelmintic activity of Mebendazole is ....
   (a) Benzoyl group   (b) Benzimidazole
   (c) Methylcarbamate   (d) Imidazole
3. Piperazine citrate is used as ....
   (a) Anthelmintic   (b) Amoebicidal
   (c) Antimalarial   (d) Metabolite antagonist

Answers :

1. (d)	2. (c)	3. (a)

Answer the Following Questions:

1. Give a brief account on Anthelmintics with suitable examples.
2. How would you classify Anthelmintics on the basis of chemical structures? Give suitable examples.
3. Describe the synthesis, uses and mechanism of action of Mebendazole.
4. What is Invermectin? Discuss its mechanism of action.
5. Classify Helminths with suitable examples.
6. How would you synthesize the following drugs?
   (a) Diethylcarbamazine citrate, (b) Mebendazole
7. Give the structures, chemical names and the uses of :
   (a) Albendazole, (b) Thiabendazole, (c) Oxamniquine, (d) Diethylcarbamazine citrate.
8. Classify anthelmintics with suitable examples.   ∎∎∎

chapter ... 11

SULPHONAMIDES AND SULPHONES

♦ LEARNING OBJECTIVES ♦

After completing this sub-unit the students should be able:

- *To study definition and history of sulphonamide drugs.*
- *To study mode of action and SAR of sulphonamides.*
- *To study detail classification of sulphonamides with examples.*
- *To study various sulphonamide drugs with their MOA and uses.*
- *To study Folate reductase inhibitor drugs.*
- *To study different sulphone drugs with their MOA and uses.*
- *To learn the synthetic scheme of some selective sulphonamides.*

11.1 INTRODUCTION

The term sulphonamides are employed as a generic name for the derivatives of para amino benzene sulphonamide (sulphanilamide). The sulphonamide drugs were the first effective chemotherapeutic agents to be employed systemically for the prevention and treatment of bacterial infections in humans. The sulphonamides are bacteriostatic antibiotics with a wide spectrum action against most Gram-positive bacteria and many Gram-negative organisms.

11.2 HISTORY OF SULPHA DRUGS

Sulphanilamide, was first synthesized by Gelmo in 1908 as an intermediate in the study of azo dyes. Surprisingly it was many years before its therapeutic value was actually ascertained. Gerhard Domagk in 1935 screened a number of these azo-dyes for their antibacterial effects and observed that they were active against *streptococci*.

In 1935, a German firm prepared a red dye 4-sulphonamide-2', 4'-diamino-benzene or *p'*-sulphonyl chrysoidine, and after three years Domagk suggested significant curative properties of this compound and named it *Prontosil*. Actually it was found to be the metabolic product of Prontosil, which is responsible for antibacterial activity, and this has given the initiation to develop sulphonamides as antibacterial agents.

$$H_2N-\text{⟨benzene⟩}(NH_2)-N=N-\text{⟨benzene⟩}-SO_2NH_2 \longrightarrow H_2N-\text{⟨benzene⟩}-SO_2NH_2$$

Prontosil → **Sulphanilamide**

Fuller (1937) further substantiated and confirmed by isolating 'free sulphonamide' from the blood and urine of subjects being treated with Prontosil. In 1937, two British researchers prepared 'sulphapyridine' that was indeed the first and foremost structural analogue of 'sulphanilamide'. This particular compound proved to be a grand and tremendous success in curing pneumonia. This magnificent discovery, in fact, paved the flood gates for the synthesis and screening of hundreds of derivatives of sulphanilamide, but only a few have retained the glory of being potent medicinal compounds.

Sulphonamides are selective drugs used to treat urinary tract infections, bacterial respiratory infections, and gastrointestinal (GI) infections.

11.3 MODE OF ACTION

Sulphonamides are structure analogues and competitive antagonists of Para-Amino Benzoic Acid (PABA). They compete with PABA for the bacterial enzyme dihydropteroate synthase, thereby preventing the incorporation of PABA into dihydrofolic acid, the immediate precursor of folic acid. This leads to an inhibition of bacterial folic acid synthesis and *de novo* synthesis of purines and pyrimidines, ultimately resulting in cell growth arrest and cell death.

Synergistic effect is obtained by a combination of trimethoprim. The compound trimethoprim is a potent and selective inhibitor of microbial dihydrofolate reductase, the enzyme that reduces dihydrofolate to tetrahydrofolate. The simultaneous administration of sulphonamide and trimethoprim blocks the pathway of cell-wall synthesis sequentially.

Uses and Spectrum of Action of the Sulphonamide:

Sulphonamides inhibit Gram-positive and Gram-negative bacteria, nocardia, *Chlamydia trachomotitis* and some protozoa. They also inhibit some enteric bacteria, such as *E.coli* and *Klebsiella, Salmonella, Shigella* and *Enterobacter* spp. They are infrequently used as single agents and useful in some urinary tract infections because of their high excretion fraction through the kidney.

Despite the tremendous ability of sulphanilamide to effect cures of pathogenic bacteria, its benefits were often offset by the propensity of the drug to cause severe renal damage by crystallizing in the kidneys (crystalluria).

11.4 STRUCTURE ACTIVITY RELATIONSHIP OF SULPHONAMIDES

$$H_2N \underset{4}{-} \overset{5\quad 6}{\underset{3\quad 2}{\bigcirc}} \underset{1}{-} SO_2NHR$$

The major features of SAR of sulphonamides include the following:

1. Sulphanilamide skeleton is the minimum structural requirement for antibacterial activity.

2. The amino and sulphonyl groups on the benzene ring are essential and should be in 1 and 4 position.

3. The N-4 amino group could be modified to be prodrugs, which are converted to free amino function *in-vivo*.

4. Sulphur atom should be directly linked to the benzene ring.

5. Replacement of benzene ring by other ring systems or the introduction of additional substituents on it decreases or abolishes its activity.

6. Exchange of the $-SO_2NH$ group by $-CONH$ reduces the activity.

7. On N-1-substituted sulphonamides, activity varies with the nature of the substituent at the amino group. With substituents imparting electron rich characters to SO_2 group, bacteriostatic activity increases.

8. Heterocyclic substituents lead to highly potent derivatives, while sulphonamides, which contain a single benzene ring at N-1 position, are considerably more toxic than heterocyclic ring analogues.

9. The free aromatic amino groups should reside para to the sulphonamide group. Its replacement at ortho or meta position results in compounds devoid of antibacterial activity.

10. The active form of sulphonamide is the ionized, maximum activity that is observed between the pKa values 6.6 - 7.4.

11. Substitutions in the benzene ring of sulphonamides produce inactive compounds.

12. Substitution of free sulphonic acid $(-SO_3H)$ group for sulphonamido function destroys the activity, but replacement by a sulphinic acid group $(-SO_2H)$ and acetylation of N-4 position retains back the activity.

11.5 CLASSIFICATION OF SULPHONAMIDES

Sulphonamides can be classified in various ways:

(A) On the basis of the Site of Action:

- **Sulphonamides for general infection:** Sulphanilamide, Sulphapyridine, Sulphadiazine, Sulphamethoxacine, Sulphamethoxazole.

- **Sulphonamides for urinary tract infections:** Sulphisoxazole, Sulphathiazole.

- **Sulphonamides for intestinal infections:** Phthalylsulphathiazole, Succinyl sulphathiazole, Sulphasalazine.

- **Sulphonamides for local infections:** Sulphacetamide, Mafenide, Silver sulphadiazine.

- **Sulphonamides for dermatitis:** Dapsone, Solapsone.

- **Sulphonamides in combination:** Trimethoprim with Sulphamethoxazole.

(B) On the basis of the Pharmacokinetic Properties:

- **Poorly absorbed sulphonamides (locally acting sulphonamides):** Sulphasalazine, Phthalylsulphathiazole, Sulphaguanidine, Salicylazosulphapyridine, Succinyl sulpha-thiazole.

- **Rapidly absorbed and rapidly excreted (systemic sulphanamides):** Sulpha-methoxazole, Sulphisoxazole, Sulphadiazine, Sulphadimidine, Sulphafurazole, Sulphasomidine, Sulphamethiazole, Sulphacetamide, Sulphachlorpyridazine.

- **Topically used sulphonamides:** Sulphacetamide, Mafenide, Sulphathiazole, Silver sulphadiazine.

(C) On the basis of the Pharamacological Activity:

- **Antibacterial agents:** Sulphadiazine, Sulfisoxazole.

- **Drugs used in dermatitis:** Dapsone.

(D) On the basis of the Duration of Action:

- **Extra long-acting sulphonamides (half-life greater than 50 hours):** Sulphasalazine, Sulphaclomide, Sulphalene.

- **Long-acting sulphonamides (half-life greater than 24 hours):** Sulphadoxine, Sulphadimethoxine, Sulphamethoxy pyridazine, Sulphamethoxydiazine, Sulpha-phenazole, Sulphamethoxine.

- **Intermediate-acting sulphonamides (half-life between 10–24 hours):** Sulphasomizole, Sulphamethoxazole.

- **Short-acting sulphonamides (half-life less than 20 hours):** Sulphamethiazole, Sulphisoxazole.

- **Injectables (soluble sulpha drugs):** Sulphafurazole, Sulphadiazine, Sulpha-methoxine.

(E) On the basis of the Chemical Structure:

- **N-1 substituted sulphonamides:** Sulphamethizole, Sulphisoxazole, Sulphamethoxaole, Sulphadiazine, Sulphacetamide, Sulphapyridine, Sulphamethazine (Sulphadimidine).

- **N-4 substituted sulphonamides (prodrugs):** Prontosil.

- **Both N-1 and N-4 substituted sulphonamides:** Sulphasalazine, Succinyl sulpha-thiazole, Phthalylsulphathiazole.

- **Miscellaneous:** Mefenide sodium.

11.6 DRUG PROFILE

1. Sulphamethizole:

Sulphamethizole

- Sulphamethizole is a broad-spectrum sulphanilamide and a synthetic analog of para-aminobenzoic acid (PABA) with antibacterial property.
- It is chemically, 4-amino-N-(5-methyl-1,3,4-thiadiazol-2-yl)benzenesulphonamide.
- It has the general properties and mode of action of sulphonamides

Uses:

- Sulphamethizole is employed in the treatment of coliform infections of the urinary tract.

2. Sulphisoxazole:

Sulphisoxazole

- Sulphisoxazole is a broad-spectrum, short-acting sulphanilamide and a synthetic analog of para-aminobenzoic acid (PABA) with antibacterial property.
- It is chemically, 4-amino-N-(3,4-dimethyl-1,2-oxazol-5-yl)benzenesulphonamide.
- It has the general properties and mode of action of sulphonamides.

Uses:

- Sulphisoxazole acts against a wide range of Gram-negative and Gram-positive organisms.
- It is used in the treatment of urinary tract infections.

3. Sulphamethazine (Sulphadimidine):

Sulphamethazine

- Sulphamethazine is a sulphonamide consisting of pyrimidine with methyl substituents at the 4- and 6-positions and a 4-aminobenzenesulphonamido group at the 2-position.
- It is chemically, 4-amino-N-(4,6-dimethylpyrimidin-2-yl)benzenesulphonamide.
- It has the general properties and mode of action of sulphonamides.

Uses:

- Sulphamethazine acts as an anti-infective agent, a carcinogenic agent, a ligand, an antibacterial drug and an antimicrobial agent.
- It is less effective in meningeal infection because of its poor penetration into the cerebrospinal fluid.

4. Sulphacetamide:

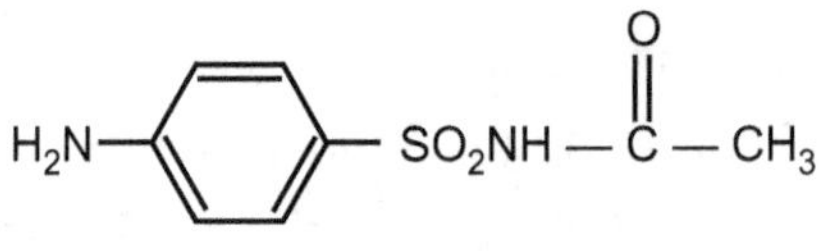

$$H_2N-\text{C}_6H_4-SO_2NH-\overset{\overset{\displaystyle O}{\|}}{C}-CH_3$$

Sulphacetamide

- Sulphacetamide is a broad spectrum synthetic sulphanylacetamide derivative with bacteriostatic activity.
- It is chemically, N-(4-aminophenyl)sulphonylacetamide.
- It has the general properties and mode of action of sulphonamides.

Uses:

- Sulphacetamide has a role as an antimicrobial agent, an anti-infective agent, dihydropteroate synthase inhibitor and an antibacterial drug.
- It is used as an anti-infective topical agent to treat skin infections and as an oral agent for urinary tract infections.

5. Sulphapyridine:

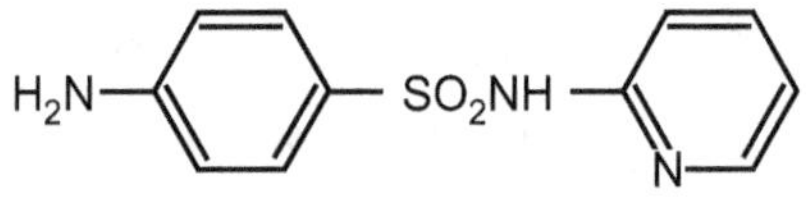

$$H_2N-\text{C}_6H_4-SO_2NH-\text{(pyridin-2-yl)}$$

Sulphapyridine

- Sulphapyridine is a short-acting sulphonamide, consisting of pyridine with a 4-aminobenzenesulphonamido group at the 2-position.
- It is also by-product of the non-steroidal anti-inflammatory drug sulphasalazine.
- It is chemically, 4-amino-N-pyridin-2-yl-benzenesulphonamide.
- It has the general properties and mode of action of sulphonamides.

Uses:

- Sulphapyridine acts as an anti-infective agent, a dermatologic drug, a xenobiotic, an environmental contaminant and a drug allergen.
- It is mainly used in the treatment of dermatitis herpetiformis for such patients who do not give positive response to dapsone.
- It is also effective in pneumonia.
- Though it is more potent than sulphanilamide, it is more toxic and has been replaced by sulphadiazine.

6. Sulphamethoxazole:

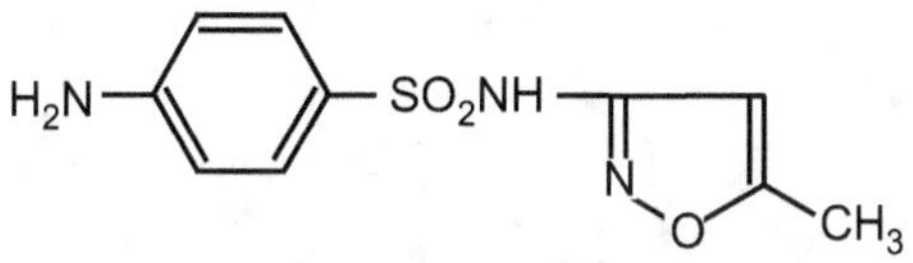

Sulphamethoxazole

- Sulphamethoxazole is a sulphonamide bacteriostatic antibiotic that is most commonly used in combination with trimethoprim as the drug "Bactrim".

- It is an isoxazole (1,2-oxazole) compound having a methyl substituent at the 5-position and a 4-aminobenzenesulphonamido group at the 3-position.

- It is chemically, 4-amino-N-(5-methyl-1,2-oxazol-3-yl)benzenesulphonamide.

- It has the general properties and mode of action of sulphonamides.

Uses:

- Sulphamethoxazole is used in the treatment of bacterial infections.

- It has a role as an antibacterial agent, an anti-infective agent, an antimicrobial agent, an environmental contaminant, a xenobiotic and a drug allergen.

7. Sulphadiazine:

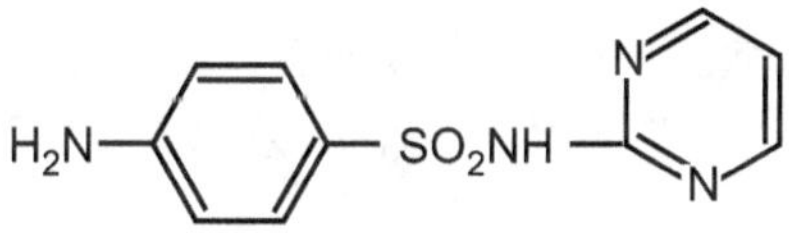

Sulphadiazine

- Sulphadiazine is a synthetic pyrimidinyl sulfonamide derivative with short-acting bacteriostatic activity.

- It is a sulphonamide consisting of pyrimidine with a 4-aminobenzenesulphonamido group at the 2-position.

- It is chemically, 4-amino-N-pyrimidin-2-yl-benzenesulphonamide.

- It has the general properties and mode of action of sulphonamides.

Uses:

- Sulphadiazine is used in the therapy of mild-to-moderate infections due to sensitive organisms.

- It has a role as an antimicrobial agent, an anti-infective agent, an antiprotozoal drug, a xenobiotic, an environmental contaminant and a drug allergen.

- It is also used in the treatment of canceroids and rheumatic fever.

- It is used in combination with pyrimethamine to treat toxoplasmosis in patients with acquired immunodeficiency syndrome and in newborns with congenital infections.

8. Mefenide Acetate:

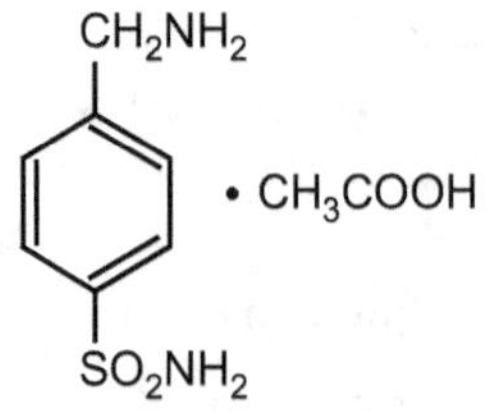

$$CH_2NH_2$$ — (benzene ring) — SO_2NH_2 · CH_3COOH

Mefenide Acetate

- Mefenide acetate is a homologue of the sulphanilamide molecule.
- It is chemically, acetic acid; 4-(aminomethyl)benzenesulphonamide.
- It is not a true sulphonamide as it is not inhibited by PABA.
- Its antibacterial action involves a mechanism that differs from that of true suphonamide-type compounds.

Uses:

- Mafenide acetate is bacteriostatic against many Gram-negative and Gram-positive organisms, including *Pseudomonas aeruginosa* and certain strains of anaerobes.
- It is used alone or with antibiotics in the treatment of infected wounds.
- It is used in the treatment and cure of gas gangrene.
- It is also effective against *Clostridium welchii* on topical application.

9. Sulphasalazine:

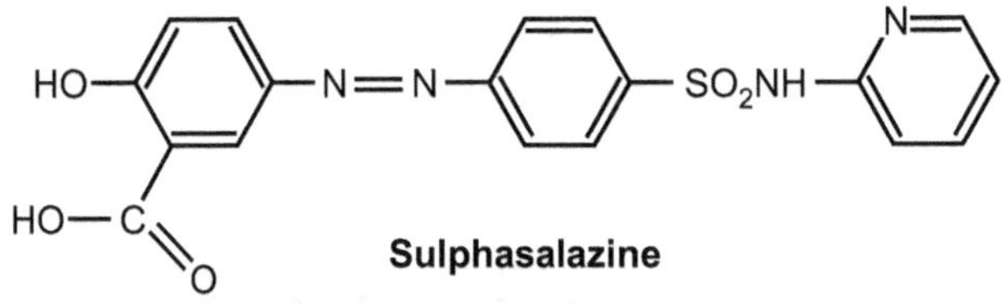

Sulphasalazine

- Sulphasalazine undergoes reductive metabolism by gut bacteria, converting the drug into sulphapyridine and 5-amino salicylic acid, which are active components.
- It is chemically, 2-hydroxy-5-[[4-(pyridin-2-yl-sulphamoyl)phenyl]diazenyl]benzoic acid.
- The metabolite (sulfphapyridine) has mode of action of sulphonamides.

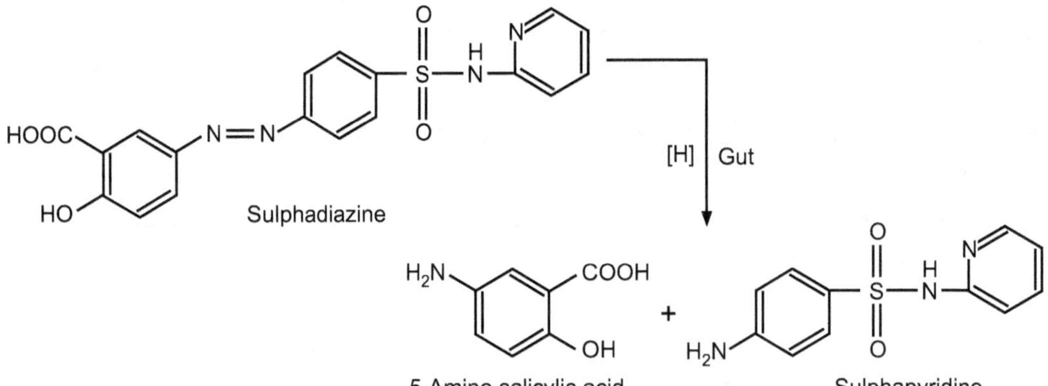

Sulphadiazine

[H] | Gut

5-Amino salicylic acid
(Mesalamine)

Sulphapyridine

Uses:

- Sulphasalazine has a role as a non-steroidal anti-inflammatory drug, an anti-infective agent, a gastrointestinal drug, and a drug allergen.

- It is an anti-inflammatory agent used extensively in chronic, long term therapy of inflammatory bowel disease.

- It is used in the treatment of ulcerative colitis.

11.7 FOLATE REDUCTASE INHIBITORS

A dihydrofolate reductase inhibitor (DHFR inhibitor) is a molecule that inhibits the function of dihydrofolate reductase enzyme which carries out the conversion of dihydrofolate to tetrahydrofolate leading to the inhibition of DNA synthesis and cell growth.

Dihydrofolate reductase is present in mammalian cells as well as bacterial cells, but mutation over millions of year have resulted in a significant difference in structure between the two enzymes such that trimethoprim recognized and inhibits the bacterial enzyme more strongly. In fact, trimethoprim is 100000 times more active against the bacterial enzyme.

11.7.1 Drug Profile

1. Trimethoprim:

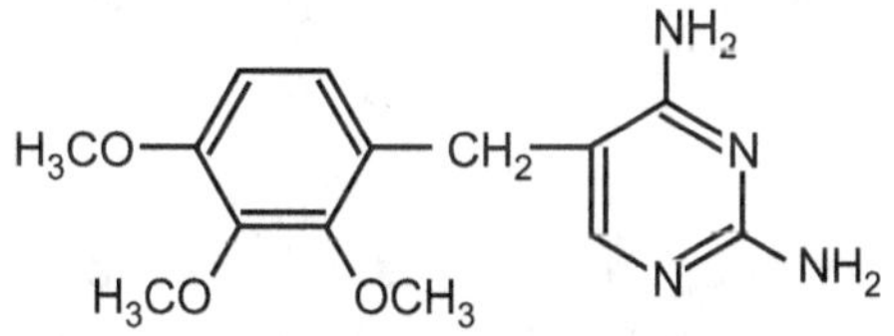

Trimethoprim

- Trimethoprim is a synthetic derivative of trimethoxybenzyl-pyrimidine with anti-bacterial and antiprotozoal properties.

- It is chemically, 5-[(3,4,5-trimethoxyphenyl)methyl]pyrimidine-2,4-diamine.

- It is an inhibitor of bacterial dihydrofolate reductase. It binds tightly to the bacterial enzyme, blocking the production of tetrahydrofolic acid from dihydrofolic acid.

- The antibacterial activity of this agent is potentiated by sulphonamides.

Uses:

- Trimethoprim is used only for the treatment of uncomplicated urinary tract infections.

2. Co-trimoxazole:

- Co-trimoxazole is an antibacterial drug composed of two active principles, sulphamethoxazole and trimethoprim.

- Co-trimoxazole is generally bactericidal; it acts by sequential blockade of folic acid enzymes in the synthesis pathway.

- The sulphamethoxazole component inhibits formation of dihydrofolic acid from para-aminobenzoic (PABA), whereas trimethoprim inhibits dihydrofolate reductase.

- It consists of 1 part trimethoprim to 5 parts sulphamethoxazole. It can be given by mouth or intravenously.

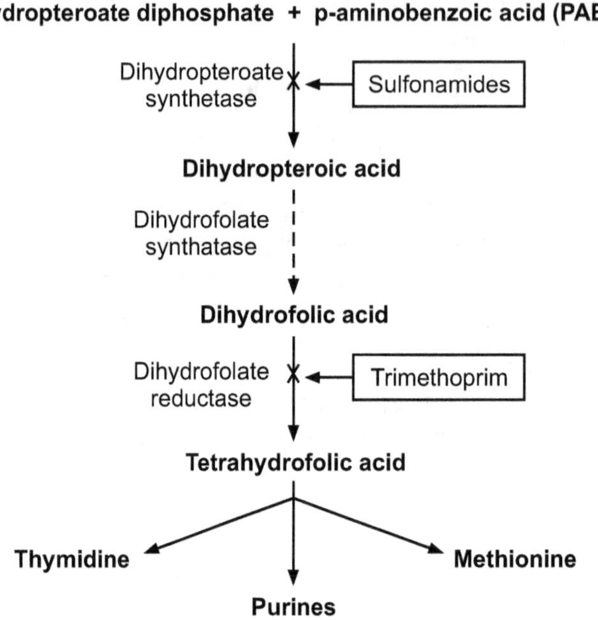

Uses:

- Co-trimoxazole (Trimethoprim with sulphamethoxazole) is a fixed antibiotic combination (*synergistic action*) that is widely used for mild-to-moderate bacterial infections and as prophylaxis against opportunistic infections.

- It is a drug combination with broad-spectrum antibacterial activity against both Gram-positive and Gram-negative organisms.

- It is used for urinary tract infections, methicillin resistant *Staphylococcus aureus* skin infections, travelers' diarrhea, respiratory tract infections, and cholera.

- It may be used both to treat and prevent *pneumocystis pneumonia* and toxoplasmosis in people with HIV/AIDS.

11.8 SULPHONES

A large number of diphenylsulphone analogues have been developed for the treatment of leprosy. Incidentally one such member chemically known as 4, 4'-diaminodiphenyl sulphone (dapsone) exhibited prophylactic activity against resistant *P. falciparum*.

Dapsone in conjunction with pyrimethamine has been effectively used in the treatment of malaria due to chloroquine resistant *P. falciparum*. Its mechanism of action is very much similar to that of sulphanilamide. It is employed profusely in the treatment of both *lepromatous* and *tuberculoid* types of leprosy. However, in combination with rifampin, it is regarded as the 'drug of choice' in the chemotherapy of leprosy. Besides, the combination with clofazimine affords a similar therapeutic effect.

The 'drug' is the most preferred 'sulphone' because of the two cardinal facts, such as:

(a) cost-effective; and

(b) equally efficacious to other sulphones.

Interestingly, when combined with trimethoprim, it is found to exert almost identical activity as trimethoprim-sulfamethoxazole in the plausible treatment of *Pneumocystis carinii* pneumonia. Also used with pyrimethamine for treatment of malaria.

11.8.1 Drug Profile

1. Dapsone:

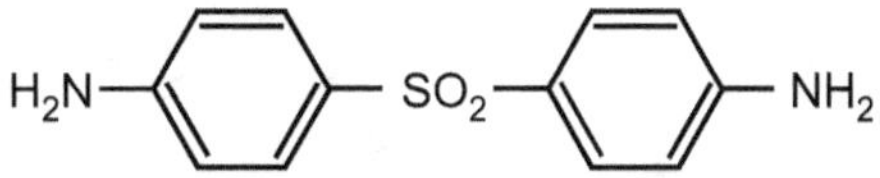

$$H_2N - \text{C}_6H_4 - SO_2 - \text{C}_6H_4 - NH_2$$

Dapsone

- Dapsone is a synthetic derivative of diamino-sulphone with anti-bacterial and anti-inflammatory properties.

- It is chemically, 4-(4-aminophenyl)sulphonylaniline.

- It has the general properties and mode of action of sulphonamides.

- It is active against a wide range of bacteria, but is mainly employed for its actions against *Mycobacterium leprae.*

Uses:

- Dapsone is used as folic acid synthesis inhibitor in the treatment of leprosy and nocardiosis.

- It also has a role as an antimalarial, an anti-infective agent and an anti-inflammatory drug.

SYNTHESIS

1. Sulphacetamide:

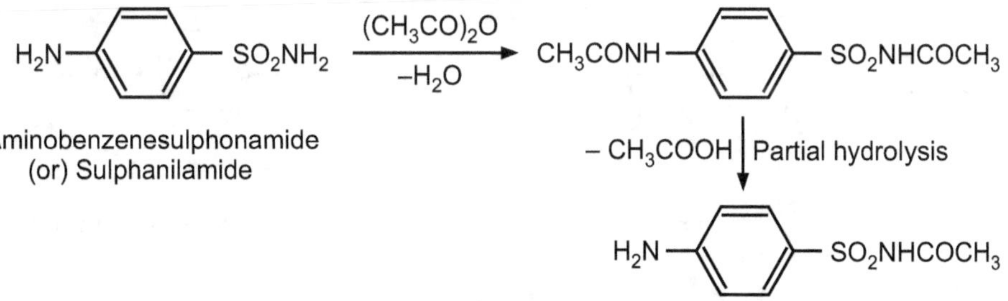

$$H_2N - \text{C}_6H_4 - SO_2NH_2 \xrightarrow[-H_2O]{(CH_3CO)_2O} CH_3CONH - \text{C}_6H_4 - SO_2NHCOCH_3$$

4-Aminobenzenesulphonamide
(or) Sulphanilamide

$$- CH_3COOH \downarrow \text{Partial hydrolysis}$$

$$H_2N - \text{C}_6H_4 - SO_2NHCOCH_3$$

Sulphacetamide

2. Sulphamethoxazole:

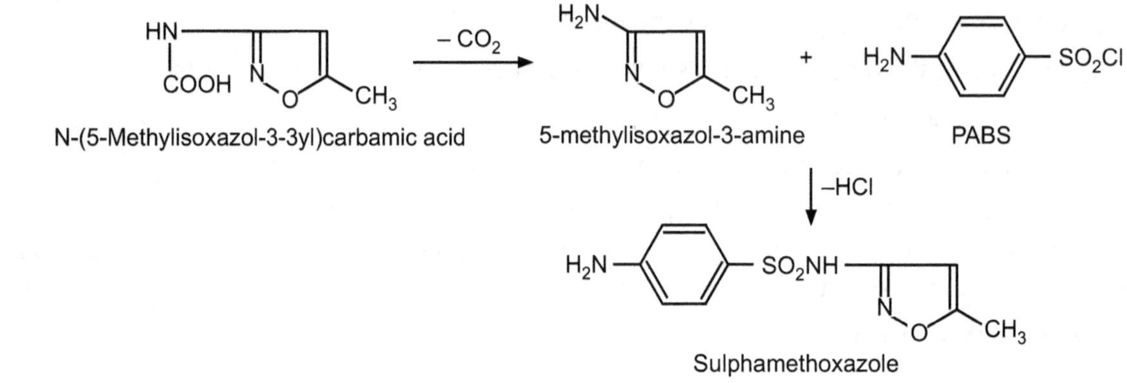
HN
COOH
N
O
CH3
– CO2
H2N
N
O
CH3
+
H2N
SO2Cl
N-(5-Methylisoxazol-3-3yl)carbamic acid
5-methylisoxazol-3-amine
PABS
–HCl
H2N
SO2NH
N
O
CH3
Sulphamethoxazole

3. Trimethoprim:

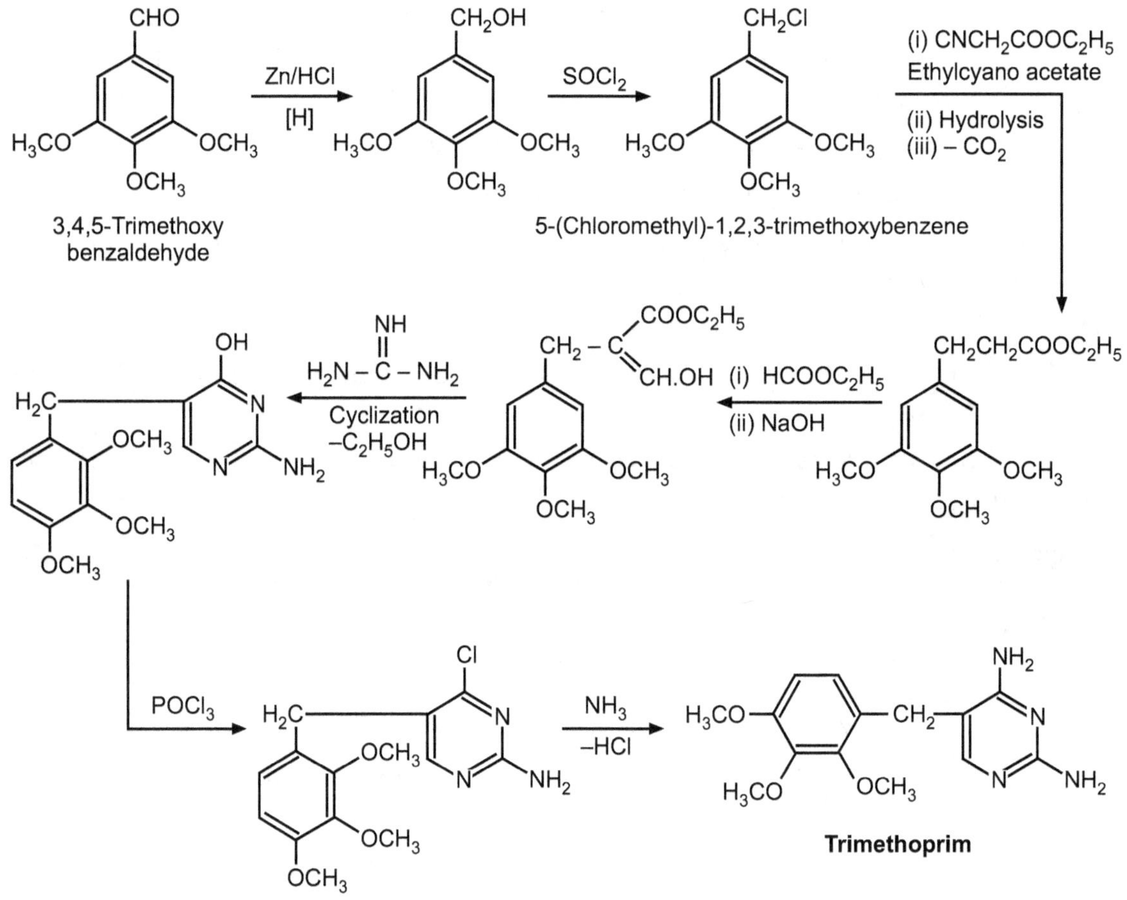
CHO
H3CO
OCH3
OCH3
Zn/HCl
[H]
CH2OH
SOCl2
CH2Cl
(i) CNCH2COOC2H5
Ethylcyano acetate
(ii) Hydrolysis
(iii) – CO2
3,4,5-Trimethoxy benzaldehyde
5-(Chloromethyl)-1,2,3-trimethoxybenzene
CH2CH2COOC2H5
(i) HCOOC2H5
(ii) NaOH
COOC2H5
CH2 – C
CH.OH
NH
H2N – C – NH2
Cyclization
–C2H5OH
OH
H2C
N
N
NH2
POCl3
Cl
NH3
–HCl
CH2
NH2
Trimethoprim

4. Dapsone:

O_2N—⟨benzene⟩—Cl + Na_2S + Cl—⟨benzene⟩—NO_2

1-Chloro-4-nitrobenzene   1-Chloro-4-nitrobenzene

$\xrightarrow[\text{Condensation}]{-2\ NaCl}$

O_2N—⟨benzene⟩—SO_2—⟨benzene⟩—NO_2 $\xleftarrow[\text{Chromic acid}]{(O)}$ O_2N—⟨benzene⟩—S—⟨benzene⟩—NO_2

bis (4-nitrophenyl)sulphane

(H) | Sn/HCl

H_2N—⟨benzene⟩—SO_2—⟨benzene⟩—NH_2

Dapsone

SYNTHESIS

Multiple Choice Questions:

1. Sulphasalazine is a prodrug that is activated in the instestine by bacterial enzyme. The enzyme responsible is ....

    (a) Azo reductase   (b) Cholinesterase

    (c) Gluconyl transferase   (d) Amylase

2. Sulpha drugs can be conveniently estimated using the reagent ....

    (a) 4,4-Dithibis-(2-nitrobenzoic acid)

    (b) Tris-(hydroxyl methyl) amino-methane sodium nitrate

    (c) N-(1-naphthyl) ethylenediamine

    (d) N-ethylacidamide

3. Sulphonamide tragedy was due to its combination with ....

    (a) Penicillin   (b) Streptomycin

    (c) Diethylene glycol   (d) Bicarbonate

4. Sulphonamides block the synthesis of ....

    (a) PABA   (b) DFA

    (c) DHFA   (d) TFA

5. Which of the following statement refers is true?

    (a) Sulphanilamide is soluble in water.

    (b) Sulphonamides are retained in urine before excretion.

    (c) The terminal amino function is not required for activity.

    (d) Sulphonamides are useful for antitubercular therapy.

6. Sulphonamide is structurally similar to ………
    (a) Para amino benzoic acid   (b) Para amino salicylic acid
    (c) Para amino piperonic acid   (d) Benzoic acid

7. Sulphacetamide synthesized from ………
    (a) Sulphonamide   (b) Sulphanilamide
    (c) Benzoic acid   (d) Sulphonyl chloride

8. Example for a N_1 and N_4 - substituted sulphonamides is ………
    (a) succinyl sulphathiazole   (b) sulphacetamide
    (c) sulphadiazine   (d) sulphanilamide

9. Topically used sulphonamide is ………
    (a) Sulphadoxine   (b) Sulphamethoxazol
    (c) Silver sulphadiazine   (d) Dapsone

10. Dapsone is used primarily for the treatment of ………
    (a) Tuberculosis   (b) Leprosy
    (c) Malaria   (d) Urinary tract infection

Answers :

1. (a)	2. (c)	3. (c)	4. (a)	5. (b)	6. (a)	7. (b)	8. (a)	9. (c)	10. (b)

Answer the Following Questions:

1. Classify sulphonamides on the basis of their site of action. Give the structure, chemical names and uses of one potent drug of each class.

2. Give the structures and IUPAC names of:
    (a) Sulphapyridine, (b) Sulphathiazole, (c) Sulphadiazine, (d) Dapsone.

3. How would you synthesize the following drugs?
    (a) Sulphacetamide, (b) Sulphamethoxazole, (c) Trimethoprim, (d) Dapsone.

4. Give the structures, chemical names and the uses of:
    (a) Sulphisoxazole, (b) Mefenide acetate, (c) Sulphasalazine., (d) Sulphamethizole.

5. Name the members of sulphonamides used in chemotherapy of leprosy. Discuss the synthesis of that compound.

6. Give an account of the 'mode of action of sulphonamides' with suitable examples.

7. Write in short history of sulphonamide drugs.

8. Give in brief structure activity relationship of sulphonamides.

9. Classify sulphonamides on the basis of the site of action with suitable examples.

10. Classify sulphonamides on the basis of the duration of action and chemical structure.

11. Write a brief note on Co-trimoxazole.

■■■

Unit-V

chapter ... 12

INTRODUCTION TO DRUG DESIGN AND COMBINATORIAL CHEMISTRY

♦ LEARNING OBJECTIVES ♦

After completing this sub-unit the students should be able:

- *To understand the importance of drug design and different techniques of drug design.*
- *To study the chemistry of drugs with respect to their biological activity.*
- *To study the physicochemical parameters used in Quantitative Structure Activity Relationship (QSAR) such as partition coefficient, Hammet's electronic parameter, Tafts steric parameter*
- *To know the importance of SAR of drugs. Various approaches used in drug design.*
- *To understand Prodrug concept and Computer Aided Drug Design (CADD).*
- *To study pharmacophore modeling and docking techniques.*
- *To study the concept of combinatorial chemistry and its application.*

12.1 INTRODUCTION TO DRUG DESIGN

One of the most important challenges that medicinal chemists face today is the design of new drugs with improved properties and diminished side-effects for treating human disease. Medicinal chemists began the process by taking a lead structure and then finding analogs exhibiting the preferred biological activities. Next, they used their experience and chemical insight to eventually choose a nominee analog for further development. This process is difficult, expensive and took a long time. The conventional methods of drug discovery are now being supplemented by shortest approaches made possible by accepting the molecular processes involved in the original disease. In this view, the preliminary point in drug design is the molecular target which is receptor or enzyme in the body as an option of the existence of known lead structure.

Rational drug design is based on the belief that the biological properties of drugs are related to their actual structural features. 'Drug design' or 'tailor-made compound' aims at developing a drug with high degree of chemotherapeutic index and specific action. It is a logical effort to design a drug on as much a rational basis as possible, thus reducing to the minimum trial and error approach. It essentially involves the study of biodynamics of a drug besides the interaction between drug molecules and molecules composing the biological objects.

Drug design seeks to explain:

(a) Effects of biological compounds on the basis of molecular interaction in terms of molecular structures or precisely the physicochemical properties of the molecules involved.

(b) Various processes by which the drugs usually produce their pharmacological effects.

(c) How the drugs specifically react with the protoplasm to elicit a particular pharmacological response.

(d) How the drugs usually get modified or detoxicated, metabolized or eliminated by the organism.

(e) Probable relationship between biological activities with chemical structure.

In short, drug design may be considered as an integrated whole approach which essentially involves various steps, namely: chemical synthesis, evaluation for activity-spectrum, toxicological studies, metabolism of the drug, i.e., biotransformation and the study of the various metabolites formed, assay procedures, and lastly formulation and biopharmaceutics.

The 'drug design' in a broader sense implies random evaluation of synthetic as well as natural products in bioassay systems, creation of newer drug molecules based on biologically-active-prototypes derived from either plant or animal kingdom, synthesis of congeners displaying interesting biological actions, the basic concept of isosterism and bioisosterism, and finally precise design of a drug to enable it to interact with a receptor site efficaciously.

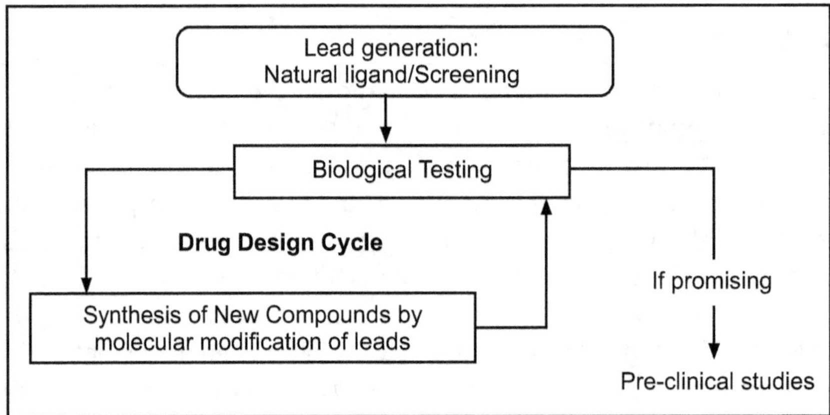

Fig. 12.1: Traditional Drug Design (Pharmacophore-based drug design)

Stages required in Drug Design and Drug Discovery:

1. Choose a disease.
2. Choose a drug target.
3. Identify a bioassay.
4. Find a 'lead compound'.
5. Isolate and purify the lead compound, if necessary.

6. Determine the structure of the lead compound.
7. Identify structure-activity relationships (SARs).
8. Identify the pharmacophore.
9. Improve target interactions.

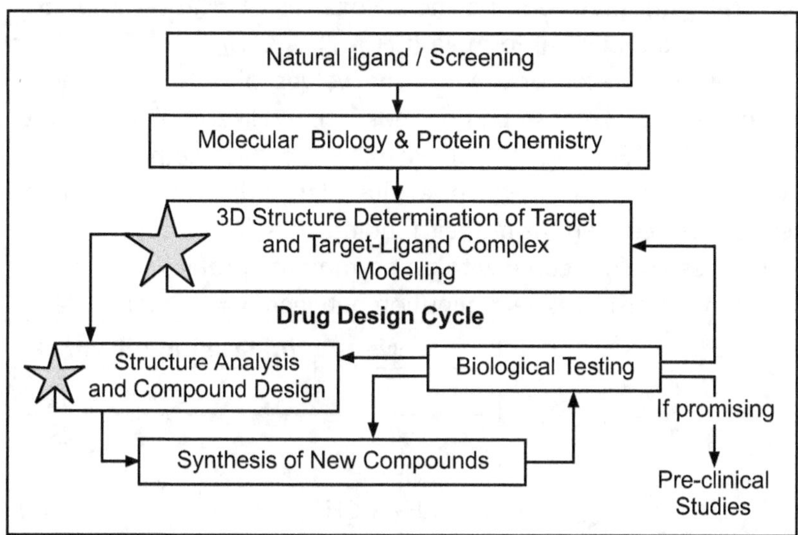

Fig. 12.2: Structure-Based Drug Design (SBDD) or Target-based approach

12.2 VARIOUS APPROACHES USED IN DRUG DESIGN

In the recent past, another terminology 'prodrugs' has been introduced to make a clear distinction from the widely used term 'analogues'. Prodrugs are frequently used to improve pharmacological or biological properties. Analogues are primarily employed to increase potency and to achieve specificity of action.

12.2.1 Design of Analogues

An analogue is normally accepted as being that modification which brings about a carbon-skeletal transformation or substituent synthesis. Analogues can also be synthesized by changing the position of substitution group. Examples: Oxytetracycline, Demclocycline, Chlortetracycline, Trans-diethylstilbesterol with regard to Oestradiol.

The term analogy, derived from the Latin and Greek analogia, is used in natural science since 1791 to describe structural and functional similarity. Extended to drugs, this definition implies that the analogue of an existing drug molecule shares chemical and therapeutic similarities with the original compound. The chemical design of analogues makes use of simple and traditional procedures of medicinal chemistry such as the synthesis of homologues, vinylogues, isosteres, positional isomers, optical isomers, transformation of ring systems, and the synthesis of twin drugs.

12.2.1.1 Analogues Produced by Homologous Variations
Homology through Monoalkylation:

Simple homologous variations applied on a neuramidase-inhibiting lead achieved a 6300-fold increase in potency.

Polymethylenic Bis-Ammonium Compounds: Hexa- and Decamethonium

Compounds having the general formula $(CH_3)_3 N^+ - (CH_2)_n - N^+(CH_3)_3$ usually show high affinity for the cholinergic receptors. When the values of n are intermediate (n = 5 or 6: penta- or hexamethonium), these compounds behave like cholinergic agonists (towards the sympathetic ganglia). For higher values (n = 10: decamethonium), the compounds become antagonists of acetylcholine (at the muscular endplate). In both cases, increasing acetylcholine levels displace them from their binding sites. While considering neuromuscular blockade, one observes again a curve with an asymmetric profile: sudden changes between n = 6 and n = 8, and then progressive diminution between n = 9 and n = 12.

Neuraminidase inhibition	
R	**IC_{50} (nM)**
H	6.300
CH_3	3.700
$CH_3 - CH_2$	2.000
$CH_3 - CH_2 - CH_2$	180
$CH_3 - CH_2 - CH_2 - CH_2$	300
$(CH_3)_2 - CH_2 - CH_2$	200
$CH_3 - CH_2 - CH(CH_3)$	10
$(CH_3 - CH_2)_2 - CH$	1
$(CH_3 - CH_2 - CH_2) - CH$	16
Cyclopentyl	22
Cyclohexyl	60
Phenyl	530

Homology in Cyclic Compounds:

Homology in cyclic compounds can dramatically change the affinity of a ligand for its target. This is illustrated by a series of cyclic ACE inhibitors related to enalapril.

ACE inhibition	IC_{50} (nM)
n = 1	19,000
n = 2	1,700
n = 3	19
n = 4	4.8

For these compounds, an almost 4000-fold increase in activity was observed in passing from the five-member to the eight-member homologue.

12.2.1.2 Analogues Produced by Vinylogy

Tolcapone was designed as an inhibitor of the enzyme Catechol O-methyl Transferase (COMT) and is useful in the L-DOPA treatment of Parkinson's disease. In avoiding the methylation of L-DOPA as well as that of dopamine, it prolongs the beneficial activities of these molecules. Catechol O-methyl transferase inhibition represents therefore a valuable adjuvant to the L-DOPA decarboxylase inhibition. Unfortunately, tolcapone exhibited severe liver damage and had to be removed from the market. The corresponding vinylogue entacapone is devoid of this side effect.

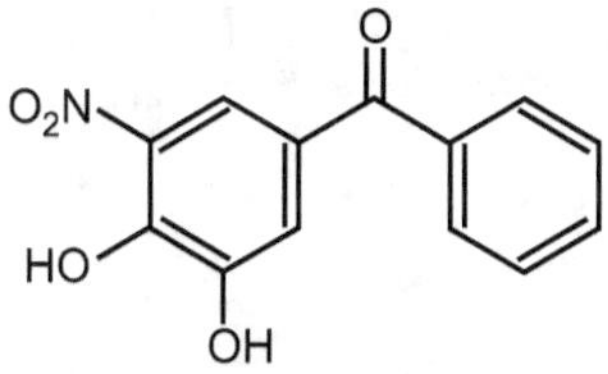

Tolcapone 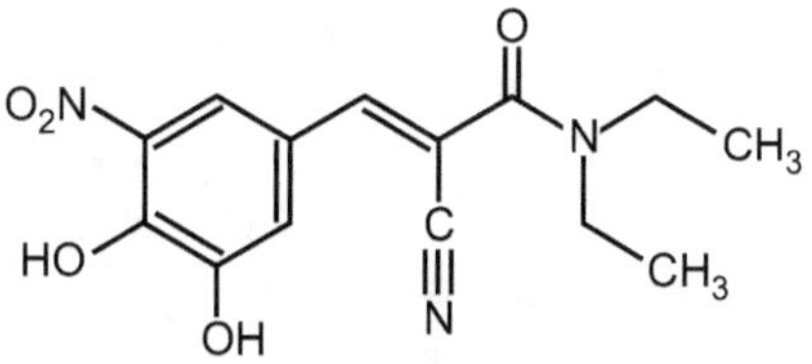   **Entacapone**

Zaprinast Benzologues:

A very convincing example of the usefulness of benzologues is provided by the synthesis of compound A, a linear benzologue of the prototypical phosphodiesterase type 5 (PDE5) inhibitor zaprinast, and its optimization to potent and selective PDE-5 inhibitors such as compound B.

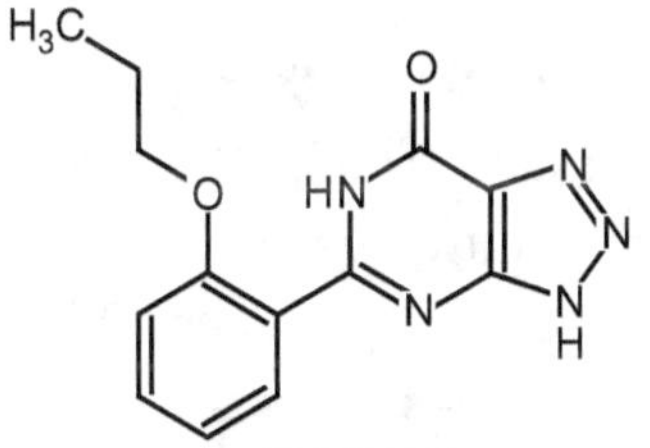

Zaprinast 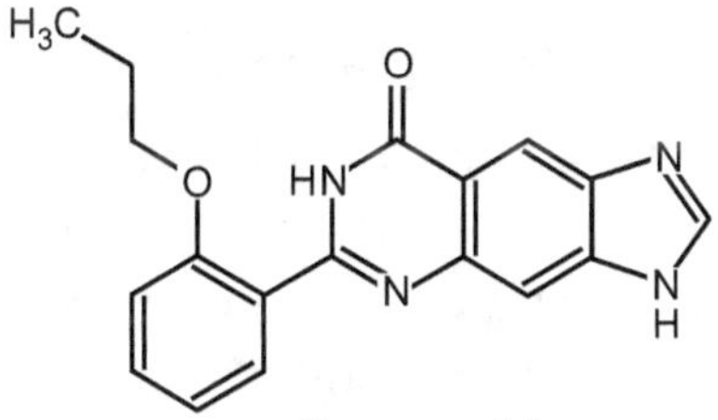   **Compound A**

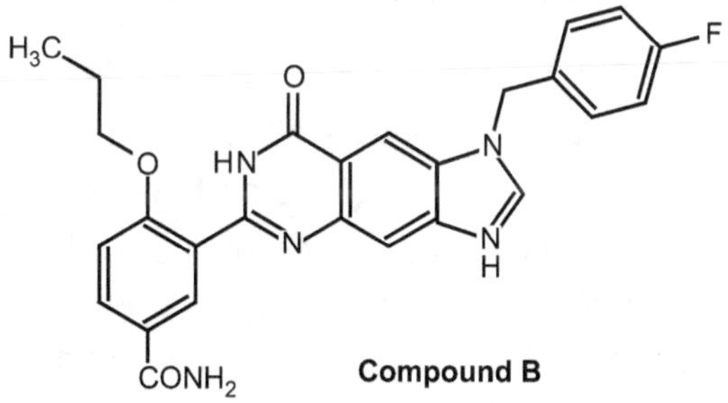

Compound B

12.2.1.3 Analogues Produced by Isosteric Variations

The Dominant Parameter is Structural:

Structural factors are important when the portion of the molecule involved in the isosteric change serves to maintain other functions in a particular geometry. That is the case for tricyclic psychotropic drugs.

Imipramine

Maprotiline

Antidepressants: $\alpha = 55 - 65°$
Neuroleptics   : $\alpha = 25°$

Chlorpromazine

Chlorprothixene

For the two antidepressants (imipramine and maprotiline), the bioisosterism is geometrical insofar that the dihedral angle 'a' formed by the two benzo rings is comparable: a = 65° for the dibenzazepine and a = 55° for the dibenzocycloheptadiene. This angle is only 25° for the neuroleptic phenothiazines and for the thioxanthenes. In these examples, the part of the molecule modified by isosterism is not involved in the interaction with the receptor. It serves only to position correctly the other elements of the molecule.

The Dominant Parameter is Electronic:

The electron-attracting nitro group in the antibiotic chloramphenicol (Table 12.1) has been replaced by other electron-attracting functions such as methyl-sulfonyl (thiamphenicol) or an acetyl (or cetophenicol). Apparently, the dominant feature is of electronic nature. Similar electronic effects are found in the benzodiazepines series in which the chlorine atom of diazepam can be exchanged with a bromine (bromazepam) or with a nitro group (nitrazepam).

Table 12.1: Isosteric replacements in the amphenicol family

Compound	X	Y
Chloramphenicol	$- NO_2$	$- CH - CH_2$
Thiamphenicol	$CH_3 - SO_2 -$	$- CH - Cl_2$
Cetophenicol	$CH_3 - CO -$	$- CH - Cl_2$

The Dominant Parameter is Lipophilicity:

Typical examples of lipophilic analogues of prototypes are eptastigmine (N-heptyl-physostigmine), derived from physostigmine by replacement of the N-methyl group by n-heptyl group.

$R = CH_3$ Physostigmine
$R = n\text{-}C_7H_{15}$ Eptastigmine

Nipecotic acid

12.2.1.4 Positional Isomers Produced as Analogues

In a series of non-peptide corticotropin-releasing factor 1 (CRF1), scientists from Neurocrine observed a dramatic change in affinity simply by shifting one nitrogen atom of the pyrimidine ring.

Ki = 30 nM   Ki > 10,000 nM

12.2.1.5 Optical Isomers Produced as Analogues

Due to their almost identical chemical structure, enantiomers represent a subtle class of analogues. Often in a pair of enantiomers, the desired biological activity is concentrated in only one enantiomer. Then, the passage from a recemic mixture to the pure active eutomer – which is usually termed "recemic switch" – can produce an improved drug. However, in some cases and despite their similar constitution, both enantiomers can have totally different pharmacodynamic or pharmacokinetic profiles.

S-(–)-levamisole   **R-(+)-dexamisole**

12.2.1.6 Analogues Produced by Ring Transformations

When active molecules contain cyclic systems, these can be opened, expanded, contracted, and modified in many other ways, or even abolished. Conversely, non-cyclic molecules can be cyclized, attached to, or included in ring systems. Two interesting examples are found in cyclic analogues of β-blockers. Cyclization to the morpholine yields the antidepressant viloxazine (mode 1), whereas cyclization to chromanols (mode 2) yields the potassium channel blocker cromakalim.

Viloxazine

Cromakalim

12.2.1.7 Twin Drugs

The search for cationic cholinergic agents has led to numerous twin drugs. The bis-quaternary ammonium salts hexamethonium and decamethonium are potent blockers in ganglia and in neuromuscular junctions, respectively. Other neuromuscular blocking agents such as succinyl and sebacyl dicholines can be regarded as pure acetylcholine twin drugs.

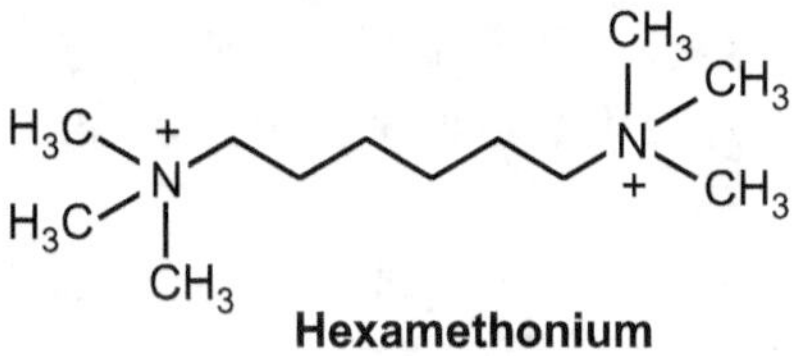

Hexamethonium

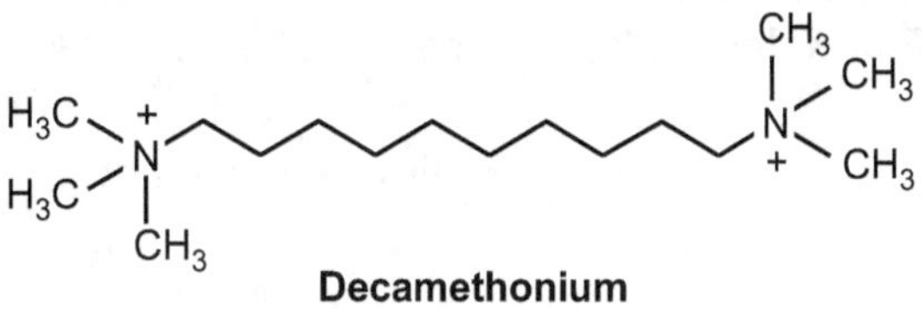

Decamethonium

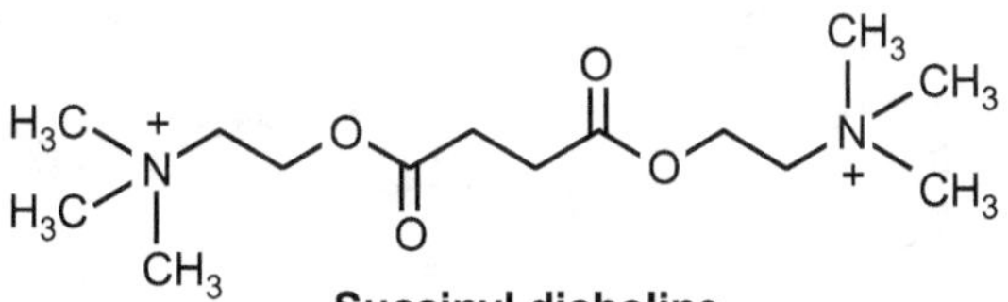

Succinyl dicholine

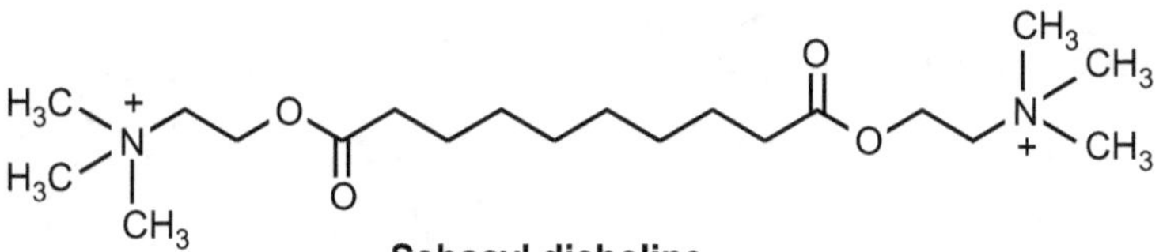

Sebacyl dicholine

12.2.2 Design of Prodrugs

The term prodrug is applied to either an appropriate derivative of a drug that undergoes *in-vivo* hydrolysis to the parent drug, e.g., testosterone propionate, chloramphenicol palmitate and the like ; or an analogue which is metabolically transformed to a biologically active drug, for instance: phenylbutazone undergoes *in-vivo* hydroxylation to oxyphenbutazone.

12.2.3 Classification of Prodrugs

1.   Carrier linked prodrugs: Active drug is covalently linked to an inert carrier or transporter moiety. They have enhanced lipophilicity due to attached carrier. The active drug is released by hydrolytic cleavage, either chemically or enzymatically.

2.   Bioprecursors: These are inert molecules obtained by chemical modification of the drug, but do not contain a carrier. Such a molecule has the same lipophilicity as the parent drug and is bioactivated generally by redox biotransformation, only enzymatically. e.g. NSAID –nabumetone (relafen) -arthritis.

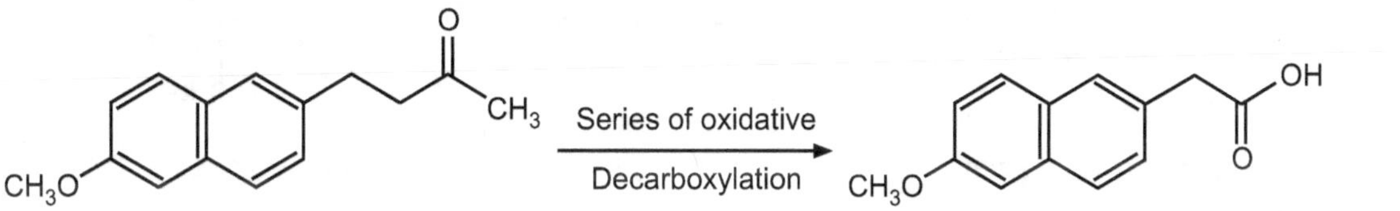

Series of oxidative

Decarboxylation

Active form of the drug that inhibits prostaglandin biosynthesis by cyclooxygenase

3.   Mutual Prodrugs: The prodrug comprises of two pharmacologically active agents coupled together to form a single molecule such that each acts as the carrier for the other.

Examples: (i) Benorylate is mutual prodrug of NSAIDs aspirin and paracetamol.

(ii) Emcyt is a mutual prodrug containing estramustine and nornitrogen mustard linked to each other.

Estermustine Sodium Phosphate
Emcyt-Pharmacia & Upjohn

Sodium phosphate
and
Carbon dioxide

Nomitrogen mustard

Aziridine

Actual alkylating species

12.2.4 Applications of Prodrugs:

1. Prodrugs to improve patient acceptability
2. Enhancing drug solubility
3. Enhancing drug absorption and distribution
4. Site specific drug delivery
5. Sustained drug action

1. Pharmaceutical Applications/Prodrugs to Improve Patient Acceptability:

(a) Improvement of taste:

- Bitter taste of the drug.
- Unsuitable for preparation of suspension.
- Reduce the solubility of the drug in the saliva.

Lipase

Chloramphenicol palmitate

Chloramphenicol

(b) Improvement of odour:

- The odor of the compound depends upon its vapor pressure. e.g. ethyl mercaptan is a foul smelling liquid of boiling point 35 °C. It is converted into its phthalate ester, diethyldithio-isophthalate ester which is odourless and has higher boiling point. (Used in the treatment of Tuberculosis).

$$O=C-SC_2H_5$$

Diethyldithio-isophthalate $\xrightarrow{\text{Thioesterase}}$ CH_3CH_2SH Ethyl mercaptan

(c) Reduction of gastric irritation:

- Increased stimulation of acid secretion.
- Interference with the protective mucosal layer.

Parent drug	Prodrug
Salicylic Acid	Aspirin
Diethyl stibesterol	Fosfestrol
Phenyl butazone	N-methyl piperazine
Oleandrin	Olendrine

(d) Reduction of pain on injection:

- Drug precipitates or penetrates into the surrounding tissues.
- The solution of Clindamycin is strongly acidic, alkaline or alcoholic. Clindamycin-2'-phosphate ester decreases the pain at the site of injection.

Clindamycin-2'-phosphate ester $\xrightarrow{\text{Phosphatase}}$ Clindamycin

2. Enhancement of Solubility and Dissolution Rate:

- Dissolution is the rate limiting step in the absorption of drug.
- Parenteral and ophthalmic formulations of such agents require agent having better solubility and dissolution.

(a)

Esterases →

Methylprednisolone succinate ester

R = H prednisolone (corticosteroid)
R = CH$_3$ methyl prednisolone

(b)

Amidases →

Amino acid amide of benzocaine

Benzocaine (local anesthetic)

3. Prodrugs for Improved Absorption and Distribution:

- Ampicillin when administered orally only about 40% of dose is absorbed. Therefore, ampicillin when presented in the form of its esters has increased absorption.
- **Example:** Pivampicilline and Becampicillin prodrugs for improved absorption and distribution.

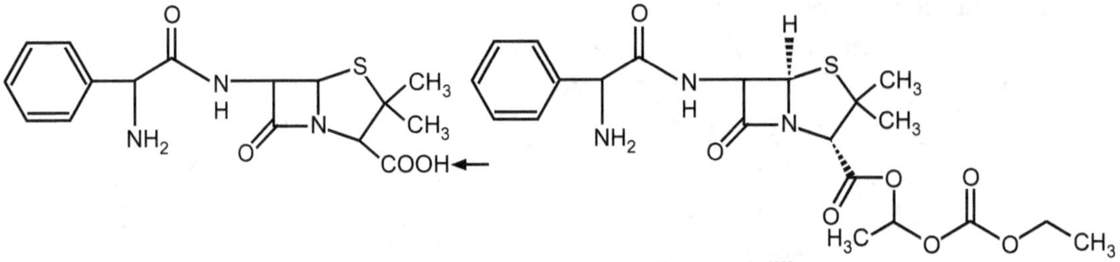

Becampicillin

4. Prodrugs for Site Specificity:

- Diethylstilbesterol diphosphate shows site specificity in case of breast cancer treatment.

Phosphatase

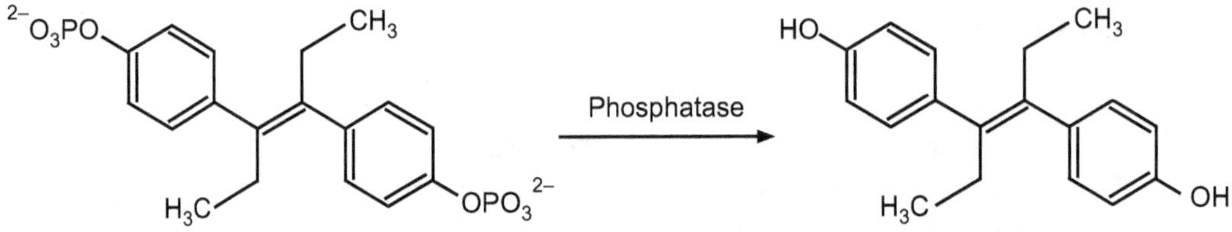

Diethylstilbestrol diphosphate

Diethylstilbestrol
(breast cancer treatment)

5. Prodrugs for Stability (First-pass Metabolism):

- Propranolol rapidity does to first pass metabolism but its hemisuccinate salt increases the stability.

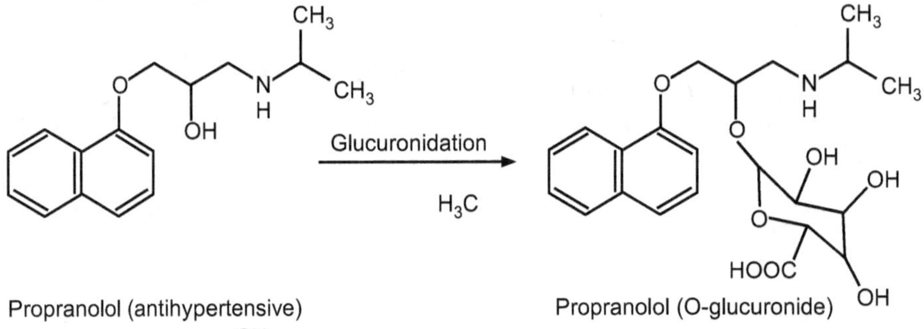

Glucuronidation

Propranolol (antihypertensive)

Propranolol (O-glucuronide)

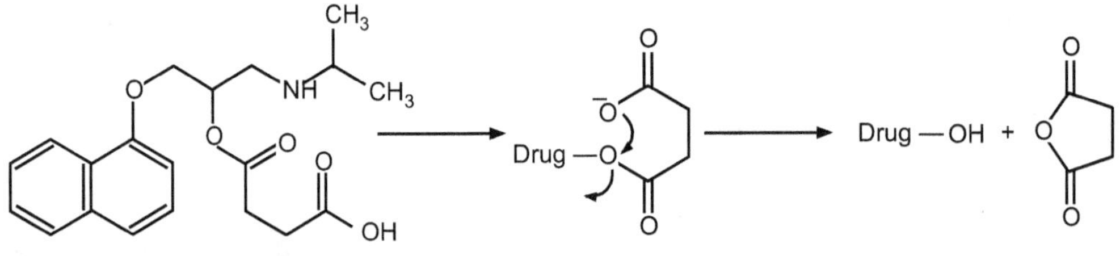

Drug—O

Drug—OH +

Propranolol hemisuccinate

6. Prodrugs for Slow and Prolonged Release:

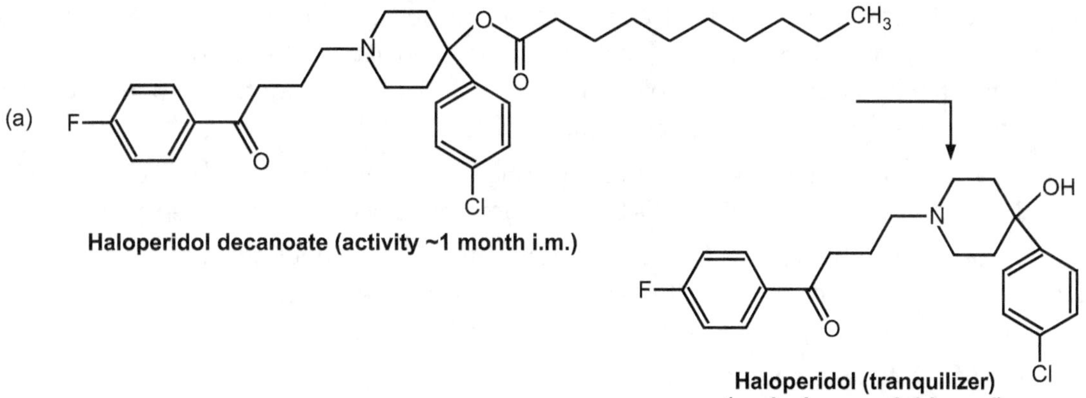

(a)

Haloperidol decanoate (activity ~1 month i.m.)

Haloperidol (tranquilizer)
(peak plasma ~ 2-6 hr oral)

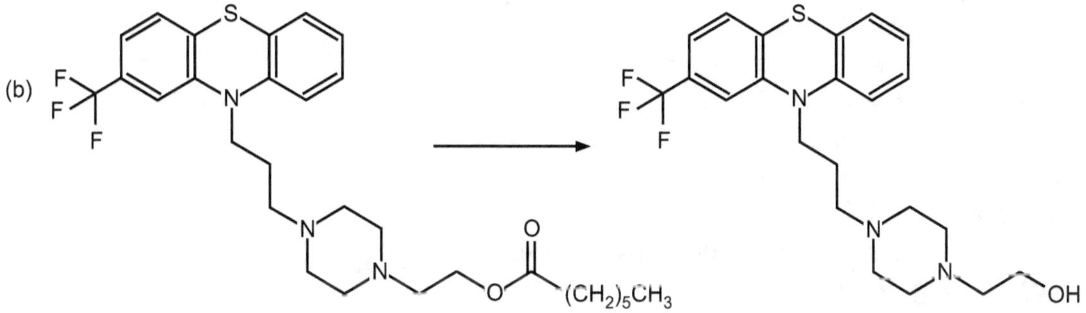

(b)

Fluphenazine enanthate
(duration of activity ~1 month)

Fluphenazine (antipsychotic)
(duration of activity 6-8 hrs)

7. Prodrugs to minimize toxicity:

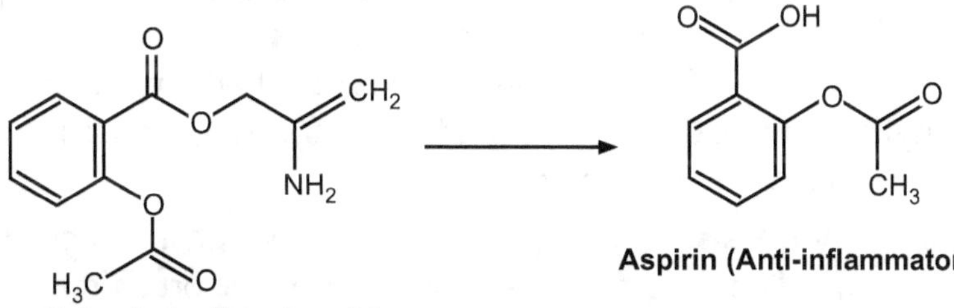

Aspirin (Anti-inflammatory)

Ester derivative of aspirin
(without gastric irritation)

12.2.5 Design of Lead and Lead Discovery

In 'drug design' as the vital process of envisioning and preparing specific new molecules that can lead more efficiently to useful drug discovery. This may be considered broadly in terms of two types of investigational activities. These include:

(a) Exploration of leads, which involves the search for a new lead and

(b) Exploitation of leads, that requires the assessment, improvement and extension of the lead.

It is a chemical compound obtained from natural or synthetic sources that possesses a particular biological activity. A lead can be characterized as a compound that has some desirable biological activity, not extremely polar or lipophilic, and not containing toxic or reactive functional groups. Often, molecular weight (< 350) and lipophilicity (log P < 3) are considered as the most obvious characteristics of a drug-like lead.

The lead should also have a series of congeners that modulate biological activity, indicating that further structural modification will improve selectivity and potency.

Drug design can be achieved by exploration of the lead compounds, which involves the search for a new lead or exploitation of the existing leads to produce more active compounds with less toxicity than the original lead compound.

Sources of finding lead compound:

(a) Screening of natural products:
- The plant kingdom
- The microbial world
- The marine world
- Animal sources
- Venoms and toxins

(b) Medical folklore.

(c) Screening synthetic compound libraries.

(d) Existing drugs:
- 'Me too' drugs, **Example:** Captopril.
- Enhancing a side effect. **Example:** Sulphonamides and sulphonyl ureas.

(e) Starting from the natural ligand or modulator:
- Natural ligands for receptors – Adrenalin, nor – adrenalin.
- Natural substrates for enzymes – enkephalins.
- Enzyme products as lead compounds – Product of an enzyme catalysed reaction – L-benzyl succinic acid (Carboxypeptidase catalysed hydrolysis).
- Natural modulators as lead compounds.

(f) Combinatorial synthesis: It is an automated solid phase procedure aimed at producing as many different structures as possible in as short a time as possible.

(g) Computer aided design.

(h) Serendipity and the prepared mind.

Example: Cisplatin, Ampicillin.

(i) Computerised searching for structural database: Database mining.

(j) Designing lead compounds by NMR.

Example:
- **Sulphanilamide:** Isolated from the degradation of prontosil or synthesized chemically and acts as antibacterial agent.

Sulphanilamide $\xrightarrow[10°C]{NaNO_2/HCl}$ Diazotized sulphanilamide + P-aminophenyldiamine

Sulphanilamide $\xleftarrow[\text{(in-vivo)}]{\text{Reduction}}$ Prontosil

- **Lead compound from natural sources:** Morphine from opium, cocaine from coca leaves, and quinine from the bark of cinchona tree.

Morphine

Morphine
(Schaumann's Model)

Pethidine
(Meperidine)

12.2.6 Factors Governing Drug Design

A few cardinal factors governing the efficacy towards the evaluation of drug design include:

(a) The smaller the expenditure of human and material resources involved to evolve a new drug of a particular value, the more viable is the design of the program.

(b) Experimental animal and clinical screening operations of the new drugs.

(c) Relationships between chemical features and biological properties need to be established retrospectively.

(d) Quantitative structure-activity relationships (QSARs) vary to an appreciable extent in depth and sophistication based on the nature of evaluation of structure or activity. A purposeful relation of structural variables must include steric factors, electronic features of component functional groups and, in general, the molecule as a whole.

(e) The trend to synthesize a huge number of newer medicinal compounds indiscriminately for exploratory evaluation still prevail which exclusively reflects the creative genuineness and conceptual functions of a highly individualized expression of novelty by a medicinal chemist.

(f) Introduction of functional groups in a molecule that need not essentially resemble metabolites, but are capable of undergoing bonding interactions with important functional groups of biochemical components of living organisms affords an important basis for exploration.

(g) Disease etiologies and various biochemical processes involved prove useful.

12.2.7 Rational Approach to Drug Design

A rational approach to drug design may be viewed from different angles, namely:

1. **Quantum Mechanical Approach:**

   Quantum mechanics (or wave mechanics) is composed of certain vital principles derived from fundamental assumptions describing the natural phenomena effectively. The properties of protons, neutrons and electrons are adequately explained under quantum mechanics. The electronic features of the molecules responsible for chemical alterations form the basis of drug molecule phenomena.

2. **Molecular Orbital Approach:**

   Based on the assumption that the electrons present in molecules seem to be directly linked with orbitals, engulfing the entire molecule sets forth the molecular orbital theory. The molecular orbital approach shows dependence on electronic charge as evidenced by the study of three volatile inhalation anaesthetics, and also on molecular conformation as studied with respect to acetylcholine by such parameters as bond lengths and angles including torsional angles.

   Molecular orbital calculations are achievable by sophisticated computers, and after meticulous interpretations of results the molecular structure in respect of structure-activity analysis is established.

3. **Molecular Connectivity Approach:**

   This approach establishes the presence of structural features like cyclization, unsaturation skeletal branching, and the position and presence of heteroatom in molecules with the aid of a series of numerical indices. For example: an index was determined to possess a correlative factor in the SAR study of amphetamine-type hallucinogenic drugs.

   Molecular connectivity approach has some definite limitations, such as, electronegativity variance between atoms, non-distinguishable entity of cis-trans isomerism.

4. **Linear Free-Energy Approach:**

   This method establishes the vital link between the proper selections of physicochemical parameters with a specific biological phenomenon. However, such a correlation may not guarantee and allow a direct interpretation with regard to molecular structure, but may positively offer a possible clue towards the selection of candidate molecules for synthesis.

12.2.8 Drug-Design: The Method of Variation

Under this method a new drug molecule is developed from a biologically active prototype. The various advantages are as follows:

(a) At least one new compound of known activity is found.

(b) The new structural analogues even if not superior may be more economical.

(c) Identical chemical procedure is adopted and hence, considerable economy of time, library and laboratory facilities.

(d) Screening of a series of congener (i.e., member of the same gene) gives basic information with regard to pharmacological activity.

(e) Similar pharmacological technique for specific screening may be used effectively. The cardinal objectives of the method of variation are:

- To improve potency.
- To modify specificity of action.
- To improve duration of action.
- To reduce toxicity.
- To effect ease of application or administration or handling.
- To improve stability.
- To reduce cost of production.

Once the molecular structure of the compound in question is drawn on the drawing board, one takes into consideration such information as the following:

(a) Variation of functional groups and their proximity to one another.

(b) Various probable rotational and spatial configurations.

(c) Possibility of steric hindrance between various portions of the molecule in different configurations in space.

(d) Probability of electronic interactions between various portions of the molecule including such matters as inductive and mesomeric effects, hyper-conjugation, ionizability, polarity, possibility of chelation, asymmetric centres and zwitterion formation.

The application of the method of variation, depending on the considerations enumerated above, is exploited in two different manners to evolve a better drug. The two main approaches for this goal can be indicated as:

1. Drug design through disjunction and
2. Drug design through conjunction.

1. Drug Design through Disjunction:

Disjunction comes in where there is the systematic formulation of analogues of a prototype agent, in general, towards structurally simpler products, which may be viewed as partial or quasieplicas of the prototype agent.

The method of disjunction is usually employed in three different manners, namely:

(i) Unjoining of certain bonds;

(ii) Substitution of aromatic cyclic system for saturated bonds; and

(iii) Diminution of the size of the hydrocarbon portion of the parent molecule.

Example: The extensive study on the estrogenic activity of oestradiol via drug design through disjunction ultimately rewarded in the crowning success of the synthesis and evaluation of trans-diethylstilbesterol.

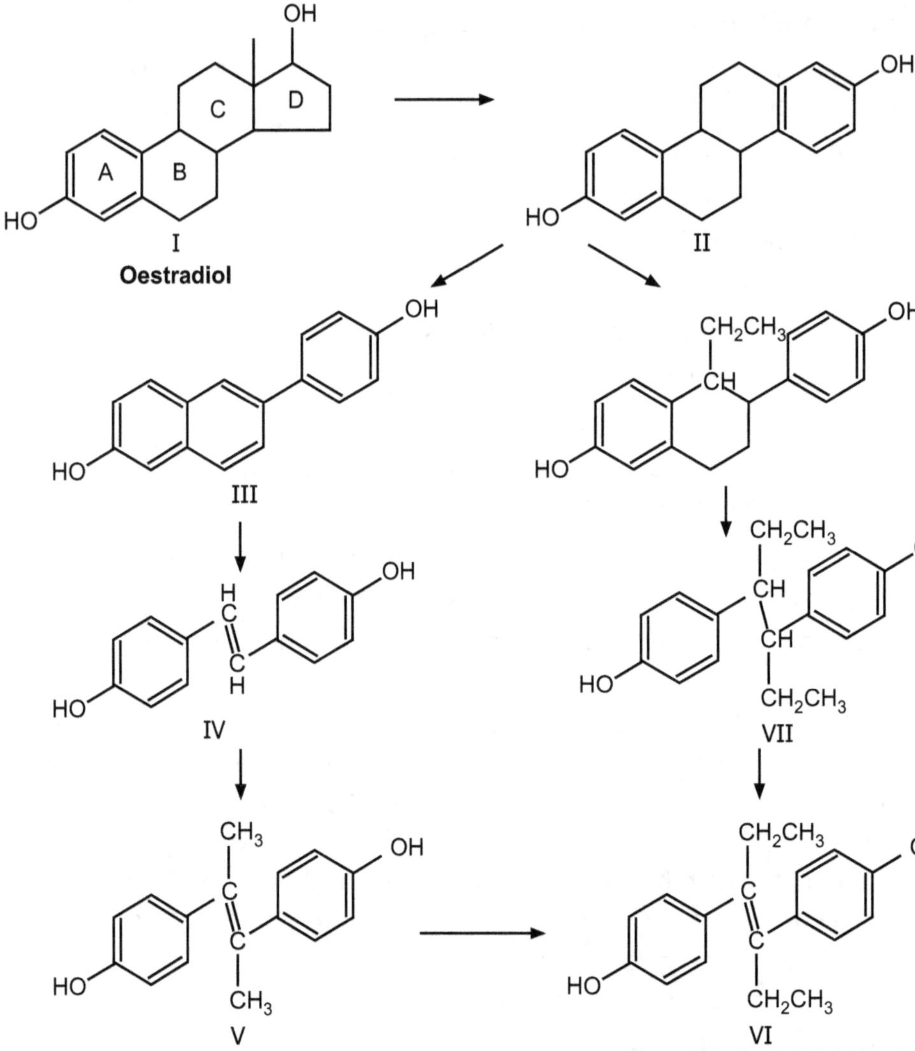

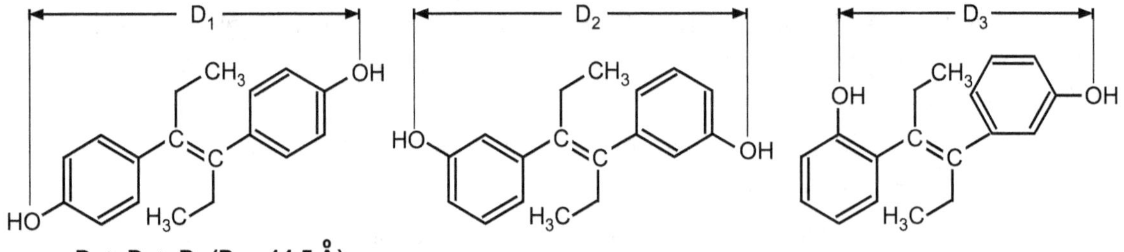

$D_1 > D_2 > D_3$ (D_1 = 14.5 Å)

2. Drug Design through Conjunction:

This is known as the systematic formulation of analogues of a prototype agent, in general, towards structurally more complex products, which may be viewed as structures embodying, in a general or specific way, certain or all of the features of the prototype.

In this type of drug-design, the main principle involved is the 'principle of mixed moieties'. A drug molecule is essentially made up with two or more pharmacophoric moieties embedded into a single molecule.

Example: Ganglionic blocking agent –its development is based on the principle of mixed moieties.

The principle of mixed moieties actually involve the conjunction of two or more different types of pharmacophoric moieties within a single molecule.

Acetylcholine is an effective postganglionic parasympathetic stimulant in doses that afford no appreciable changes in the ganglionic function; whereas hexamethonium possesses only a slight action at postganglionic parasympathetic endings in doses that produce a high degree of ganglionic blockade.

The 'drug discovery process' may be categorized into four distinct heads, namely:

(i)   Target identification and selection,

(ii) Target optimization,

(iii) Lead identification, and

(iv) Lead optimization.

12.2.9 Receptors

The drug molecules which exert some chemical influence on one or more constituents of the cells to produce a pharmacological response are known as receptors.

12.2.9.1 Types of Receptors

Receptors elicit many different types of cellular effect. Some of them are very rapid, that is, those involved in synaptic transmission, operating within milliseconds, and other receptors for hormones that operate after hours and days. There are four types of receptors.

1. Ligand-gated ion channels.

2. G-protein-coupled receptors.

3. Kinase-linked receptors.

4. Nuclear receptors.

1. **Ligand-gated ion channels:** The ligand-gated ion channels are also known as ionotropic receptors. These are membrane proteins with a similar structure to other ion channels, but incorporating a ligand-binding site.

   Examples: Nicotinic acetylcholine receptor, GABA-A receptor, and glutamate receptor of N-methyl-D-aspartic acid (NMDA).

2. **G-protein-coupled receptors:** These are also called metabotropic receptors or seven-trans membrane spanning receptors that act through a second messenger, which elicits an action. Second messengers usually are cyclic adenosine monophosphate (cAMP) and inositol trisphosphate.

   Examples: Muscarinic receptors, β-adrenergic receptors, serotonin receptors and opioid receptors.

3. **Kinase-linked or enzyme-linked receptors:** These constitute extracellular ligand-binding domain that is linked to an intracellular domain by a single transmembrane helix. In many cases, the intracellular domain is enzymatic in nature.

4. **Nuclear receptors:** The nuclear receptors regulate the gene transcriptions, are located in the cytosol, and migrate to the nuclear compartment when a ligand is present. The receptor protein is inherently capable of binding to specific genes. These include the receptors of glucocorticoids and thyroid hormone.

12.2.9.2 Theories of Receptors

1. **Occupation Theory:** Occupation theory was proposed by Gaddum and Clark. The theory states that the intensity of pharmacological effect is directly proportional to the number of receptors occupied by the drug. The pharmacological response of a drug molecule depends on the amount of dose, the total number of receptors available, and its intrinsic activity that can be expressed as $K_1[R] \times [A]$.

   where $\quad K_1 =$ Association constant

   $\quad\quad R =$ Concentration of the receptors not occupied by drugs

   $\quad\quad A =$ Concentration of drug molecules or dose

2. **Rate Theory:** The rate theory explains that the pharmacological activity is a function of the rate of association and dissociation of a drug with the receptor and is not the function of the number of occupied receptors.

$$\frac{K_1[A]\,([r] - [RA])}{[r]} = \frac{K_2\,[RA]}{[r]}$$

$$\text{or Rate of receptor occupation} = \frac{K_2}{1} + \frac{RA}{[A]}$$

   When the response is proportional to the number of receptors occupied.

3. **Induced Fit Theory:** It is proposed by Koshland to give explanation for the action of enzymes and substrates. It explains that the receptor (enzyme) need not necessarily exist in the same conformation that is required to bind the drug (substrate). As the drug approaches the receptor, a conformational change is induced for binding, which initiates the pharmacological activity.

   Example: Acetylcholine interacts with the regulating protein and alters the normal forces that stabilize the structure of the protein and thereby producing a transient rearrangement in membrane structure and a consequent change in its ion regulating property.

4. **Macromolecular Perturbation Theory:** According to this theory, the drug interaction with a receptor leads either to specific conformational perturbations (SCPs) or to nonspecific conformational perturbations (NSCPs). An SCP will produce a specific response from an agonist in which the drug possesses intrinsic activity. In NSCP, no stimulant action, but antagonistic or blocking action may be produced.

5. **Activation – Aggregation Theory:** According to this theory, even in the absence of drugs, a receptor is in a state of dynamic equilibrium between an activated form, which is responsible for biological responses and an inactive form. Agonists shift, the equilibrium to activated form and antagonists shift the equilibrium to inactivated form.

12.2.9.3 Forces involved in Drug Receptor Interaction

1. **Covalent Bonding:** Covalent bonds are the one which are produced by a strong energy. These are produced only when an irreversible antagonist inactivates the receptors.

   Example: Acetylcholinesterase is irreversibly inactivated by a number of phosphate esters (organophosphorus compounds includes pesticides). The nitrogen mustards are irreversible inhibitors of certain receptors.

2. **Dipole-Dipole and Ion-Dipole Interactions:** It is associated with electrostatic bonding. Molecules in which there is a partial charge separation between adjacent atoms or functional groups can interact either with each other or with ions.

3. **Hydrogen Bonding:** It forms a weak (energy from 7 to 40 KJ/mol) and easily breaking bond. Since drugs contain hydroxyl, amino, carboxyl, and carbonyl groups, it can form H-bonds with the receptors. H-bonding is a type of dipole-dipole interaction formed between the proton of a group X-H (X-is an electronegative atom) and other electronegative atoms (Y) containing pairs of non-bonded electrons.

4. **Electrostatic Bonding:** The opposite charged compound will interact with the opposite charged part of the receptor. The positively charged quaternary N-acetylcholine may be attracted to the negative charge of an ionized carboxyl group in the receptor.

5. **Charge Transfer Complex:** A dipole-dipole interaction is produced and a charge transfer complex is formed when any molecule with electron-donating property comes near the electron-accepting group.

6. **Hydrophobic Forces:** In the presence of non-polar molecules, the surrounding water molecules orient themselves, and therefore, are in a high-energy state, when two non-polar receptor groups (one from the drug and another from the receptor) come together.

7. **Van der Waal's or London Dispersion Forces:** Atoms in non-polar molecular structure have a temporary non-symmetrical distribution of electron density, which results in the generation of a temporary dipole that creates an intermolecular attraction called Van der Waal's force. However, this is a weak bond.

12.2.9.4 Factors affecting the Drug-Receptor Interaction:

1. **Isosterism:** Groups of atoms that possess similar physical or chemical properties of a molecule due to similarity in size, electronegativity, or stereochemistry are referred to as isosteres. The existence of such groups in molecules is termed as isosterism.

2. **Steric Features of a Drug:** The drug must possess stereoselective property to initiate a response at a particular receptor. For example, trans-diethylstilbesterol is oestrogenic, while cis-isomer is almost inactive.

3. **Optical isomerism:** Enantiomers, asymmetry, and chirality are important concepts to give better receptor interaction with drugs.

12.2.10 Computer Aided Drug Design

Computer aided drug design (CADD) involves all the computer-assisted techniques that are used to discover, design, and optimize biologically active compounds with putative use as a drug having the desired structure and properties. The rational drug design processes have changed the way in which potential new drugs are discovered.

The rational drug design process starts with an understanding of the fundamental physiological and biochemical aspects of the disease or target, rather than random screening process. One method to bring about cost effectiveness in drug design process is by applying both the knowledge of mechanistic basis of a target disease and molecular characteristics of the compounds to have an effect on diseases state. This approach to therapeutic development is called rational drug design approach.

CADD is a specialized branch, that covers computational methods of calculation, and graphics techniques, gives information about drug-receptor interactions. Computational resources and other software technologies like information technology, information management, and databases, provide the infrastructure for bioinformatics. On the scientific side, bioinformatics methods are used extensively in molecular biology, genomics, proteomics, and in CADD research.

Bioinformatics supports CADD research in the following aspects:

- Virtual high-throughput screening
- Sequence analysis
- Homology modelling
- Similarity searches
- Drug lead optimization
- Physicochemical modelling
- Drug bioavailability and bioactivity

Advantages of CADD:

CADD methods and bioinformatics tools offer significant benefits for drug discovery programs.

- **Cost saving:** The cost of drug discovery and development has reached $800 million for a single drug to be successfully brought into the market. Recently, many pharmaceutical industries are focusing the CADD to reduce this cost burden.

- **Time-to-market:** The predictive power of CADD can reduce the time period for drug development and optimization and avoids potential 'dead-end' compound on final stage. It can get drugs to the market more quickly and cost effectively.

- **Insight:** The molecular graphics technique of CADD gives information about drug-receptor interaction and atomic scale binding properties to particular ligand or protein. It may give new ideas for researcher to modify the drug compounds for improved fit. Therefore, CADD and bioinformatics together are a powerful combination in drug research and development.

12.3 PHYSICOCHEMICAL PARAMETERS USED IN QUANTITATIVE STRUCTURE-ACTIVITY RELATIONSHIP (QSAR)

Several strategies involved a change in shape such that the new drug had a better 'fit' for its target binding site. Other strategies involved a change in functional groups or substituents such that the drug's pharmacokinetics or binding site interactions were improved. These later strategies often involved the synthesis of analogues containing a range of substituents on aromatic or hetero aromatic rings or accessible functional groups. The number of possible analogues that could be made is infinite if we were to try and synthesize analogues with every substituent and combination of substituents possible. Therefore, it is clearly advantageous if a rational approach can be followed in deciding which substituents to use. The quantitative structure-activity relationship (QSAR) approach has proved extremely useful in tackling this problem.

The QSAR approach attempts to identify and quantify the physicochemical properties of a drug and to see whether any of these properties has an effect on the drug's biological activity. By quantifying physicochemical properties, it should be possible to calculate in advance what the biological activity of a novel analogue might be. There are two advantages to this. Firstly, it allows the medicinal chemist to target efforts on analogues which should have improved activity and, thus, cut down the number of analogues that have to be made. Secondly, if an analogue is discovered which does not fit the equation, it implies that some other feature is important and provides a lead for further development.

In the simplest situation, a range of compounds is synthesized in order to vary one physicochemical property (e.g. log P) and to test how this affects the biological activity (log 1/C). A graph is then drawn to plot the biological activity on the y-axis versus the physicochemical feature on the x-axis.

Draw the best possible line through the data points on the graph through linear regression analysis by the least squares method. If we draw a line through a set of data points, most of the points will be scattered on either side of the line. The best line will be the one closest to the data points. To measure how close the data points are, vertical lines are drawn from each point. These verticals are measured and then squared in order to eliminate the negative values. The squares are then added up to give a total (the sum of the squares).

The equation of the straight line will be $y = k_1 x + k_2$, where k_1 and k_2 are constants. By varying k_1 and k_2, different equations are obtained until the best line is obtained. This whole process can be done speedily using relevant software. The next stage in the process is to see whether the relationship is meaningful. The regression or correlation coefficient (r) is a measure of how well the physicochemical parameters present in the equation explain the observed variance in activity. For a perfect fit $r = 1$, in which case the observed activities would be the same as those calculated by the equation. Such perfection is impossible with biological data and so r values greater than 0.9 are considered acceptable.

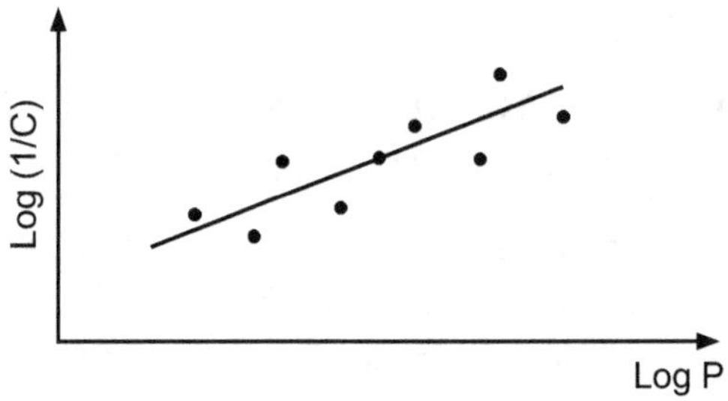

Fig. 12.3: Biological activity versus log P

The regression coefficient is often quoted as r^2, in which case values over 0.8 are considered a good fit. If r^2 is multiplied by 100, it indicates the percentage variation in biological activity that is accounted for the physicochemical parameters used in the equation. Thus, r^2 value of 0.85 signifies that 85% of the variation in biological activity is accounted for by the parameters used. There are dangers in putting too much reliance on 'r', as the value obtained takes no account of the number of compounds (n) involved in the study and it is possible to obtain higher values of 'r' by increasing the number of compounds tested. Therefore, another statistical measure for the goodness of fit should be quoted alongside 'r'. This is the standard error of estimate or the standard deviation (s). Ideally, 's' should be zero, but this would assume there were no experimental errors in the experimental data or the physicochemical parameters. In reality, 's' should be small, but not smaller than the standard deviation of the experimental data. It is therefore necessary to know the later to assess whether the value of 's' is acceptably low.

Statistical tests called Fisher's F-tests are often quoted. These tests are used to assess the significance of the coefficients k for each parameter in the QSAR equation. Normally, 'p' values (derived from the F-test) should be less than or equal to 0.05 if the parameter is significant. If this is not the case, the parameter should not be included in the QSAR equation.

Many physical, structural, and chemical properties have been studied by the QSAR approach, but the most common are hydrophobic, electronic, and steric properties. This is because it is possible to quantify these effects. Hydrophobic properties can be easily quantified for complete molecules or for individual substituent. However, it is more difficult to quantify electronic and steric properties for complete molecules, and this is only really feasible for individual substituents.

Consequently, QSAR studies on a variety of totally different structures are relatively rare and are limited to studies on hydrophobicity. It is more common to find QSAR studies being carried out on compounds of the same general structure, where substituents on aromatic rings or accessible functional groups are varied. The QSAR study then considers how the hydrophobic, electronic, and steric properties of the substituents affect biological activity. The three most studied physicochemical properties are now considered in some detail.

12.3.1 Partition Coefficient

The hydrophobic character of a drug can be measured experimentally by testing the drug's relative distribution in an n-octanol/water mixture. Hydrophobic molecules will prefer to dissolve in the n-octanol layer of this two-phase system, whereas hydrophilic molecules will prefer the aqueous layer. The relative distribution is known as the partition coefficient (P) and is obtained from the following equation:

$$P = \frac{\text{Concentration of drug in n-octanol}}{\text{Concentration of drug in aqueous solution}}$$

Hydrophobic compounds have a high P value, whereas hydrophilic compounds have a low P value.

Varying substituents on the lead compound will produce a series of analogues having different hydrophobicities and, therefore, different P values. By plotting these P values against the biological activity of these drugs, it is possible to see if there is any relationship between the two properties. The biological activity is normally expressed as 1/C, where C is the concentration of drug required to achieve a defined level of biological activity. The reciprocal of the concentration (1/C) is used, as more active drugs will achieve a defined biological activity at lower concentration. The graph is drawn by plotting log (1/C) versus log P. In studies where the range of the log P values is restricted to a small range (e.g. log P = 1 – 4), a straight line graph is obtained (Fig.12.3) showing that there is a relationship between hydrophobicity and biological activity. Such a line would have the following equation:

$$\log \left(\frac{1}{C}\right) = - k_1 \log P + k_2$$

A straight-line relationship between log P and biological activity is observed in many QSAR studies because the range of log P values studied is often relatively narrow. For example, the study carried out on serum albumin binding was restricted to compounds having log P values in the range 0.78 – 3.82. If these studies were to be extended to include compounds with very high log P values, then we would see a different picture. The graph would be parabolic, as shown in Fig. 12.4. Here, the biological activity increases as log P increases until a maximum value is obtained. The value of log P at the maximum (log P_0) represents the optimum partition coefficient for biological activity. Beyond that point, an increase in log P results in a decrease in biological activity.

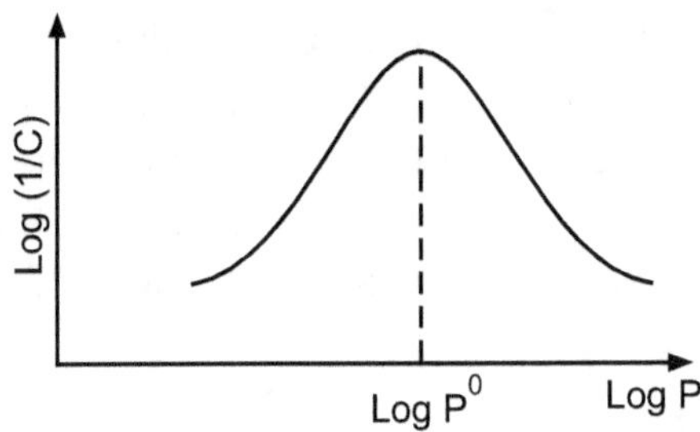

Fig. 12.4: Parabolic curve of log (1/ C) vs. log P

If the partition coefficient is the only factor influencing biological activity, the parabolic curve can be expressed by the equation:

$$\log\left(\frac{1}{C}\right) = -k_1 (\log P)^2 + k_2 \log P + k_3$$

Note that the $(\log P)^2$ term has a minus sign in front of it. When P is small, the $(\log P)^2$ term is very small and the equation is dominated by the log P term. This represents the first part of the graph where activity increases with increasing P. When P is large, the $(\log P)^2$ term is more significant and eventually 'overwhelms' the log P term. This represents the last part of the graph where activity drops with increasing P. k_1, k_2, and k_3 are constants and can be determined by a suitable software program.

There are relatively few drugs where activity is related to the log P factor alone. Such drugs tend to operate in cell membranes where hydrophobicity is the dominant feature controlling their action. The best example of drugs which operate in cell membranes is the general anesthetics. Although they also bind to GABA-A receptors, general anesthetics are thought to function by entering the central nervous system (CNS) and 'dissolving' into cell membranes where they affect membrane structure and nerve function. In such a scenario, there are no specific drug receptor interactions and the mechanism of the drug is controlled purely by its ability to enter cell membranes (i.e. its hydrophobic character). The general anesthetic activity of a range of ethers was found to fit the following parabolic equation:

$$\log\left(\frac{1}{C}\right) = -0.22 (\log P)^2 + 1.04 \log P + 2.16$$

According to this equation, anaesthetic activity increases with increasing hydrophobicity (P), as determined by the log P factor. The negative $(\log P)^2$ factor shows that the relationship is parabolic and that there is an optimum value for log P (log P_0) beyond which increasing hydrophobicity causes a decrease in anaesthetic activity. With this equation, it is now possible to predict the anaesthetic activity of other compounds, given their partition coefficients. However, there are limitations. The equation is derived purely for anaesthetic ethers and is not applicable to other structural types of anaesthetics. This is generally true in QSAR studies. The procedure works best if it is applied to a series of compounds which have the same general structure.

The substituent hydrophobicity constant (π)

Partition coefficients can be calculated by knowing the contribution that various substituents make to hydrophobicity. This contribution is known as the substituent hydrophobicity constant (π) and is a measure of how hydrophobic a substituent is relative to hydrogen. The value can be obtained as follows. Partition coefficients are measured experimentally for a standard compound, such as benzene, with and without a substituent (X). The hydrophobicity constant (π_X) for the substituent (X) is then obtained using the following equation:

$$\pi_X = \log P_X - \log P_H$$

where P_H is the partition coefficient for the standard compound and P_X is the partition coefficient for the standard compound with the substituent.

A positive value of π indicates that the substituent is more hydrophobic than hydrogen; a negative value indicates that the substituent is less hydrophobic. The π values for a range of substituents are shown in Table 12.2. These π values are characteristic for the substituent and can be used to calculate how the partition coefficient of a drug would be affected if these substituents were present. The 'P' value for the lead compound would have to be measured experimentally, but, once that is known, the 'P' value for analogues can be calculated quite simply.

As an example, consider the log P values for benzene (log P = 2.13), chlorobenzene (log P = 2.84), and benzamide (log P = 0.64). Benzene is the parent compound, and the substituent constants for Cl and $CONH_2$ are 0.71 and −1.49 respectively. Having obtained these values, it is now possible to calculate the theoretical log P value for meta-chloro benzamide:

$$\log P_{(chloro\ benzamide)} = \log P_{(benzene)} + \pi_{Cl} + \pi_{CONH_2}$$
$$= 2.13 + 0.17 + (-1.49)$$
$$= 1.35$$

The observed log P value for this compound is 1.51.

QSAR equations relating biological activity to the partition coefficient 'P' have already been described, but there is no reason why the substituent hydrophobicity constant π cannot be used in place of P if only the substituents are being varied. The equation obtained would be just as relevant as a study of how hydrophobicity affects biological activity. That is not to say that 'P' and π are exactly equivalent - different equations would be obtained with different constants.

Table 12.2: Values of π for a range of substituents

Group	CH₃	t-Butyl	OH	OCH₃	CF₃	Cl	Br	F
π (aliphatic substituents)	0.50	1.68	– 1.16	0.47	1.07	0.39	0.60	– 0.17
π (aromatic substituents)	0.52	1.68	– 0.67	– 0.02	1.16	0.71	0.86	0.14

Most QSAR equations have a contribution from P or from π, but there are examples of drugs for which they have only a slight contribution. For example, a study on antimalarial drugs showed very little relationship between antimalarial activity and hydrophobic character.

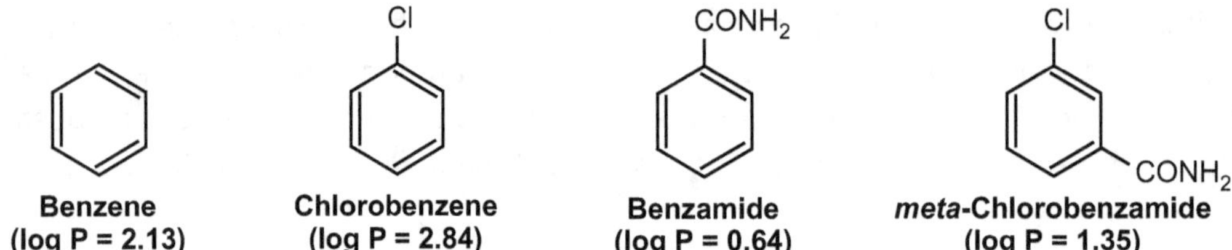

Benzene
(log P = 2.13)

Chlorobenzene
(log P = 2.84)

Benzamide
(log P = 0.64)

***meta*-Chlorobenzamide**
(log P = 1.35)

12.3.2 Hammet's Electronic Parameter

The electronic effects of various substituents will clearly have an effect on a drug's ionization or polarity. This, in turn, may have an effect on how easily a drug can pass through cell membranes or how strongly it can interact with a binding site. It is, therefore, useful to measure the electronic effect of a substituent.

As far as substituents on an aromatic ring are concerned, the measure used is known as the Hammett substituent constant (σ). This is a measure of the electron withdrawing or electron-donating ability of a substituent, and has been determined by measuring the dissociation of a series of substituted benzoic acids compared with the dissociation of benzoic acid itself.

Benzoic acid is a weak acid and only partially ionizes in water An equilibrium is set up between the ionized and non-ionized forms, where the relative proportion of these species is known as the equilibrium or dissociation constant K_H (the subscript H signifies that there are no substituents on the aromatic ring). When a substituent is present on the aromatic ring, this equilibrium is affected. Electron-withdrawing groups, such as a nitro group, result in the aromatic ring having a stronger electron-withdrawing and stabilizing influence on the carboxylate anion, and so the equilibrium will shift more to the ionized form. Therefore, the substituted benzoic acid is a stronger acid and has a larger K_X value (X represents the substituent on the aromatic ring). (Fig. 12.5)

If the substituent 'X' is an electron-donating group such as an alkyl group, then the aromatic ring is less able to stabilize the carboxylate ion. The equilibrium shifts to the left indicating a weaker acid with a smaller K_X value. (Fig. 12.5)

The Hammett substituent constant (σ_X) for a particular substituent (X) is defined by the following equation:

$$K_H = \frac{[PhCO_2^-]}{[PhCO_2H]}$$

Benzoic acids containing electron-withdrawing substituents will have larger K_X values than benzoic acid itself (K_H) and, therefore, the value of σ_X for an electron withdrawing substituent will be positive. Substituents such as Cl, CN, or CF_3 have positive σ values.

Benzoic acids containing electron-donating substituents will have smaller K_X values than benzoic acid itself and, hence, the value of σ_X for an electron-donating substituent will be negative. Substituents such as $-CH_3$, $-CH_3CH_2$, and t-butyl have negative values of σ. The Hammett substituent constant for H is zero.

$$\sigma_X = \log \frac{K_X}{K_H} = \log K_x - \log K_H$$

The Hammett substituent constant takes into account both resonance and inductive effects. Therefore, the value of σ for a particular substituent will depend on whether the substituent is meta or para. This is indicated by the subscript m or p after the σ symbol. For example, the nitro substituent has $\sigma_p = 0.78$ and $\sigma_m = 0.71$. In the meta position, the electron-withdrawing power is due to the inductive influence of the substituent, whereas at the para position inductive and resonance both play a part and so the σ_p value is greater. For the hydroxyl group $\sigma_m = 0.12$ and $\sigma_p = -0.37$. At the meta position, the influence is inductive and electron-withdrawing. At the para position, the electron donating influence due to resonance is more significant than the electron-withdrawing influence due to induction.

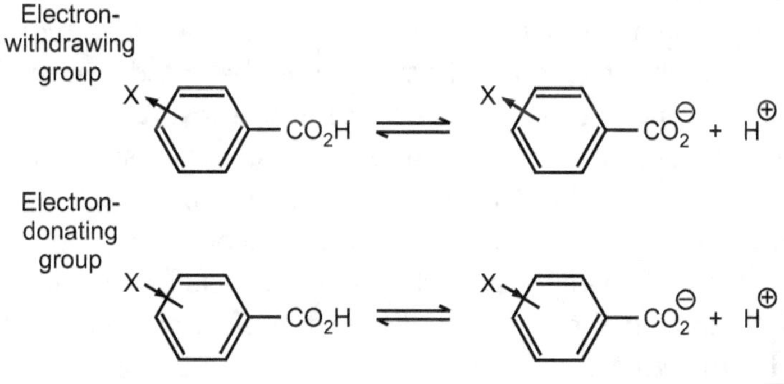

Fig. 12.5: Position of equilibrium dependent on substituent group X

meta nitro group - electronic influence on R is inductive

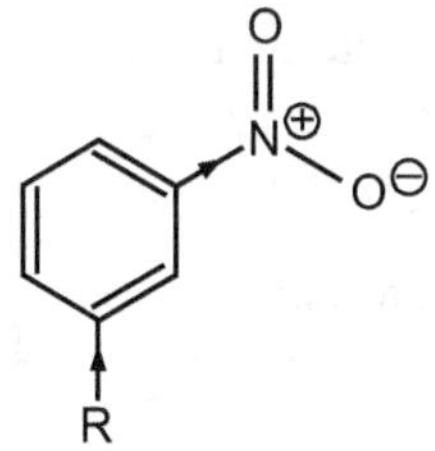

para nitro group - electronic influence on R is due to inductive and resonance effects

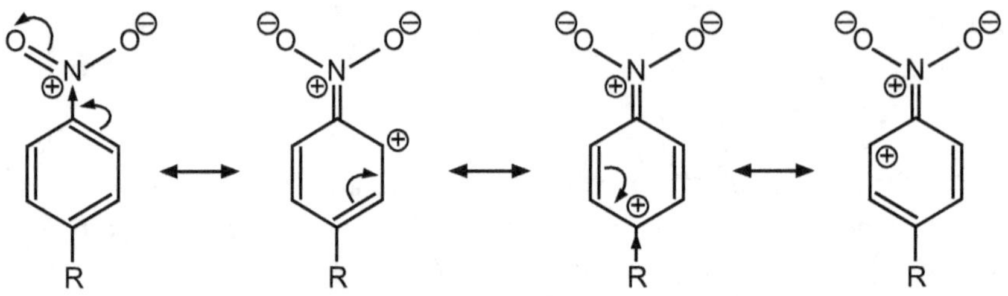

Fig. 12.6: Substituent effects of a nitro group at the meta and para-positions

meta hydroxyl group - electronic influence on R is inductive

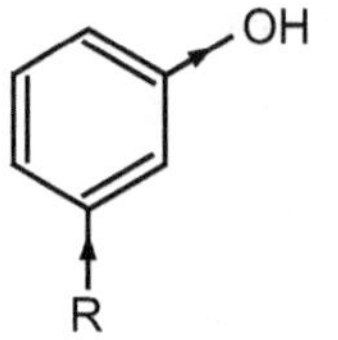

para hydroxyl group - electronic influence on R is dominated by resonance effects

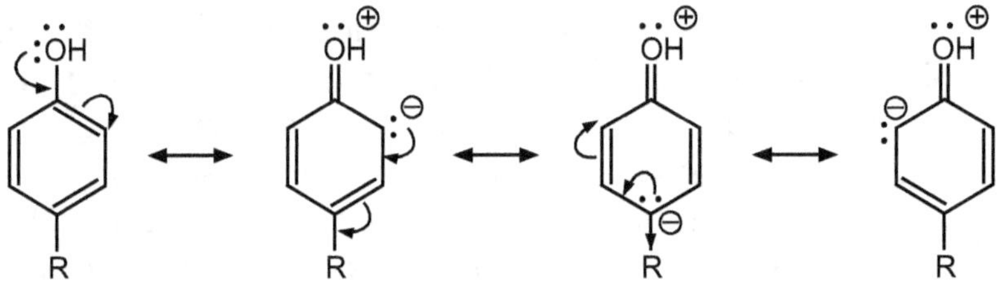

Fig. 12.7: Substituent effects of a phenol at the meta and para positions

There are limitations to the electronic constants described so far. For example, Hammett substituent constants cannot be measured for ortho substituents as such substituents have an important steric, as well as electronic effect. It should be noted that the inductive effect is not the only factor affecting the rate of hydrolysis. The substituent may also have a steric effect. For example, a bulky substituent may shield the ester from attack and lower the rate of hydrolysis. It is, therefore, necessary to separate out these two effects. This can be done by measuring hydrolysis rates under both basic and acidic conditions. Under basic conditions, steric and electronic factors are important, whereas under acidic conditions only steric factors are important. By comparing the rates, values for the electronic effect (σ_I), and the steric effect (E_S) can be determined.

12.3.3 Tafts Steric Parameter

The bulk, size, and shape of a drug will influence how easily it can approach and interact with a binding site. A bulky substituent may act like a shield and hinder the ideal interaction between a drug and its binding site. Attempts have been made to quantify the steric features of substituents by using Taft's steric factor (E_s).

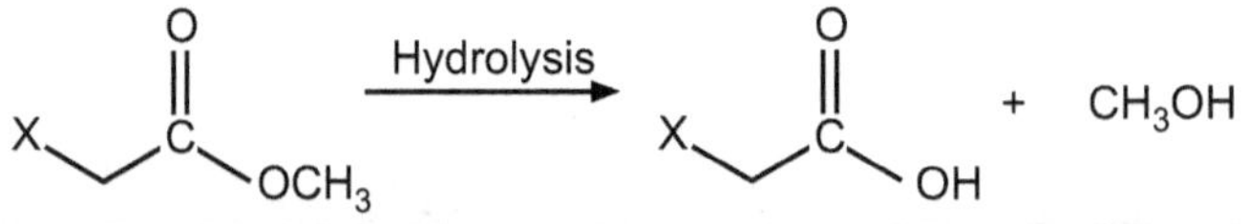

The value for E_s can be obtained by comparing the rates of hydrolysis of substituted aliphatic esters against a standard ester under acidic conditions. Thus,

$$E_S = \log k_X - \log k_O$$

where k_X represents the rate of hydrolysis of an aliphatic ester bearing the substituent X and k_O represents the rate of hydrolysis of the reference ester. The substituents that can be studied by this method are restricted to those which interact sterically with the tetrahedral transition state of the reaction and not by resonance or internal hydrogen bonding. For example, unsaturated substituents which are conjugated to the ester cannot be measured by this procedure. Examples of E_s values are shown in Table 12.3. Note that the reference ester is X = Me. Substituents such as H and F, which are smaller than a methyl group, result in a faster rate of hydrolysis ($k_X > k_O$), making E_s positive. Substituents which are larger than methyl reduce the rate of hydrolysis ($k_X < k_O$), making E_s negative. A disadvantage of E_s values is that they are a measure of an intramolecular steric effect, whereas drugs interact with target binding sites in an intermolecular manner. For example, consider the E_s values for i-Pr, n-Pr, and n-Bu. The E_s value for the branched isopropyl group is significantly greater than that for the linear n-propyl group since the bulk of the substituent is closer to the reaction centre. Extending the alkyl chain from n-propyl to n-butyl has little effect on E_s. The larger n-butyl group is extended away from the reaction centre and so has little additional steric effect on the rate of hydrolysis. As a result, the E_s value for the n-butyl group undervalues the steric effect which this group might have if it was present on a drug approaching a binding site.

Table 12.3: Values of E_s for various substituents

Substituent	H	F	CH_3	CH_3-CH_2	n-Pr	n-Bu	i-Pr	i-Bu	Cyclopentyl
E_S	1.24	0.78	0	−0.07	−0.36	−0.39	−0.47	−0.93	−0.51

12.3.4 Hansch Analysis

In a situation where biological activity is related to only one physicochemical property, a simple equation can be drawn up. The biological activity of most drugs, however, is related to a combination of physicochemical properties. In such cases, simple equations involving only one parameter are relevant only if the other parameters are kept constant. In reality, this is not easy to achieve and equations which relate biological activity to a number of different parameters are more common. These equations are known as Hansch equations and they usually relate biological activity to the most commonly used physicochemical properties (log P, π, σ, and a steric factor). If the range of hydrophobicity values is limited to a small range, then the equation will be linear, as follows:

$$\log \left(\frac{1}{C}\right) = k_1 \log P + k_2 \sigma + k_3 E_S + k_4$$

If the log P values are spread over a large range, then the equation will be parabolic for the same reasons:

$$\log \left(\frac{1}{C}\right) = -k_1 (\log P)^2 + k_2 \log P + k_3 \sigma + k_4 E_S + k_5$$

The constants $k_1 - k_5$ are determined by computer software in order to get the best fitting equation. Not all the parameters will necessarily be significant. For example, the adrenergic blocking activity of β-halo-arylamines was related to π and σ and did not include a steric factor. This equation tells us that biological activity increases if the substituents have a positive π value and a negative σ value. In other words, the substituents should be hydrophobic and electron donating.

When carrying out a Hansch analysis, it is important to choose the substituents carefully to ensure that the change in biological activity can be attributed to a particular parameter. There are plenty of traps for the unwary. Take, for example, drugs which contain an amine group. One of the studies most frequently carried out on amines is to synthesize analogues containing a homologous series of alkyl substituents on the nitrogen atom (i.e. Me, Et, n-Pr, n -Bu). If activity increases with the chain length of the substituent, is it due to increasing hydrophobicity, increasing size, or both? If we look at the π and MR values of these substituents, we find that both sets of values increase in a similar fashion across the series and we would not be able to distinguish between them (Table 12.4). In this example, a series of substituents would have to be chosen where π and MR are not correlated. The substituents H, Me, OMe, NHCOCH$_2$, I and CN would be more suitable.

$$\log \left(\frac{1}{C}\right) = 1.22\,\pi - 1.59\,\sigma + 7.89$$

$$(n = 22,\ r^2 = 0.841,\ s = 0.238)$$

β-Halo-arylamines

Fig. 12.8: QSAR equation for β-halo-arylamines

Table 12.4: Values for π and MR for a series of substituents

Substituent	H	Me	Et	n-Pr	n-Bu	OMe	NHCONH$_2$	I	CN
π	0.00	0.56	1.02	1.50	2.13	− 0.02	−1.30	1.12	− 0.57
MR	0.10	0.56	1.03	1.55	1.96	0.79	1.37	1.39	0.63

Hansch approach became the most popular approach in QSAR. The high-dimensional QSAR analyses (3D, 4D, and 5D) are developed to avoid pitfalls of classical method and to create the hypothetical drug receptor model.

Advantages of QSAR:

1. It gives quantifying the relationship between structure and activity with their physicohemical property basis.

2. Possible to make predictions of designed compounds before the chemical synthesis of novel analogues.

3. It may help to understand the interactions between functional group of designed molecules and their activity of target enzyme or protein.

Disadvantages of QSAR:

1. Due to biological data experimental error it may give false correlations.
2. If training set of molecules is less, the data may not reflect the complete property and it cannot be used to predict the most active compounds.
3. In some 3D QSAR study ligands binding receptor or protein may not be available in that case the common approach result may not represent the reality.
4. Cannot expect that the QSAR works all the time give successful applications.

The Craig Plot:

Although tables of π and σ factors are readily available for a large range of substituents, it is often easier to visualize the relative properties of different substituents by considering a plot where the y-axis is the value of the σ factor and the x-axis is the value of the π factor. Such a plot is known as a Craig plot. The example shown in Fig. 12.9 is the Craig plot for the σ and π factors of para-aromatic substituents. There are several advantages to the use of such a Craig plot.

- The plot shows clearly that there is no overall relationship between π and σ. The various substituents are scattered around all four quadrants of the plot.

- It is possible to tell at a glance which substituents have positive π and σ parameters, which substituents have negative π and σ parameters, and which substituents have one positive and one negative parameter.

- It is easy to see which substituents have similar π values. For example, the ethyl, bromo, trifluoro methyl, and trifluoro methyl sulfonyl groups are all approximately on the same vertical line on the plot. In theory these groups could be interchangeable on drugs where the principal factor affecting biological activity is the π factor. Similarly, groups which form a horizontal line can be identified as being isoelectronic or having similar σ values (e.g. CO_2H, Cl, Br, I).

- The Craig plot (Fig. 12.9) is useful in planning which substituents should be used in a QSAR study. In order to derive the most accurate equation involving π and σ, analogues should be synthesized with substituents from each quadrant. For example, halogen substituents are useful representatives of substituents with increased hydrophobicity and electron-withdrawing properties (positive π and positive σ), whereas an OH substituent has more hydrophilic and electron-donating properties (negative π and negative σ). Alkyl groups are examples of substituents with positive π and negative σ values, whereas acyl groups have negative π and positive σ values.

- Once the Hansch equation has been derived, it will show whether π or σ should be negative or positive in order to get good biological activity. Further developments would then concentrate on substituents from the relevant quadrant. For example, if the equation shows that positive π and positive σ values are necessary, then further substituents should only be taken from the top right quadrant.

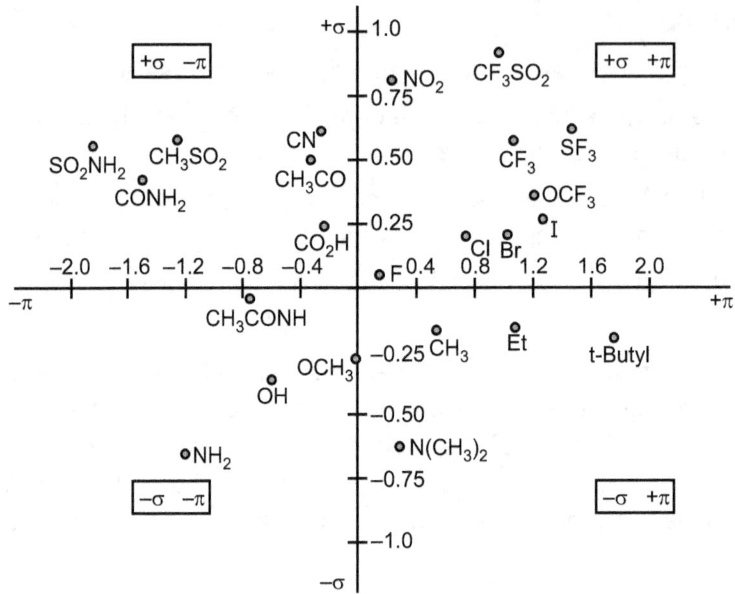

Fig. 12.9: Craig plot comparing the values of σ and π for various substituents

The Topliss Scheme:

A Topliss scheme is a 'flow diagram' which allows such a procedure to be followed. There are two Topliss schemes, one for aromatic substituents (Fig. 12.10) and one for aliphatic side-chain substituents (Fig. 12.11). The schemes were drawn up by considering the hydrophobicity and electronic factors of various substituents, and are designed such that the optimum substituent can be found as efficiently as possible. They are not meant to be a replacement for a full Hansch analysis, however. Such an analysis would be carried out in due course, once a suitable number of structures have been synthesized.

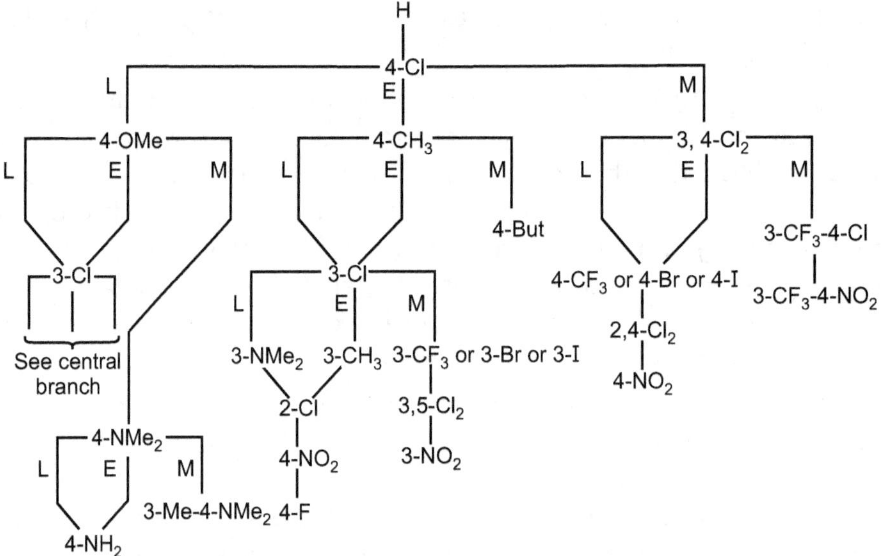

Fig. 12.10: Topliss scheme for aromatic substituents.

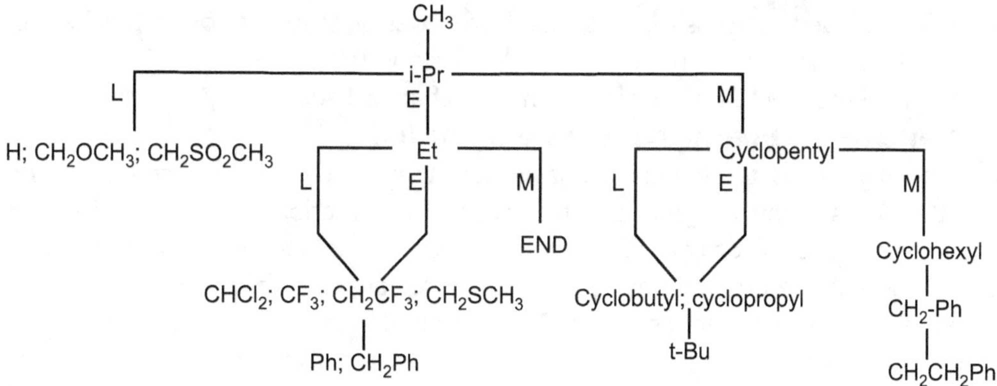

Fig. 12.11: Topliss scheme for aliphatic side-chain substitute

12.4 PHARMACOPHORE MODELLING

Pharmacophore term and concept was first introduced in 1909 by Ehrlich, who defined the pharmacophore as 'A molecular framework that carries (phoros) the essential features responsible for a drug's (pharmacon) biological activity'. The methodology of pharmacophore has remained unchanged from several decades, but has simultaneously reached advancements by introduction of computational methods. Pharmacophore model is 'an ensemble of steric and electronic features that is necessary to ensure the optimal supramolecular interactions with a specific biological target and to trigger (or block) its biological response'. This model helps the medicinal chemist to understand chemical features of the active site. The protocol of structure-based Pharmacophore modeling involves a scrutinization of the complementary chemical features of the active site and association with spatial relationships, and a subsequent pharmacophore model assembly with selected features. This study minimizes the work of medicinal chemist and helps him to select and optimize the lead molecule. There are several softwares like DS visualizer®, ligand scout® etc. Ligand-based pharmacophore modeling is a key computational strategy which facilitates drug discovery in case of absence of a macromolecular target structure. It is usually carried out by extracting common chemical fetures of ligands in the form of 3D structures which shows interactions with macromolecular target. The pharmacophore concept was rapidly used for rational drug design approaches and has now been routinely incorporated into virtual screening strategy.

Scopes of Pharmacophore Modelling:

- The concept is very efficient in the absence of a 3D molecular structure for a particular receptor of therapeutic interest.
- Drug discovery and designing of ligands become easy task for a medicinal chemist.
- Ligand-based drug design is based on the principle of similarity, which explains if there are similarity in ligand structures, then it is possible that they may exhibit similar physical, chemical and biological properties. This approach depends on a principle, which states that structurally similar compounds are more likely to exhibit

similar properties. Thus, ligand-based drug design appears to be the best choice, based on which several molecules can be designed.

- It can aid the identification of the common chemical and biological features.

12.4.1 Methods for Pharmacophore Generation

There are two ways to deduce a pharmacophore: direct- and indirect- methods. The direct method uses both the ligand and the receptor information, while the indirect method employs only a collection of ligands. Indirect methods are generally used by the medicinal chemists because there are very less crystal structures available of receptors. However, the direct methods are useful for researchers to re-explore the structures of known proteins. A pharmacophore model is a versatile tool for lead molecule discovery and development.

12.4.2 Steps in Identifying a Pharmacophore

In general, all the algorithms for pharmacophore identification use the following six steps for pharmacophore modelling:

1. Input
2. Conformational search
3. Feature extraction
4. Structure representation
5. Pattern identification
6. Scoring

1. **Inputs required for Pharmacophore Identification:** A diversified set of ligands should be collected and should be used for pharmacophore identification. This data will help the chemist to use a wide varieties of ligands for development of a suitable lead.

2. **Conformational Search:** The rotation along the carbon-carbon single bond leads to several conformational structures. These conformations lead to formation of several scaffolds with varied energy levels. The conformation with minimum energy level is considered to be the best one and the other are synchronized in similar manner.

3. **Feature Extraction:** All the atomic, electronic and function based features of the molecule should critically studied before performing the pharmacophore modelling.

4. **Structure Representation:** The complete structure is critically studied for all the features and the basic properties should always be kept aside.

5. **Pattern Identification:** There are various stages involved in identification of common features of pharmacophore as:

    (a) **The constructive stage:** This identifies pharmacophore candidates that are common among the most active set of ligands. This is done by comparing the common characteristics of the set of ligands.

    (b) **The subtractive stage:** It involves removal of those pharmacophore candidates constructed in the earlier stage that are also present in more than half of the least active ligands.

    (c) **The optimization stage:** This involves several attempts to improve the scoring pattern of the pharmacophore molecules that have passed subtractive stages.

6. **Scoring:** In this step scoring based on the results obtained were performed. This helped the medicinal chemist to understand the structure of useful and substantial ligands and pharmacophores.

12.5 MOLECULAR DOCKING

The molecular docking is a well known computational technique which predicts interaction between two molecules (ligand and receptor). This technique incorporates algorithm like Monto Carlo Stimulation, molecular dynamics, fragment based search which helps the chemist to predict the interactions between drugs and receptors. The molecular docking study is used to determine interaction of two molecules and detects the best orientation of ligand which formed a complex with overall minimum energy. The small molecule known as ligand tends to attach or fit within protein cavity which is usually predicted by search algorithm. The complete activity of protein-ligand complex activates after the macromolecule only if ligand had bound to the active site. The binding is measured as binding affinity and energy. These binding interaction values help the medicinal chemist to understand and scrutinize the ligands. Freely available softwares like pymol, rasmol can be used for visualization. The softwares like Schrodinger, bovia, V-Life, autodock, Glide etc. can be used for docking the ligands and proteins.

Different Types of Interactions:

Interaction between particles is defined as the "Force between molecules contained by particles". These forces are divided into four categories:

- **Electrostatic forces:** These are the forces with electrostatic origin due to the charges residing in the matter. The most common interactions are charge-charge, charge-dipole and dipole-dipole.
- **Electrodynamic forces:** The most widely known is the Van der Waals interactions.
- **Steric forces:** Steric forces are generated when atoms in different molecules come into very close contact with one another and start affecting the reactivity of each other. The resulting forces can affect chemical reactions and the free energy of a system.
- **Solvent-related forces:** These are forces generated due to chemical reactions between the solvent and the protein or ligand. Examples are hydrogen bonds (hydrophilic interactions) and hydrophobic interactions. The changes in protein and ligand are necessary for successful docking.

Molecular docking divided into two separate sections:

1. **Search algorithm:** The search algorithm determines all possible conformations for given complex (protein-protein, protein-ligand) in environment. The position and orientation of both molecules are related to each other. It also calculates the energy of resulting complex of each interaction.

The different types of algorithms used for docking analysis are given below:-

- Molecular dynamics
- Monte Carlo methods
- Genetic algorithms
- Fragment-based methods
- Point complementary methods
- Distance geometry methods
- Systematic searches

2. **Scoring function:** It is a mathematical method used to predict the strength of non-covalent interactions called as binding affinity between the two molecules they have been docked. The scoring function has also been developed to predict the strength of other type of intermolecular interaction.

   For example:

   - **Empirical scoring function of any docking program:**

     Fitness = v dw + H-bond + Elect

   - **Binding Energy:**

     $\Delta G_{bind} = \Delta G_{v\ dw} + \Delta G_{H\text{-}bond} + \Delta G_{elect} + \Delta G_{conform} + \Delta G_{tor} + \Delta G_{sol}$

Types of Docking:

1. **Lock and Key or Rigid Docking:** In rigid docking the geometry of receptor and ligand is fixed during docking.

2. **Induced Fit or Flexible Docking:** The both ligand and side chain of protein are flexible and energy for different conformations of ligand fit into protein is calculated. For induced fit docking, the main chain is also moved to incorporate the conformational changes of the protein upon ligand binding. Though it is time consuming and computationally expensive, this method can evaluate many different possible conformations which make it more exhaustive and possibly simulate real life phenomenon and hence trustworthy.

12.6 COMBINATORIAL CHEMISTRY

Combinatorial chemistry is a technique through which large numbers of structurally distinct molecules may be synthesized at a time and submitted for high throughput screening (HTS) assay. Combinatorial chemistry is one of the recent methodologies developed by researchers in the pharmaceutical industry to reduce the time and costs associated with producing successful and competitive new drugs. By accelerating the process of biologically active compounds, this method is having a profound effect on all the branches of chemistry, especially on drug discovery. Through the rapidly evolving technology of combinatorial chemistry, it is now possible to produce compound libraries to screen for novel bioactivities. This powerful new technology has begun to help pharmaceutical companies to find novel drug candidates quickly, save significant money in preclinical development costs, and ultimately change their fundamental approach to drug discovery.

12.6.1 Principles of Combinatorial Chemistry

The key of combinatorial chemistry is that a large range of analogues are synthesized using the same reaction conditions and the same reaction vessels. In this way, the organic chemist can synthesize hundreds or thousands of compounds at one time instead of preparing only a few by a traditional methodology. For example, compound A would have been reacted with compound B to give product AB, which would have been isolated after reaction, work up and purification.

Conventional Reaction: $A + B \Upsilon \rightarrow A - B$

In contrast to this approach, combinatorial chemistry offers the potential to make every combination of a compound A_1 to A_n with compound B_1 to B_n. The range of combinatorial techniques is highly diverse, and these products could be made individually in a parallel or in mixtures, using either solution or solid-phase techniques. Whatever be the technique used, the common denominator is that productivity has been amplified beyond the levels that have been routine for the last hundred years. The origin of combinatorial chemistry lies in the use of solid supports for peptide synthesis. By coupling the growing peptide to a solid support, such as a polystyrene bead, it is possible to use excess reagents and so ensure that the reaction proceeds to completion. Any excess reagent is simply washed away. In the original applications of solid-phase chemistry to peptide synthesis, the goal was generally the synthesis of a single molecular target. A key breakthrough was the recognition that this methodology could be used to generate large number of molecules using a scheme known as **split–mix technique**. This technique starts with a set of reagents (which we may also refer to as monomers), each of which is coupled to the solid support. These are then mixed together and divided into equal-sized aliquots for reaction with the second reagent. The products from this reaction are reacted with the third reagent, and so on. If the number of reagents at each step are n_1, n_2, n_3, etc., then the total number of molecules produced is the product is $(n_1\, n_2\, n_3)$. The size of the library, thus, increases exponentially with the number of reagents - hence the use of the term 'combinatorial'.

Combinatorial Synthesis:

$$A(1 - n) + B(1 - n) \rightarrow A(1 - n) - B(1 - n)$$

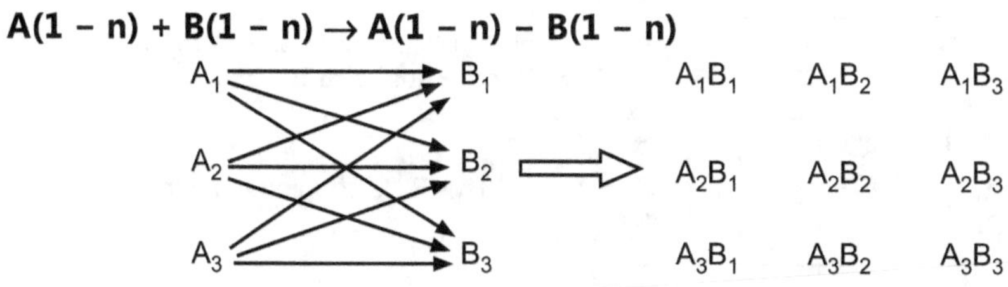

Fig. 12.12: Combinatorial synthesis

Salient Features: The various salient features of 'combinatorial chemistry' are as enumerated under:

1. **Chemical diversity of products:** Useful libraries of 'reactive' chemical functional moieties invariably give rise to the chemical diversity of products which shall be duly screened for respective biological activity.

2. Chemistry involved is not only graceful and stylish, but also comparatively simple; whereby a few 'same reactions' could suffice in yielding thousands of drug molecules in a specific congeneric series.

3. Invariably, one makes use of the solid-state synthetic techniques to allow the desired growth of drug molecules upon polymer support.

4. The 'chemical reactions' involved in (2) and (3) above must fulfil three vital and important criteria, such as:
   (i)   Clean reaction,
   (ii) Reproducible reaction, and
   (iii) High yielding reaction.

5. 'Robotics' have been employed profusely to cut down the 'effective cost of synthesis' drastically.

12.6.2 Concept and Applications of Combinatorial Chemistry

1. Combinatorial Synthesis Split-Pool-Method:

- Developed for combinatorial peptide synthesis in 1988 to obtain large libraries more easily.
- Compounds bound to resin beads (solid-supported chemistry).
- Also termed "divide, couple and recombine synthesis" in regard to the technical routine applied.
- Currently the most popular method for generating large libraries of compound mixtures.
- Resulting library can be described as "one bead, one compound" type.

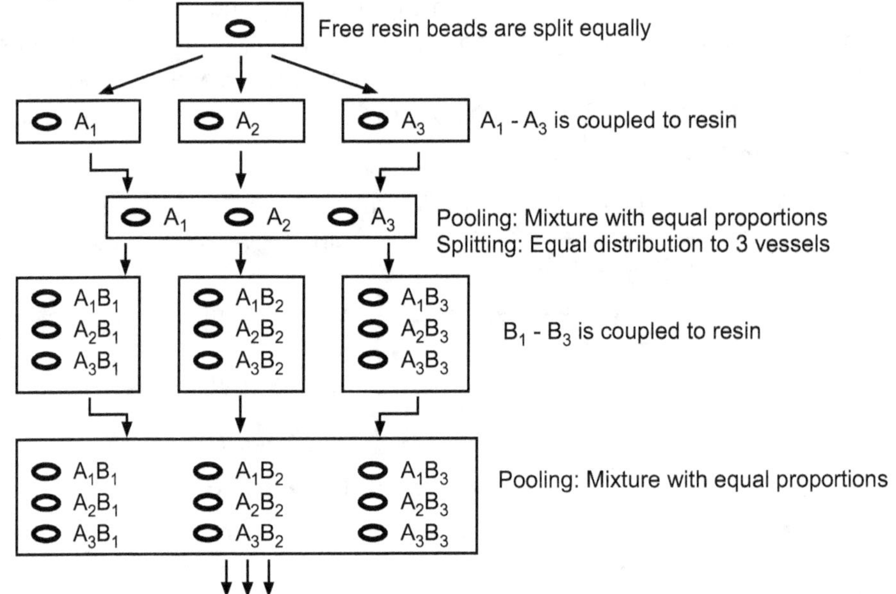

Fig. 12.13: Combinatorial synthesis split-pool-method

2. Parallel Synthesis:

In parallel synthesis, a reaction is carried out in a series of wells such that each well contains a single product. This method is a 'quality rather than quantity' approach and is often used for focused lead optimization studies.

Advantages:

1. Simple analysis, compound structure known at any time, biological evaluation simplified, purification by simple chromatography.

Disadvantages:

1. More cost and labour intensive: Many more single reactions needed.

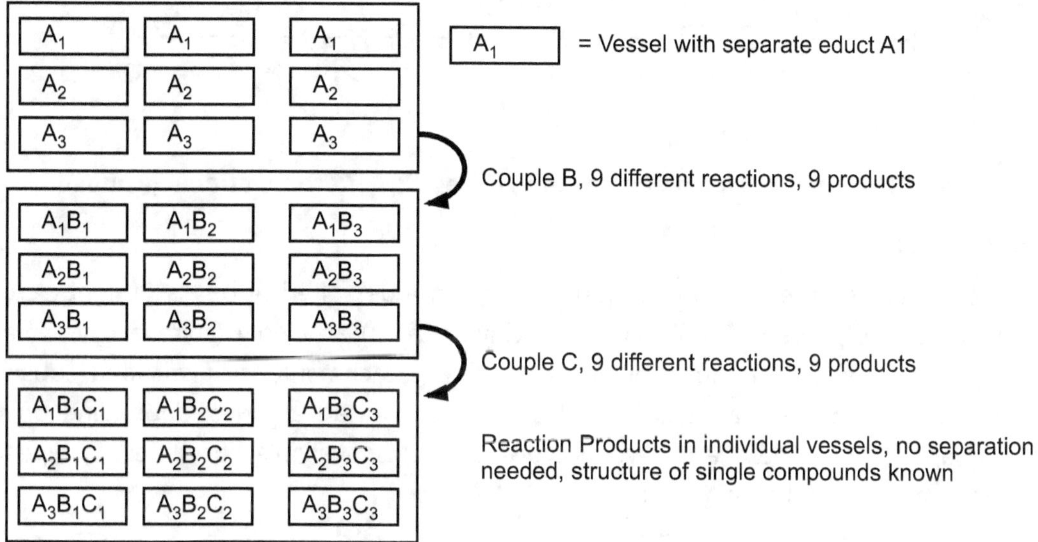

Fig. 12.14: Parallel synthesis

12.6.3 Solid Phase and Solution Phase Synthesis

1. Combinatorial Synthesis on Solid Phase:

In 1963, Merrifield pioneered the solid phase synthesis (SPS) work, which earned him a nobel prize. Merrifield's SPS concept was first applied for a developed biopolymer, recently it has spread in every field where organic synthesis is involved. Now-a-days, many academic laboratories and pharmaceutical companies focused on the development of the technologies and chemistry suitable for SPS. This resulted in the impressive outbreak of combinatorial chemistry, which profoundly changed the approach to new drugs, new catalyst, or new natural discovery.

The utilization of solid support for the organic synthesis relies on three inter-connected requirements. These are as follows:

1. A cross-linked, insoluble polymeric material should be inert to the condition of synthesis.

2. The linking substrate (linker) to the solid phase that permits selective cleavage of some or all the products from the solid support during synthesis for analysis of the extent of reaction(s) and ultimately to give the final product of interest.

3. The chemical protection strategy must allow selective protection and deprotection of reactive groups.

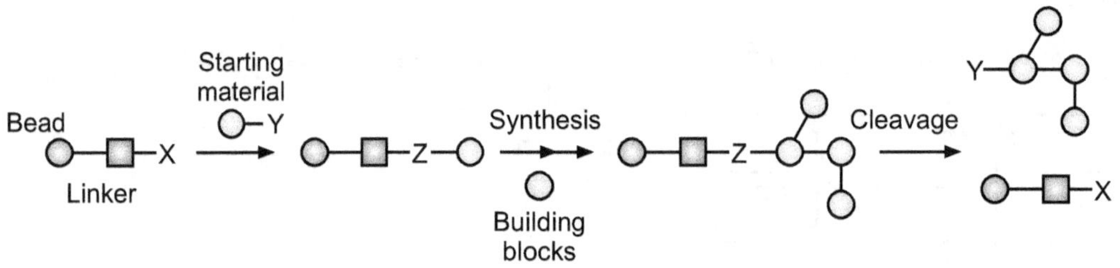

Fig. 12.15: The principles of an anchor/linker. X, Y, Z are functional groups

Resins for SPS:

In solid phase synthesis, resin supports for SPS include spherical beads of lightly cross-linked gel type polystyrene (GPS) (1%–2% divinylbenzene) and poly (styrene-oxyethylene) graft copolymers, which are functionalized to allow attachment of linkers and substrate molecules. Each of these materials has advantages and disadvantages, depending on the particular application. There are several types of resins available for different types of reactions, as mentioned below.

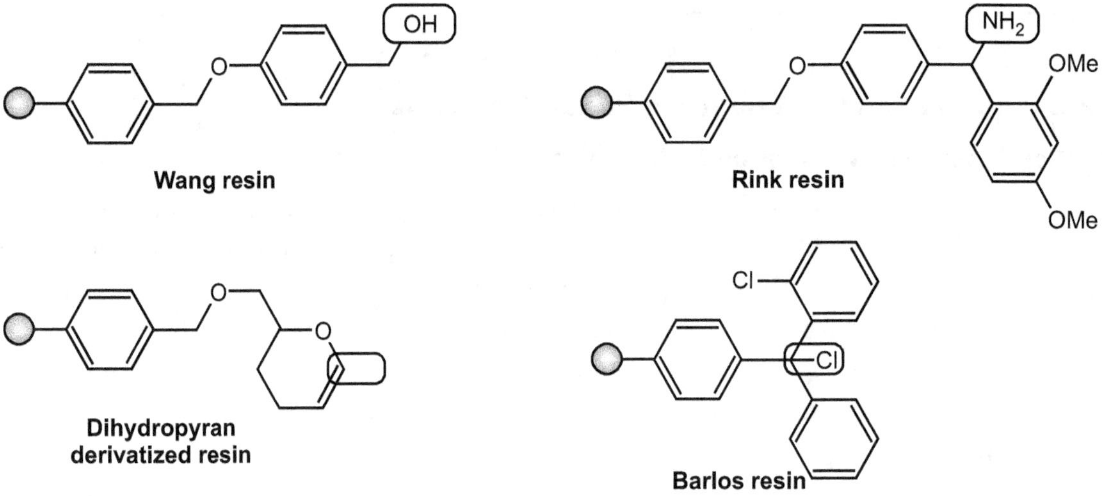

Fig. 12.16: Types of resin with the linkage point circled

Advantages of Solid Support Reagents:

1. Solid-supported reagents are easily removed from reactions by filtration.
2. Excess reagents can be used to drive reactions to completion without introducing difficulties in purification.
3. Recycling of recovered reagents is economical, environmentally - sound and efficient.
4. Ease of handling is especially important when dealing with expensive or time-intensive catalysts, which can be incorporated into flow reactors and automated processes.
5. Finely tune chemical properties by altering choice of support and its preparation.
6. Toxic, explosive, and noxious reagents are often more safely handled when contained on solid support.
7. Reagents on solid-support react differently, mostly more selectively, than their unbound counterparts.

Disadvantages of Solid Support Reagents:

1. Some reagents may not interact well with solid support.
2. Ability to recycle reagents on solid support is not assured.
3. Reactions may run more slowly due to diffusional constraints.
4. Polymeric support materials can be very expensive to prepare.
5. Stability of the support material can be poor under harsh reaction conditions.
6. Side reactions with the polymer support itself may occur.

2. Combinatorial Synthesis on Solution Phase:

When combinatorial chemistry first emerged, the initial focus was on solid-phase approaches due to the many advantages. Solution chemistry was not regarded as being suitable for combinatorial chemistry because of the often tedious isolation and purification.

The main problem of solution phase combinatorial synthesis is to obtain pure products. The significance of purity varies with the purpose for which a combinatorial library is produced (search for new lead compounds vs. lead optimization). It was first used for easily synthesized compound classes (amides, sulfonamides, ureas, heterocycles).

In recent years, a number of technologies have emerged for solution chemistry, so that in many cases it became an alternative to solid-phase synthesis. Presently, solution-phase combinatorial synthesis is attracting more interest because of some advantages.

Advantages:

1. Many more reactions are optimised in solution phase.
2. All reactive groups of the starting materials are available for structural modifications.
3. No limitations of the thermal or chemical stability of the resin or the linker.

4. Synthesis is shorter by one or two steps. Reactions in solution often need considerably less time.

5. Reactions that involve insoluble components are confined to solution-phase.

6. Reactions can conveniently be followed by simple means (TLC, NMR, UV).

7. In general, the reaction volumes in relation to the amount of product are smaller.

QUESTIONS

Multiple Choice Questions:

1. Which of the following is a QSAR method used manually?

    (a) Hansch approach   (b) Fujita ban approach

    (c) Free Wilson approach   (d) Topliss appraoach

2. Which one of the following is not used in QSAR?

    (a) Molecular connectivity index   (b) Molecular similarity index

    (c) Topological surface area   (d) Partition coefficient

3. QSAR method involves ....

    (a) Target structure   (b) Target properties

    (c) Ligand structure   (d) Ligand properties

4. Sigma is the measure of substituents ....

    (a) Inductive effect   (b) Resonance effect

    (c) Both (a) and (b)   (d) Mesomeric effect

5. Molar refractivity is .... parameter.

    (a) Hydrophobic   (b) Electronic

    (c) Steric   (d) None of these

6. What is the symbol π in a QSAR equation?

    (a) The hydrophobicity of the molecule.

    (b) The electronic effect of a substituent.

    (c) The substituent hydrophobicity constant.

    (d) A measure of the steric properties for a substituent.

7. What does MR represent in a QSAR equation?

    (a) Molar refractivity is a steric factor.

    (b) Molar refractivity is an electronic factor.

(c) Molar refractivity is a hydrophobic factor.

(d) Molar refractivity is a stereoelectronic factor.

8.   What software programme is used to determine the Verloop steric parameter?

(a) Alchemy

(b) Chem3D

(c) Sterimol

(d) ChemDraw

9.   What does a negative value of σ signify for a substituent?

(a) It is electron donating.

(b) It is electron withdrawing.

(c) It is neutral.

(d) It is hydrophobic.

10. Which of the following statements is untrue when comparing 3D QSAR with conventional QSAR?

(a) Only drugs of the same structural class should be studied by 3D QSAR or QSAR.

(b) 3D QSAR has a predictive quality unlike QSAR.

(c) Experimental parameters are not required by 3D QSAR, but are for QSAR.

(d) Results can be shown graphically in 3D QSAR, but not with QSAR.

11. What value does the regression coefficient have for a perfect fit?

(a) 0.1

(b) 1

(c) 10

(d) 100

12. Dynamic combinatorial chemistry is an alternative method of producing compounds other than the classic mix and split method. Which of the following statements is true about dynamic combinatorial chemistry?

(a) The target should be absent from the reaction flask.

(b) There is no scope for amplification.

(c) It is necessary to 'freeze' the equilibrium reaction to identify active compounds.

(d) The reactions involved should be irreversible.

13. What is meant by a scaffold?

(a) The lead compound.

(b) The carbon skeleton of a compound.

(c) The core structure of a molecule that is common to a series of compounds.

(d) The pharmacophores.

14. What is meant by a privileged scaffold?

    (a) A scaffold that is present in a wide range of drugs with different activities.

    (b) A scaffold that is easily synthesized.

    (c) A scaffold that is patented.

    (d) A scaffold that is free of side effects.

15. Which of the following statements is true?

    (a) Drugs and drug targets generally have similar molecular weights.

    (b) Drugs are generally smaller than drug targets.

    (c) Drugs are generally larger than drug targets.

    (d) There is no general rule regarding the relative size of drugs and their targets.

16. What does the symbol P represent in a QSAR equation?

    (a) pH   (b) plasma concentration

    (c) partition coefficient   (d) prodrug

17. For the determination of partition coefficient the non-aqueous solvent usually chosen is ....

    (a) 1-octanol   (b) 2-octanol

    (c) 3-octanol   (d) 4-octanol

18. What is the term used for small molecules that bind to different regions of a binding site?

    (a) Epimers   (b) Isomers

    (c) Isotopes   (d) Epitopes

19. Combinatorial and parallel synthesis can be useful at various stages of the drug design / development process. Which of the following is not such a stage?

    (a) Finding a lead compound

    (b) Optimising a lead compound

    (c) Structure determination of the lead compound

    (d) Structure-activity relationships of the lead compound

20. What is meant by a linker or an anchor?

    (a) The bond which links a molecule to a solid support.

    (b) A reactive functional group on the solid support which allows a molecule to be attached to the solid support.

(c) A molecular unit which is attached to the solid support and which contains a reactive functional group that allows attachment of a starting material.

(d) The functional group on the starting material which is used to attach the molecule to the solid support.

21. Which of the following statements regarding linkers is wrong?

(a) The link between the molecule and the solid support must be stable to the reaction conditions used in the synthesis.

(b) The link between the molecule and the solid support must be easily cleaved under specific conditions.

(c) The choice of linker used depends on the functional groups available on the first molecule to be attached.

(d) The linker must be on the outer surface of the resin bead if a molecule is to become attached to it.

22. What is meant by a scaffold?

(a) The lead compound.

(b) The carbon skeleton of a compound.

(c) The core structure of a molecule that is common to a series of compounds.

(d) The pharmacophores.

23. What is meant by a privileged scaffold?

(a) A scaffold that is present in a wide range of drugs with different activities.

(b) A scaffold that is easily synthesized.

(c) A scaffold that is patented.

(d) A scaffold that is free of side effects.

24. Which of the following statements is true with respect to scaffolds?

(a) The scaffold should be large to allow a wide variation of substituents.

(b) The scaffold should not be capable of forming any binding interactions with the target.

(c) Substituents should be localized at particular regions of the scaffold.

(d) Similar functional groups on the scaffold should be capable of being varied independently of each other.

25. What is meant by de novo drug design?

   (a) The synthesis of a compound from simple starting materials.

   (b) The design of the synthesis required to generate a novel range of structures.

   (c) The design of a novel drug based on molecular modeling studies of a binding site.

   (d) The modification of a drug based on molecular modeling studies into how it binds to its target binding site.

Answers :

1. (d)	2. (b)	3. (d)	4. (c)	5. (c)	6. (c)	7. (a)	8. (c)	9. (a)	10. (a)
11. (b)	12. (c)	13. (c)	14. (a)	15. (b)	16. (c)	17. (a)	18. (d)	19. (c)	20.(c)
21. (d)	22. (c)	23. (a)	24. (d)	25. (c)					

Answer the following questions:

1.   Describe the various approaches of lead discovery.
2.   Write in detail about computer aided drug design (CADD).
3.   Define QSAR and explain about Hansch analysis.
4.   Write in detail about the steps involved in the QSAR studies.
5.   What is combinatorial chemistry? Write its application in the drug discovery.
6.   Write a note on combinatorial synthesis on solid phase.
7.   What is pro-drug? Write their classification based on the functional group.
8.   What are the advantages of prodrugs? Explain with suitable examples.
9.   Write a note on bioprecursor prodrugs.
10. Justify the following statements:

   (a) Drug design aims at developing a drug with high degree of chemotherapeutic index and specific action.

   (b) From the practical view-point it is the 'Exploitation of Leads' wherein rational approaches to Drug-design have been mostly productive with fruitful results.

11. Discuss the various 'factors governing drug-design'.
12. Elaborate the 'rational approach to drug design' with regard to Quantum Mechanics (or Wave Mechanics), Molecular Orbital Theory, Molecular Connectivity and Linear Free-Energy Concepts.
13. Enumerate the various cardinal objectives of 'The Methods of Variation' giving appropriate examples.
14. The first synthetic oestrogen trans-diethyl stilbesterol came into existence by applying the principle of 'drug-design through disjunction' from 'oestradiol'. Explain.

15. 'Tailoring of Drugs' is the outcome of unique blend of skill involving various configurational and stereochemical changes attributing its flexibility and overall dimension. Explain.

16. Discuss the various possible approaches in designing newer drugs by applying variation of a 'biologically active prototype'.

17. Differentiate the basic concepts of 'analogues' and 'prodrugs' with the help of suitable examples of parent drug molecule(s).

18. Why the geometrical isomer trans-diethyl stilbesterol exhibit higher oestrogenic activity than the cis-isomer?

19. Discuss the specific role of absorption, distribution, excretion and biotransformation (i.e., metabolism) to enable a 'drug' to reach the 'active site'.

20. Discuss the following two categories with regard to calculation of affinity:
    (a) Binding energetics and comparisons
    (b) Multiple binding modes

21. Write short notes on the following:
    (i)   Components of bonding affinity
    (ii) Simulations and the thermodynamic cycle
    (iii) Ligand-receptor recognition

22. Write a comprehensive essay on the Unknown Receptor Sites with special emphasis upon the following aspects:
    (a) Pharmacophore Vs binding site models
    (b) Molecular comparisons
    (c) Searching for similarity

23. Give a detailed account on the 'Predictive ADME'. Expatiate your answer with appropriate explanations/examples.

24. What do you mean by Molecular Modeling? What are two major aspects of Molecular Modeling? Explain.

25. Discuss briefly Molecular Mechanics and Quantum Mechanics, the two methodologies associated with Molecular Modeling.

26. Describe the following aspects with regard to the Known Receptor Sites with suitable explanations/examples:
    (a) 3D structure of Macromolecular Targets
    (b) Structure-Based drug design
    (c) Major Steps in Structure Based Drug Design
    (d) Ligand Receptor Recognition
    (e) Active Site for a Target Molecule.

27. Give a comprehensive account on : "Characterization of Site in Molecular Modeling". Give suitable examples to support your answer.

28. What do you understand by 'Design of Legends'? Discuss the following aspects in an elaborated manner:
    (a) Visually assisted design
    (b) 3D-Database
    (c) De Novo design.

29. Give a brief account on the 'Divide and Rule' Concept in Design of Ligands.

30. Describe the various methodologies for DOCKING.

31. What are the different types of receptors existing? Describe them with suitable examples.

32. What are the different forces involved in drug receptors interaction? Explain any two of them.

33. Explain the various factors affecting the drug-receptor interaction.

34. Write in detail about computer aided drug design (CADD).

■■■

INDEX

■■■

OUR UPCOMING BOOKS
As Per PCI Regulations Third Year (Semester VI)

- **Medicinal Chemistry III :** S.G. Walode
- **Medicinal Chemistry III :** K.G. Bothara
- **Practical Medicinal chemistry III :** S.G. Walode
- **Pharmacology III :** Dr. S. V. Tembhurne
- **Pharmacology III :** K.G. Bothara
- **Practical Pharmacology III :** Dr. Arjun Patra
- **Herbal Drug Technology :** Vaibhav shinde, Ms. K. S. Bodas, S.B. Gokhale
- **Practical Herbal Drug Technology :** Vaibhav Shinde, Ms. K. S. Bodas, S.B. Gokhale
- **Biopharmaceutics and Pharmacokinetics :** Sunil bakliwal
- **Pharmaceutical Biotechnology :** Dr. Chandrakant Kokare
- **Medicinal Chemistry III :** Dr. Abhishek Tiwari
- **Pharmacology III :** Dr. Rupesh Gautam, Dr. Kalpesh Gour
- **Herbal Drug Technology :** Dr. Versha Tiwari, Dr. Vikash Sharma
- **Biopharmaceutics and Pharmacokinetics :** Hari Kumar
- **Pharmaceutical Biotechnology :** Dr. Khush Yadav, Mr. Rajiv Saxena, Ms. Satinder Kaur, Garima Joshi
- **Quality Assurance :** Bhupender Sing Tomar, Dr. Pawan Jhalwal, Surajpal verma
- **Medicinal Chemistry III :** Vibha Chandan Patil, Dr Chandrashekhar Narajji
- **Medicinal Chemistry III :** Mr. Mayur S. Jain, Mr. Mayur R. Bhurat, Sanjay A. Nagdev, Dr. Md. Rageeb Md. Usman
- **Practical Medicinal Chemistry III :** Dr. Sunita T. Patil, Dr. Md. Rageeb Md. Usman, Dr. Parloop A. Bhatt
- **Pharmacology III :** Dr. Manjunatha. P. Mudagal
- **Practical Pharmacology III :** Dr. Manjunatha. P. Mudagal
- **Herbal Drug Technology :** Kuntal Das
- **Herbal Drug Technology :** Dr. Santram Lodhi, Dr. Md. Rageeb Md. Usman, Dr. Tushar A. Deshmukh, Mr. Vaibhav M. Darvhekar
- **Practical Herbal Drug Technology :** Prof. Md. Rageeb Md. Usman, Prof. Vaibhav M. Darvhekar, Prof. (Dr.) Akhila S., Prof. (Dr.) Vijay Kumar D.
- **Biopharmaceutics and Pharmacokinetics :** Dr. B. Prakash Rao
- **Pharmaceutical Biotechnology :** Kuntal Das
- **A Practical Book Of Medicinal Chemistry (Combined Book Sem. IV & VI)**
  Dr. Abhishek Tiwari, Dr. Rajeev Kumar

■■■